Cancer Immunotherapy

Volume 2

Series Editor
Matthias Theobald
III Department of Internal Medicine
Johannes Gutenberg University of Mainz
Mainz, Germany

Each volume of the series Cancer Immunotherapy will focus on one specific cancer covering scientific aspects as well as clinical applications including clinical trials and new drugs once immunotherapy for these cancers has reached the clinic.

Markus Moehler • Friedrich Foerster
Editors

Immune Strategies for Gastrointestinal Cancer

Springer

Editors
Markus Moehler
First Department of Medicine, Research Center for Immunotherapy (FZI)
University Cancer Center Mainz, University Medical Center of the Johannes Gutenberg University Mainz
Mainz, Germany

Friedrich Foerster
First Department of Medicine
University Cancer Center Mainz, University Medical Center of the Johannes Gutenberg University Mainz
Mainz, Germany

ISSN 2662-8384 ISSN 2662-8392 (electronic)
Cancer Immunotherapy

ISBN 978-3-031-39943-5 ISBN 978-3-031-39944-2 (eBook)
https://doi.org/10.1007/978-3-031-39944-2

This Springer imprint is published by the registered company Springer Nature Switzerland AG
The registered company address is: Gewerbestrasse 11, 6330 Cham, Switzerland

Immunotherapy in GI Cancers: Introduction

In the twenty-first century, the coming-of-age of immunotherapy has been the most relevant development for the field of cancer medicine. Particularly the class of immune checkpoint inhibitors has produced astonishing results in clinical trials in various (neo-)adjuvant or metastatic settings across numerous cancer entities. Consequently, the Nobel Assembly at Karolinska Institutet awarded the 2018 Nobel Prize in Physiology or Medicine to James P. Allison and Tasuku Honjo for their "discovery of cancer therapy by inhibition of negative immune regulation." The most prominent checkpoint inhibitors are atezolizumab, durvalumab, ipilimumab, nivolumab, and pembrolizumab, which have been commercially highly successful, generating more than 20 billion USD in sales in 2022.

While immunotherapy has produced impressive results in cancers such as non-small-cell lung cancer and melanoma, it has unfortunately been less effective in gastrointestinal (GI) cancers. In fact, initial results of clinical trials testing checkpoint inhibitors as monotherapy or in combination with chemotherapy in unselected patients with metastatic GI cancers were disappointing. However, it has become clear that selected patient populations present excellent responses, such as metastatic colon cancer patients with microsatellite instability which has led to the approval of pembrolizumab by the U.S. Food and Drug Administration and the European Medicines Agency in the first-line setting and of nivolumab and ipilimumab in the second-line setting. Many indications have followed since, giving patients with biliary tract, esophageal, gastroesophageal, gastric cancer, and hepatocellular carcinoma access to immunotherapy. This has ensued changes in the treatment landscape of these diseases at an unprecedented scale and speed.

Current and future clinical trials are exploring different kinds of immunotherapy in various settings both alone and in combination with other treatments, which will have a strong impact on the management of patients with GI cancers in the future. Their success will depend on patient selection and study design. Innovative combinations will most likely create the greatest value.

This book aims to provide the reader with an overview of the current standard-of-care of patients with GI cancers paying particular attention to the current role of immunotherapy. In addition, the perspective chapters offer the reader an outlook on the future of immunotherapy for the different entities including forms of treatment that are currently at an early stage of clinical development.

In the rapidly developing world of cancer immunotherapy, it may seem inadequate to use the medium of a book, which can only capture the knowledge and ideas as at the time of writing. However, given the multitude of therapies in clinical development for the different GI cancer entities, we deemed it overdue to assemble a book devoted to the current roles and future potentials of immunotherapy in the treatment of GI cancers.

We have been very fortunate to gather a circle of highly distinguished authors who share their expert knowledge and experience in the following chapters. We owe them a great debt of gratitude for their contributions and their commitment in bringing this book to life.

Cancer immunotherapy is currently one of the most exciting topics in medicine and will most likely remain so in the coming years. We are confident it will deliver on its promise of improving the treatment options and the prognosis of GI cancer patients. Our book has attempted to capture this enthusiasm for making it an insightful and worthwhile read. We truly hope that you, the readers, will be inspired by it and that it will help to strengthen your motivation for clinical research and daily practice.

First Department of Medicine
University Medical Center of the
Johannes Gutenberg University Mainz
Mainz, Germany

Friedrich Foerster
Markus Moehler

Contents

Part I

Role of the Tumor Microenvironment

An Overview of the Tumor Microenvironment and Response to Immunotherapy in Gastrointestinal Malignancies

Cameron J. Herting and Gregory B. Lesinski

Contents

Abstract

The activity of the immune system under homeostasis and disease states is governed by complex interactions of cells both through direct cell–cell contact and the secretion of soluble immunomodulatory factors. In cancer, the tumor microenvironment is increasingly being recognized as a key mediator of these interactions. The tumor microenvironment consists of a diverse milieu of malignant and stromal cells that typically constitute the tissue, as well as both tissue-resident immune cells and those that infiltrate from the circulation. It is now clear that

C. J. Herting · G. B. Lesinski (✉)
Department of Hematology and Medical Oncology, Winship Cancer Institute, Emory University, Atlanta, GA, USA
e-mail: gregory.b.lesinski@emory.edu

Cancer Immunotherapy (2021)

https://doi.org/10.1007/13905_2021_1,

Published Online: 14 August 2021

defining factors that govern the balance between heterogeneous cell populations within the microenvironment can advance our understanding of disease progression across different malignancies. In addition, this knowledge can be leveraged to improve clinical outcomes in patients with tumors that are traditionally refractory to immunotherapy. As the development of immunotherapeutic anticancer modalities has accelerated over the past decade, it has become abundantly clear that we must investigate and understand these interactions to rationally design effective treatment regimens. In this chapter, we will outline the major players within the tumor microenvironment across prevalent gastrointestinal malignancies. Emphasis will be placed on cell types, such as fibroblasts, that play a substantial role in shaping the dynamic microenvironment of gastrointestinal cancers. We will also describe the differential response of selected gastrointestinal cancers to immunotherapy and illustrate how the microenvironment influences these responses. This chapter will provide the reader with a fundamental overview of the tumor microenvironment and immunotherapy in gastrointestinal malignancies.

Keywords

Cancer · Fibroblast · Gastrointestinal · Immunotherapy · Inflammation · Macrophage · Microenvironment · T cell

1 An Overview of Gastrointestinal Malignancies

Cancer is ubiquitously present within all tissues of the human body. Depending on the location of origin, tumors present with variable severity and frequency. This chapter will offer an introductory journey through the GI tract to highlight the types of tumors that are frequently found at each location. Next, we will discuss in greater detail the cellular players present within the tumor microenvironment and their relevance to immunotherapy.

The gastrointestinal tract is a series of organs that form a non-interrupted pathway from the mouth to the anus (Fig. 1). Epithelial cells line these organs and are subject to constant exposure to environmental stimuli that pass through the body via the natural digestive process. While these cells are typically well-equipped through DNA repair or apoptotic mechanisms to deal with various molecular insults, they are also susceptible to transformation, which can be further fueled by inflammatory conditions [1–3]. Organs such as the liver, gallbladder, and pancreas are also considered GI organs as they secrete enzymes into the GI tract and actively participate in digestion. Each of these organs can be afflicted with primary tumors and further can be common sites of metastatic spread of tumors from various anatomic origins. In this introduction, we will discuss the primary tumors present at each location.

The upper part of the GI tract can be defined as the mouth, esophagus, stomach, and the duodenum. For the purposes of this chapter, we will refrain from discussing

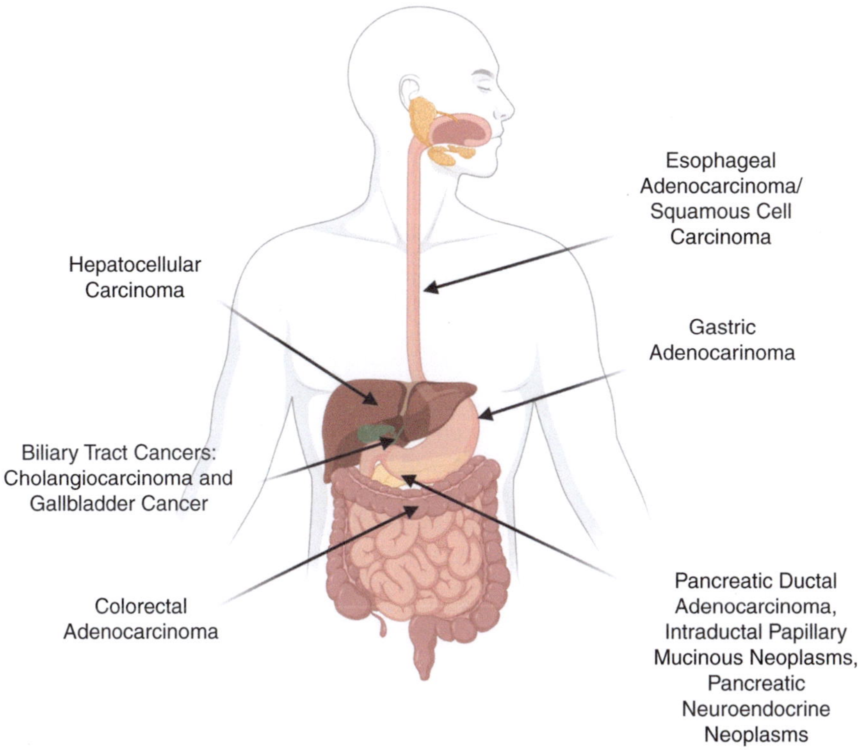

Fig. 1 Common sites of cancer development in the gastrointestinal tract. Common sites of cancer development are listed with arrows directed towards where the tumors are found. This list is meant to diagram the most frequently occurring lesions and is not a comprehensive list

cancers of the mouth. The esophagus, the first organ of the GI tract, is afflicted primarily with esophageal cancer (EC), a term that encompasses both squamous cell carcinoma and adenocarcinoma, diseases with a relatively poor 5-year survival rate of 15–20% [4]. The next location in the GI tract that is a common site for primary tumors is the stomach, where gastric cancer (GC) can arise. This disease presents a notable global health burden, landing in the top five cancers with respect to both disease incidence and cancer-related deaths [5]. Proximal to the stomach are the liver and pancreas. These organs are intimately connected to the GI tract and can also give rise to multiple individual types of cancer. Within the liver, there are two main types of primary tumors evident. First, hepatocellular carcinoma (HCC) is a cancer originating from hepatocytes, and can be driven by several factors including chronic liver inflammation from viral infection, typically with hepatitis B virus or hepatitis C virus, non-alcoholic fatty liver disease, or chronic alcohol and/or drug use [6–8]. Second, are biliary tract cancers (BTCs) which encompass cholangiocarcinoma (CCA) and gallbladder cancer, which arise in epithelial cells that constitute the biliary tree [9]. Based on anatomic location, CCA can be further divided into intrahepatic, extrahepatic, and hilar tumors. Similar to the liver, the pancreas also functions as an exocrine organ responsible for delivering digestive enzymes into the duodenum that facilitate the breakdown of food as it exits the stomach and enters the lower GI tract. The pancreas is the site of pancreatic ductal adenocarcinoma (PDAC), a cancer primarily afflicting the acinar cells responsible for producing the pancreatic digestive enzymes, intraductal papillary mucinous neoplasms (IPMN), and rare pancreatic neuroendocrine neoplasms (pNEN) that compromise only 1–2% of total pancreatic tumors [10–12]. The next location within the GI tract is the small intestine, where over forty different subtypes of tumors arise although they only account for 3–6% of total intestinal tumors. Typically these tumors are managed by operative resection with survival rate dependent on disease subtype and metastatic spread [13]. Due to the large variety of tumor subtypes, relatively small incidence, and limited information regarding tumor microenvironment and immunotherapy, we will not discuss these tumors further. The distal portion of the GI tract harbors the colon and rectum, which are frequent sites of tumorigenesis. In particular, colorectal cancer (CRC) has emerged with increasing frequency attributable to modifiable risk factors, primarily in the western world, and contributes substantially to cancer-associated mortality with near to 1 million deaths per year [14].

Cancers within the GI tract are often difficult to detect due to an absence of symptoms until late-stage disease, limited biomarkers of early stage neoplasms, and invasive as well as expensive screening tools [15]. The high mortality rates of GI malignancies, in particular PDAC, and BTC can be largely attributed to lack of detection until late-stage disease [16, 17]. By and large, surgical resection remains the only curative approach to treating these malignancies. Late-stage tumors where metastatic disease is present negate the possibility of surgical resection, thereby significantly reducing the likelihood of curing the patient. There is, however, a bit of gray area where chemotherapy can be leveraged to allow for surgical approaches to be employed. For example, in locally advanced and borderline resectable PDAC, neoadjuvant FOLFIRINOX can decrease tumor burden to a point suitable for surgical resection [18]. In total, the optimal treatment regimen for GI tumors is likely to be one that combines pharmacological and surgical therapeutic approaches. The coming years will elucidate the role that microenvironment-targeted therapies and immunotherapies play in GI oncology.

2 Key Players in the Tumor Microenvironment

The establishment of a tumor-supportive cellular microenvironment is a major factor that influences the progression and therapeutic response of GI neoplasms. The tumor microenvironment (TME) can be defined as the combination of various cell types that constitute the tumor mass. The composition of the TME varies based on tumor type and location, differs between patients, and even within different areas of single tumors. Cross-talk between tumor and stromal cells influences the development and progression of GI tumors. An intuitive way to conceptualize this was put forth by Dvorak with his description of cancer as "a wound that never heals" [19]. In essence, this description captures the dynamic environment within a tumor, where stromal cells and immune cells are constantly interacting in a manner that prevents further cell death and tissue damage. At early stages of tumor development, tumor cells secrete damage-associated molecular patterns (DAMPs), for example, interleukin-1α (IL-1α), that initiate a wound healing response [20, 21]. By late-stage disease, it is common to find a tumor microenvironment characterized by abundant immunosuppressive cell populations, extensive deposition of extracellular matrix proteins, and limited infiltration of immune cell populations with cytotoxic potential against tumors [22, 23]. This microenvironment centers around the activities of numerous stromal cell, tissue-resident immune cell, and infiltrating immune cell populations will be described herein (Fig. 2).

Perhaps the most widely studied, appreciated, and therapeutically targeted cell type within the tumor microenvironment is the cancerous cells. In tumors, the malignant cells are those with acquired mutations that drive aberrant replication [24]. These mutations can be those that activate oncogenic signaling pathways, inactivate or downregulate tumor suppressor genes, alter the epigenetic landscape of the tumor cells, and more [25]. Within the tumor microenvironment, cancer cells are initially responsible for dictating how the surrounding tissue responds. In essence, the cancer cells secrete factors that drive how the nearby cells within the tissue, and immune cells from the periphery, initially respond. For example, in PDAC cancer cells produce factors including transforming growth factor-β (TGF-β), interleukin-1α/β (IL-1α/β), fibroblast growth factor 2 (FGF2), and platelet-derived

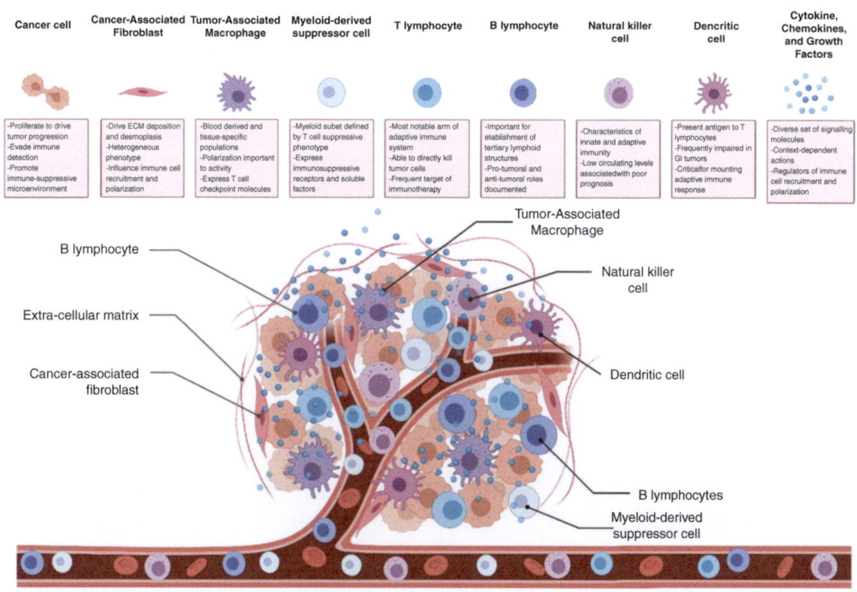

Fig. 2 Major cellular and soluble components of the tumor microenvironment in gastrointestinal malignancies. Here, the most common and well-studied cellular components of the gastrointestinal tumor microenvironment are listed. This figure is not exhaustive, and excludes cellular subsets, such as eosinophils, innate lymphoid cells, and mast cells, that may also play a role

growth factor (PDGF) that cause quiescent pancreatic stellate cells (PSCs) to activate into cancer-associated fibroblasts (CAFs) that produce substantial extracellular matrix proteins and drive the formation of PDAC-associated desmoplasia [26–29]. Further, as the tumor microenvironment is established, the stromal compartments begin secreting factors that modulate the behavior of the cancer cells. Again, considering PDAC as an example, CAFs also regulate cancer cell metabolism under conditions of glucose deprivation and secrete factors such as interleukin-6 (IL-6) and granulocyte-macrophage colony-stimulating factor (GM-CSF) that drive cancer cell invasion as well as differentiation of myeloid cells into immunosuppressive phenotypes [30–34]. Taken together, there is a clear cross-talk between cancer cells with the stromal and immune components of tumors throughout all stages of tumor development that mold the composition and behavior of the TME.

3 Cancer and Stromal Cell Cross-Talk: Role of Epithelial to Mesenchymal Transition

In addition to cancer and stromal cell cross-talk, there are intrinsic characteristics of tumor cells that are important to consider. For example, during tumor progression, it is common for cancer cells to activate transcription factors such as SNAIL and TWIST that cause the cells to undergo the epithelial to mesenchymal transition (EMT), a process that is typically observed during embryogenesis [35]. It should be noted that this is a dynamic and reversible process and cells within tumors are commonly observed on a spectrum between the two cell phenotypes [36, 37]. Specific to GI cancers, this EMT has been shown to facilitate the ability of malignant cells to resist treatment and metastasize in PDAC and CRC [38, 39]. As a result, EMT has become a notable target in a variety of malignancies [40]. An important factor that dictates the overall cancer cell phenotype and behavior is the cell of origin from which the cancer arises. In both PDAC and CRC, there exists some debate on the identity of the cell of origin and it is perhaps possible that it varies from patient to patient [41, 42]. For example, in CRC, genetic models suggest that the intestinal stem cells within the crypts of the intestinal villi are the cell of origin [43–45]. However, it has also been shown that non-stem cells within the intestine can acquire stem-like properties and serve as the cell of origin in subsets of CRC [46, 47]. In PDAC, the debate revolves around whether the ductal or acinar cells are the cell of origin. Conventional wisdom defined ductal cells as the cell of origin largely due to the morphology of tumor specimens [48, 49]. Recent work with genetically engineered mouse models, however, has shown that either cell type can be the cell of origin and that ductal-cell and acinar-cell derived tumors display distinct disease progression and morphological characteristics [50]. Future work will more conclusively characterize the roles that EMT and cell of origin play in disease progression and treatment response. It is, however, already clear that both factors play an important role in cancer cell biology.

One stromal cell type that plays a particularly important role across GI malignancies is fibroblasts. Fibroblasts are cells that make up connective tissue and are primarily responsible for producing extracellular matrix proteins under homeostatic conditions, as well as injury [51]. Activated fibroblasts in cancer are known to modulate resistance to chemotherapy, deposit large amounts of extracellular matrix proteins, drive angiogenesis, and regulate tumor progression [52]. Murine studies have established a prominent and multifaceted role for fibroblasts in the progression of both PDAC and CRC [53–55]. The relationship is more complicated than a simple model whereby CAFs support tumor growth. In fact, prior studies have shown that depletion of α-smooth muscle actin (α-SMA)-positive CAFs, or blockade of CAF-activating sonic hedgehog (SHH) signaling, leads to accelerated tumor progression in PDAC and CRC, respectively [56–58]. The role of CAFs in GI cancers is further muddled when one considers their heterogeneity. Recent work in PDAC has identified multiple different subtypes of CAFs with distinct roles and actions within the tumor microenvironment [59, 60]. The two largest phenotypically defined populations of CAFs appear to be those polarized by IL-1α and TGF-β and they appear to be associated with immune cell chemotaxis and ECM deposition, respectively [61]. Characterization of CAF heterogeneity has arguably advanced the furthest in PDAC, however is likely relevant to tumors of other anatomic origins. In addition to their cross-talk with cancer cells, CAFs also communicate with immune cell populations that are prominent in GI malignancies. For example, IL-6 produced by CAFs is known to prevent infiltration of anti-tumoral T cells in PDAC and CAF-derived IL-8 promotes accumulation and polarization of pro-tumoral M2 macrophages in CRC [62, 63]. Further, CAF-derived TGF-β has been shown to attenuate the cytotoxic potential of $CD8^+$ T cells as well as suppress natural killer (NK) cell function [63–65]. In total, CAFs are a diverse component of the tumor microenvironment in GI malignancies. They represent a heterogeneous population with both pro- and anti-tumoral properties. Ongoing work will illuminate strategies that target CAFs to enhance the efficacy of anti-tumoral immunotherapy.

4 Tumor Microenvironment: The Role of Tumor-Associated Macrophages (TAM)

Another prominent component of the tumor microenvironment in GI malignancies is tumor-associated macrophages (TAMs). TAMs can be derived from both circulating monocytes and tissue-resident macrophage populations. For example, in HCC, TAMs both infiltrate from the circulation and arise from liver-resident Kupffer cells [66, 67]. Further, tissue-resident TAMs derived from embryonic hematopoiesis play a distinct role in the progression of PDAC [68]. That is not to say that circulating TAMs do not play a role as $CCR2^+$ macrophages recruited to PDAC as well as liver metastases of CRC have been shown to contribute to resistance to chemotherapy and confer an overall poor prognosis [69, 70]. TAMs are also a heterogeneous population of cells with respect to their gene expression profile and phenotype. TAMs are often described as polarized to either M1 or M2 phenotypes, with the former considered anti-tumoral and the later pro-tumoral [71, 72]. It should be noted, however, that this polarization scheme was derived from early *in vitro* experiments comparing the response of macrophages to specific stimuli as well as their metabolic profiles in different murine strains. As a result, the polarization of macrophages in complex *in vivo* situations such as a tumor is likely much more complex than a simple M1 to M2 spectrum [73–75]. This polarization scheme, while imperfect, still offers a valuable conceptual framework considering the multifaceted role of macrophages in GI malignancies. TAMs can promote angiogenesis, drive a metastatic tumor cell phenotype, and suppress anti-tumoral T cells through expression of checkpoint molecules such as PD-L1 in CRC [76–78]. Other studies, however, have shown that increased infiltration of macrophages in CRC is associated with improved patient outcomes [79]. Transcriptional analysis of these macrophages indicates that increased levels of M1-like cells, particularly those that express high levels of immune checkpoints like PD-L1, LAG-3, and TIM-3 are responsible for this positive correlation [80, 81]. Agonism of CD11b has also been investigated as a strategy to sensitize PDAC to immunotherapy through reprogramming of innate immunity and repolarization of TAMs [82]. In total, the role of TAMs in GI cancers depends substantially on the phenotype of the cells. Considering their highly plastic nature, therapies that aim to re-educate or re-polarize TAMs as opposed to depleting them are more likely to have beneficial therapeutic effects.

5 New Interest in Cancer Immunology: Myeloid-Derived Suppressor Cells (MDSCs)

In addition to TAMs, other myeloid cell population that are of interest in cancer immunology are myeloid-derived suppressor cells (MDSCs) that, as the name suggests, are largely immunosuppressive. MDSCs were initially defined as cells sharing the CD11b and Gr-1 (Ly6C and Ly6G in mice) surface epitopes [83, 84]. The terminology MDSC arose from the observation that these cells are of myeloid origin, systemically expand in the context of cancer, and exert immune-suppressive function and were simply meant to describe the phenotype of these cells, not define a novel or distinct cell population [85]. It is now apparent that the MDSC cell subsets encompass at least two main populations, polymorphonuclear MDSCs (PMN-MDSC) and monocytic MDSCs (M-MDSC) with distinct cellular characteristics, but overlapping functions [86]. MDSCs are pathologically activated myeloid cells that arise from situations of chronic inflammation as observed in tumors [87]. Due to the aberrant and chronic activation of inflammatory pathways that are otherwise transient in nature, MDSCs mature into cells that are incapable of carrying out the normal phagocytic functions of myeloid cells, but are potent suppressors of T and NK cell-mediated cell killing [88–90]. It therefore comes as no surprise that a major role for MDSCs in the tumor microenvironment is suppression of anti-tumoral T cell immunity. MDSCs are recruited to tumors through similar chemotactic pathways to those that recruit monocyte-derived TAMs, including CCL2 and CCL5 [91, 92]. Within the tumor, MDSCs upregulate various immunosuppressive pathways and receptors through activation of HIF-1α [93]. Further, in CRC it has been demonstrated that MDSCs produce large amounts of reactive oxygen species (ROS) and nitric oxide (NO), both of which are immunosuppressive [94, 95]. MDSC can also exert immune suppression by a number of functional mediators. For example, in addition to the production of NO and ROS, or expression of inhibitory checkpoint ligands (i.e. PD-L1), they can also modulate the metabolic features of tumors through secretion of arginase, and deprivation of cysteine needed for optimal T cell function and survival [96–98]. Further, they are a prominent source of cytokines including IL-10 that can modulate dendritic cell function and antigen presentation, or IL-6 and TGF-β that modulate T cell function. In total, MDSCs are a major immunosuppressive cell type in the tumor microenvironment when considering their impact on activity of T lymphocytes and NK cells. It comes as no surprise then, that the presence of MDSCs is considered tumor-supportive in both CRC and PDAC [99, 100]. Therefore, strategies to deplete their presence, inhibit their individual functional mediators, or block their infiltration into the tumor microenvironment are suitable therapeutic avenues to target this population.

6 Adaptive Immunity in Cancer Immunotherapy

Among the most prominent cell type of relevance to mechanisms of cancer immunotherapy are T lymphocytes. T cells, so named due to their origin in the thymus, can differentiate into a multitude of phenotypic and functional subsets and represent the largest constituent of the adaptive immune system [101]. Similar to the other cell types discussed in this section, T lymphocytes are highly plastic cells with a variety of activation states governed by engagement of the T cell antigen receptor (TCR), co-stimulatory receptors, and immune checkpoint receptors [102]. All T lymphocytes are characterized by expression of the CD3 receptor [103]. This receptor is responsible for associating with the TCR and transmitting its signal via intracellular cascades within the T cell [104]. In addition to CD3, T lymphocytes can be further sub-divided by their expression of the CD4 and CD8 surface receptors that classify the cells as helper T cells and cytotoxic T cells, respectively [105, 106]. During development, progenitors from the bone marrow enter the thymus lacking expression of CD4 and CD8. They then undergo TCR rearrangement and emerge as $CD4^+CD8^+$ double-positive thymocytes that further differentiate into $CD4^+$ or $CD8^+$ cells following selection [101]. In general, $CD8^+$ T cells are those tasked with cytotoxic function while $CD4^+$ T cells facilitate this action by supporting $CD8^+$ T cell engagement with antigen-presenting cells and producing cytokines [107–109]. The process of T cell engagement and activation can be considered to be a three-step process [110]. First, the TCR engages an antigen-major histocompatibility complex (MHC) conjugate on the surface of antigen-presenting cells, leading to conformational change of the CD3 complex and thymocyte activation [111]. For complete activation, the T cell must then be co-stimulated by receptors such as CD28 [112, 113]. Following co-stimulation, T cells express cytokines such as interleukin-2 (IL-2) that drive cell proliferation and expansion [114, 115]. These general steps underlie essentially all T cell-mediated immunity in both $CD4^+$ and $CD8^+$ cells. A subset of $CD4^+$ T cells, T regulatory (T_{reg}) cells are also responsible for resolving the cytotoxic T cell response and managing T cell memory formation, largely through regulating IL-2 levels [116, 117]. T cell activity is also regulated by a variety of immune checkpoint receptors (e.g. PD-1) that are upregulated upon activation and prevent excessive adaptive immune responses [118]. These receptors will be discussed in detail in the next section discussing immunotherapy in GI malignancies.

T cell infiltration into tumors is prognostic in a variety of GI malignancies including HCC, gastric cancer, PDAC, and CRC [119–122]. By and large, these studies have shown that high amounts of T lymphocytes within tumors are associated with improved patient outcomes. Conversely, it is recognized that immunologically "cold" tumors, characterized by very limited T cell infiltration, have universally poor prognoses. This is exemplified by PDAC which is considered an immune "desert" with T cell infiltration largely limited to the tumor border and a 5-year survival rate of <10% [123]. Conversely, esophageal cancer (EC) is known to harbor larger amounts of tumor-infiltrating T cells and these have also been shown to be specific to antigens expressed by EC tumor cells including MAGE-A3 and NY-ESO-1 [124, 125]. This raises another significant point, for successful anti-tumoral T cell immunity, T cells must be able to infiltrate the tissue, they must be able to recognize a suitable tumor-associated antigen, and they must not be sufficiently restrained by checkpoint molecules or other mediators. In total, T cells represent a major tumor microenvironmental component that cancer immunotherapy often aims to manipulate.

In addition to T lymphocytes, B lymphocytes are also present in the tumor microenvironment from several GI malignancies, albeit at relatively low frequency. Their activity within the microenvironment remains somewhat controversial and incompletely defined [126–128]. For example, classical studies indicated that mice lacking B cells exhibited enhanced anti-tumor immunity when compared to those with intact B cells [129]. Further studies, including those utilizing the MC38 model of CRC, illustrated that cytotoxic T cell responses and T_H1 cytokine profiles were increased in mice lacking B cells [130]. In fact, it was even illustrated that mice lacking mature B cells were less likely to develop inflammation-associated cancer [131]. In total, these results were interpreted as evidence that B lymphocytes are largely tumor-promoting. Recent work in GI malignancies, however, is questioning these results. In patients with gastric and esophageal adenocarcinomas, immunohistochemical analysis of IGKC, a marker of a B cell subset called plasma cells, indicated that patients with increased infiltration of plasma cells had prolonged overall survival following surgical resection [132]. Similar results were obtained in CRC where a higher density of $CD20^+$ B cells and $IGKC^+$ plasma cells were both associated with improved overall survival [133]. These conflicting results beg the question, what exactly do B cells do in the tumor microenvironment?

B cells play three major roles within the tumor microenvironment. First, they serve as a subset of antigen-presenting cells, thereby facilitating T cell differentiation, expansion, and activation [134, 135]. Second, B lymphocytes in cancer immunity participate in the formation of tertiary lymphoid organs. These structures form at peripheral sites of inflammation and are characterized by separated T and B cell locations, activated dendritic cells, and generation of lymphatic vessels [136, 137].

These tertiary lymphoid structures seem to serve similar purposes to secondary lymphoid structures, such as lymph nodes, as removal of the latter does not impair formation of a memory T cell response [138]. Specific to CRC, it has been demonstrated that formation of tertiary lymphoid structures directly correlates with T cell infiltration and predicts better prognosis of early stage disease [139]. Based on these data, it might be concluded that B cells in the tumor microenvironment support antitumoral T cell immunity through formation of tertiary lymphoid structures. However, in PDAC, it has also been shown that particular B cell subsets expressing interleukin-35 (IL-35) contribute to tumor growth through polarization of TAMs to a tumor-supportive phenotype [140, 141]. This data illustrates the final role for B cells in the tumor microenvironment which is production of chemokines and cytokines. Further, the secretion of IL-35 by B cells may complement tumor-derived IL-35 that has also been noted in PDAC tumors [142]. Overall, B cells have seemingly diverse and context dependent roles within the tumor microenvironment. Further work must define these roles with greater certainty to allow for effective pharmacological targeting of this cell subset for cancer immunotherapy.

7 Natural Killer (NK) Cells as a Novel Frontier in Cancer Immunotherapy

Natural killer (NK) cells are a cell type known to bridge the adaptive and innate immune response. These large granular lymphocytes lack the ability to rearrange T cell receptor or immunoglobulin domains, like T and B cells, respectively, and instead are able to "naturally kill" target cells without priming or engagement of MHC molecules [143]. NK cells are able to recognize and kill adjacent cells that express surface makers associated with oncogenic transformation [144]. As such, NK cells are sentinel mediators of cancer immunosurveillance [145]. One example is the capability of NK cells to eliminate oncogenically transformed cells that have downregulated or eliminated expression of MHC class I. This molecule typically prevents NK cell activation through engagement of the killer cell immunoglobulin-like receptors [146, 147]. Furthermore, individuals with high levels of NK cell cytotoxicity are at reduced risk of cancer and conversely, those with defects in NK cell activity display higher rates of cancer [148, 149]. In the setting of CRC, higher levels of circulating NK cells are associated with a positive prognosis, as assessed by overall survival [150]. This epidemiological evidence strongly implies that NK cells play a pivotal role in surveillance for and elimination of malignant cells. As a result, NK cells have become a notable substrate for cell-based therapy in PDAC [151]. The common NK cell-based therapeutic modalities typically involve extracting cells, expanding them *ex vivo*, and reinfusing them into the patient. Relevant to this strategy, low levels of circulating NK cells have been tied to a lack of CXCR2 expression and low levels of *ex vivo* NK cell expansion are associated with reduced overall survival [152]. Within the tumor microenvironment, NK cells are thought to serve as a link between the innate and adaptive immune system. They secrete cytokines that modulate the activities of both dendritic cells and T cells [153, 154].

Considering the scarcity of NK cells within tumors, in some cases they constitute less than 1% of total cells, it has been challenging to study these cells and solidify the specific actions they perform and roles they play within the tumor microenvironment. Future work, likely leveraging cutting-edge single-cell technologies will further delineate the niche these cells occupy and illuminate how they can be leveraged therapeutically across GI malignancies.

8 Dendritic Cells (DCs) Link the Innate and Adaptive Immune System

Dendritic cells (DCs) play an important role as a focal point for communication between the innate and adaptive immune systems. DCs are notable for their ability to present antigen to naïve T cells and induce their activation [155]. They achieve this by continuously sampling their environment, capturing and processing foreign antigens or irregular self-antigens, and displaying these antigens to T cells with MHC molecules [156]. Further, upon exposure to a "danger" signal, for example, a peptide associated with a foreign microbe, DCs will migrate to the lymph node where they induce the expansion of T lymphocytes via engagement of co-stimulatory molecules and polarize them into either T_H1 or T_H2 cells via cytokine signals [157]. In addition to their roles in disease, DCs play a key role in tolerance through the deletion of self-reactive T cells [158]. In the context of gastrointestinal tumors, DCs appear functionally impaired, and unable to effectively induce an adaptive immune response [159, 160]. For example, in patients with both CRC and PDAC, circulating DCs are decreased compared to patients without tumors [161, 162]. In the PDAC cohort, higher levels of circulating and tumor-infiltrating DCs were associated with prolonged survival following surgical resection. Moreover, it has been shown that CRC tumor cells express immunosuppressive factors, such as 2, 3 indolamine dioxygenase (IDO), that actively dampen the ability of DCs to cross-present antigen to T cells [163]. It is clear that DCs play a critical role in establishing a sustained antitumoral adaptive immune response. By and large, however, tumors develop the capabilities to suppress DC maturation and activities, thereby enhancing their ability to escape immune detection and elimination. Future therapies should target these mechanisms to enhance DC activity within tumors, particularly in situations when T cell-targeted immunotherapy is employed.

9 Targeting the Tumor Microenvironment to Enhance Clinical Immunotherapy

The tumor microenvironment is a complex mixture of different cell types, both neoplastic and non-neoplastic as well as immune and non-immune, that largely communicate through the secretion of soluble factors. The most prominent of these factors are chemokines, cytokines, and growth factors that mediate immune cell recruitment, differentiation, and activity. There are hundreds of these factors that act in concert to coordinate these actions, a thorough discussion of which is beyond the scope of this introductory chapter. There are a few, however, that have come to prominence as key mediators of the tumor microenvironment in gastrointestinal malignancies. For example, in PDAC, interleukin-6 (IL-6) has emerged as a factor that can be secreted from stromal cells, tumor cells, or infiltrating myeloid cells [164–166]. This cytokine drives the desmoplastic stromal response and suppresses the activity of cytotoxic T cells [165, 167, 168]. Moreover, high levels of circulating IL-6 in PDAC are a predictor of poor prognosis, and IL-6 neutralization enhances the response to both chemotherapy and immunotherapy in preclinical PDAC models [62, 169, 170]. This evidence has led to the initiation of clinical trials studying the combination of IL-6 neutralizing therapy with both chemotherapy (EudraCT: 2016–000643-13) and immune checkpoint blockade (NCT04191421). Furthermore, IL-6 derived from hepatic stellate cells can drive progression of HCC and induce expansion of MDSCs [171, 172]. In addition to IL-6, the chemokine CCL2 has been identified as a key regulator of the tumor microenvironment in gastrointestinal malignancies, largely through its actions as a myeloid cell chemoattractant protein. The role of these recruited myeloid cells, however, appears to be somewhat context dependent. For example, CCL2 secreted by PDAC tumor cells following radiation therapy recruits myeloid cells to the tumor. Subsequently, these cells promote tumor proliferation and neovascularization, largely tumor-supportive actions [173]. Following CD40 agonism, however, CCL2 and interferon-gamma (IFNγ) cooperate to recruit myeloid cells that degrade the fibrotic extracellular matrix and sensitize tumors to chemotherapy [174]. Both CCL2 neutralization (NCT02732938) and CD40 agonism (NCT04130854) have been investigated in clinical trials for GI malignancies. Overall, there are a plethora of chemokines and cytokines that guide the composition and behavior of the immune microenvironment in GI malignancies. Many of these are likely to be viable therapeutic targets. Over the coming decade, it is probable that we will see the maturation of these strategies into clinically relevant modalities.

These results in total highlight that it is likely not the actions of individual chemokines and cytokines, or even the actions of individual immune cell subsets that are important in gastrointestinal malignancies. Instead, it is the overall product of these factors acting in concert to either promote or combat tumor progression. As more high-throughput technical assays, like cytometry by time of flight (CyTOF), single-cell RNA sequencing, and highly multiplexed chemokine and cytokine profiling become more widely prevalent, it is likely that we will gain a better understanding of how exactly these factors influence one another, and which factors are key orchestrators of pro-tumoral and anti-tumoral responses. Furthermore, it is possible that novel bioinformatic techniques like machine learning and artificial intelligence algorithms will usher in a new age of personalized medicine where therapeutic approaches are guided by pre-treatment assessment of circulating and tumor intrinsic chemokine, cytokine, and immune cell profiles. As it stands currently, however, we do have at least a basic understanding of the tumor microenvironment and how it dictates response to currently utilized immunotherapies. Finally, we should emphasize that this opening chapter is only meant to provide a basic framework for the reader to understand concepts presented in the remainder of the book. This is by no means a comprehensive review and there are other cellular subsets and soluble factors that are undoubtedly important components of the tumor microenvironment in GI malignancies.

10 The Tumor Microenvironment and Response to Immunotherapy in GI Malignancies

Major advances in the field of clinical oncology have been made over the past decade through the introduction and clinical approval of immunotherapeutic approaches for cancer therapy. The first reports of strategies that invoke the immune system to attack tumors span to 1891 when William B. Coley applied the idea to inject streptococcal bacteria into a patient with inoperable cancer [175]. He observed notable tumor regression and refined this strategy over the years treating nearly 1000 patients with his "Coley Toxins." This approach demonstrated success in managing the clinical progression of bone and soft-tissue sarcomas. Thankfully, the immunotherapeutic approaches used today are substantially more refined and mainly involve the direct targeting of T cell suppressive immune checkpoint molecules with antibody-based therapies. These targeted therapies have concentrated a great deal on disrupting inhibitory immune checkpoint pathways, including PD-1/PD-L1 and CTLA-4, and have illustrated variable impacts across gastrointestinal diseases. While some tumor types respond well, others illustrate negligible response. Furthermore, it has become apparent that in some cases, subsets of individual tumor types, for example, microsatellite instable CRC, are quite responsive while others are not [176]. The precise biology underpinning this variable response appears to depend on tumor cell intrinsic factors as well as factors surrounding the tumor microenvironment. For example, esophageal cancer remains largely refractory to immunotherapy [177].

Esophageal squamous cell carcinoma is slightly more responsive than adenocarcinoma, but overall response remains low. This limited response has been attributed to low expression of PD-L1 in esophageal cancer, where the cell subsets expressing this marker are of myeloid lineage, and those with >1% of these cells in the tumor display a response rate of ~25%, versus ~15% in those with <1% of these cells [178].

Similarly, ***gastric cancer*** remains minimally responsive to checkpoint blockade with the CheckMate649 trial illustrating an extension of median survival of 2.2 months to just over 1 year in patients that received nivolumab plus chemotherapy versus chemotherapy alone [179]. Overall, checkpoint blockade for gastric cancer and gastro-esophageal junction adenocarcinoma remains second- or third-line therapy following progression on standard chemotherapeutic regimens [180].

PDAC displays similarly limited response to immunotherapy. In this disease context, combination of immunotherapy with chemotherapy has been demonstrated as safe, but no notable extensions in median survival have yet been demonstrated [181, 182]. Studies of murine models of PDAC have indicated that combination of "traditional" immunotherapeutic approaches like PD-1 and CTLA-4 blockade, or cytotoxic chemotherapy, may be effective when combined with agents that target myeloid components such as CD40 agonism [183]. In fact, a recent clinical trial demonstrated the tolerability and clinical activity of combined CD40 agonism and chemotherapy in metastatic PDAC [184]. Considering the notable immunosuppressive microenvironment in PDAC, it is unsurprising that single-agent immunotherapy has proven unsuccessful. Combination therapies that simultaneously stimulate T cells while additionally remodeling the microenvironment are in preclinical development and may hold promise [185, 186]. Further, groups are investigating combining radiation with immunotherapy, various cell-therapy approaches, and oncolytic viruses in PDAC although these investigations remain at relatively early stages [187–189].

In contrast to PDAC, results in **HCC and CCA** have demonstrated more encouraging results. Single agent PD-1/PD-L1 blockade provides an objective response rate of around 5–20% in CCA [190]. Although still relatively low overall, for CCA, this disease control rate is clinically meaningful. Single agent CTLA-4 and PD-1 blockade have both only shown modest efficacy in HCC [191–194]. It should be noted that in some of these trials although a significant extension in median progression-free survival and overall survival was not observed, a favorable risk-benefit ratio was, supporting the implementation of these approaches in certain settings [194]. Moreover, combination of the anti-PD-L1 therapy atezolizumab with the vascular endothelial growth factor (VEGF) inhibitor bevacizumab has been shown to extend overall and progression-free survival relative to the standard of care sorafenib in a recent phase III clinical trial [195]. This result emphasizes that the most efficacious treatments for GI malignancies are likely to combine immunotherapy with other chemotherapeutic or biologic agents. Certainly, the rise of clinical trials testing these combinatorial approaches within the past decade illustrates the excitement the field has for these modalities.

Patients with some subsets of gastrointestinal malignancies can derive clinical benefit from immune checkpoint blockade alone. For example, patients with **CRC** largely do not respond to immunotherapy [196–198]. However, in early trials assessing PD-1 blockade in solid tumors, including CRC, it was found that a very small subset of patients derived notable clinical benefit from this approach [199]. In particular, patients with microsatellite instable/DNA mismatch repair deficient tumors (MSI-H/dMMR) display durable responses when compared to their "wildtype" counterparts [200]. These patients display tumors with higher mutational burden, thereby offering more antigens for the adaptive immune system to recognize and attack [201]. This concept has further led to the development of an immunoscore that can predict patients with CRC that will respond well to immunotherapy [202]. Moreover, MSI-H/dMMR has proven to be a positive prognostic factor for response to immunotherapy across a wide range of solid tumors [203].

11 Concluding Remarks

In total, it has become apparent over the past decade that immunotherapy offers a fundamental shift in how we treat a variety of cancers. Further, we have learned more about how tumor cell intrinsic properties (e.g. mutational burden) and tumor microenvironmental factors (e.g., extent of PD-L1-positive cells) influence response to this class of therapy. Future work will hone our understanding of these factors, in particular, interactions between microenvironmental stromal and immune cells with tumor cells, and uncover further therapeutic targets that can be leveraged to enhance the efficacy of immunotherapy in the setting of gastrointestinal tumors. Our burgeoning understanding of immunology and the receptors and soluble factors that govern the activation and polarization of immune cell subsets will also direct these efforts and provide novel modalities to advance immunotherapy for gastrointestinal cancer.

The tumor microenvironment clearly plays a role in regulating all stages of tumor development. From the earliest stages, cancer cells, the surrounding stromal cells, and tissue-resident as well as infiltrating immune cells converse through a variety of mechanisms, driving diverse microenvironmental compositions and behaviors. An easy way to conceptualize this interaction comes from considering cancer as "a wound that never heals" where the overall response to the tissue insult (cancer) is one that is characterized by tissue remodeling, scar formation, and suppression of cell-killing immune responses. Through our increased understanding of these interactions, we are constantly developing tools that allow for modulation of the composition and behavior of the tumor microenvironment to promote antitumor immunity. As this understanding matures, we will develop context-specific pharmacological approaches that combine tumor microenvironment-targeted therapies with immunotherapy to drive potential curative responses. This chapter sets the foundation for what will be discussed in detail throughout the remainder of the book. In particular, specifics regarding the tumor microenvironment, microenvironment-targeted therapies, and immunotherapies for all GI malignancies will be discussed in detail.

Acknowledgements The authors would like to thank the patients and clinicians who continue to advance the field of cancer immunotherapy through their commitment to clinical research. The figures presented here were generated with BioRender.com.

Compliance with Ethical Standards

Funding This work was supported by NIH grants R01CA208253, R01CA228406 and P30CA138292. *The content is solely the responsibility of the authors and does not necessarily represent the official views of the National Institutes of Health.*

Conflict of Interest Dr. Lesinski has consulted for ProDa Biotech, LLC and received compensation. Dr. Lesinski has received research funding through a sponsored research agreement between Emory University and Merck and Co., Bristol-Myers Squibb, Boerhinger-Ingelheim, and Vaccinex. Dr. Herting has no conflicts to disclose.

References

1. Blander JM (2016) Death in the intestinal epithelium-basic biology and implications for inflammatory bowel disease. FEBS J 283(14):2720–2730
2. Ullman TA, Itzkowitz SH (2011) Intestinal inflammation and cancer. Gastroenterology 140(6):1807–1816
3. Kulkarni MS, Yielding KL (1985) DNA damage and repair in epithelial (mucous) cells and crypt cells from isolated colon. Chem Biol Interact 52(3):311–318
4. Napier KJ, Scheerer M, Misra S (2014) Esophageal cancer: a review of epidemiology, pathogenesis, staging workup and treatment modalities. World J Gastrointest Oncol 6(5):112–120
5. Carcas LP (2014) Gastric cancer review. J Carcinog 13:14
6. Villanueva A (2019) Hepatocellular carcinoma. N Engl J Med 380(15):1450–1462
7. Benedict M, Zhang X (2017) Non-alcoholic fatty liver disease: an expanded review. World J Hepatol 9(16):715–732
8. El-Serag HB (2012) Epidemiology of viral hepatitis and hepatocellular carcinoma. Gastroenterology 142(6):1264–73.e1
9. Banales JM, Marin JJG, Lamarca A, Rodrigues PM, Khan SA, Roberts LR et al (2020) Cholangiocarcinoma 2020: the next horizon in mechanisms and management. Nat Rev Gastroenterol Hepatol 17(9):557–588
10. Adamska A, Domenichini A, Falasca M (2017) Pancreatic ductal adenocarcinoma: current and evolving therapies. Int J Mol Sci 18(7):1338
11. Machado NO, Al Qadhi H, Al Wahibi K (2015) Intraductal papillary mucinous neoplasm of pancreas. N Am J Med Sci 7(5):160–175
12. Sun J (2017) Pancreatic neuroendocrine tumors. Intractable Rare Dis Res 6(1):21–28
13. Williamson JM, Williamson RC (2014) Small bowel tumors: pathology and management. J Med Assoc Thail 97(1):126–137
14. Dekker E, Tanis PJ, Vleugels JLA, Kasi PM, Wallace MB (2019) Colorectal cancer. Lancet 394(10207):1467–1480
15. Tiwari AK, Laird-Fick HS, Wali RK, Roy HK (2012) Surveillance for gastrointestinal malignancies. World J Gastroenterol 18(33):4507–4516
16. Orth M, Metzger P, Gerum S, Mayerle J, Schneider G, Belka C et al (2019) Pancreatic ductal adenocarcinoma: biological hallmarks, current status, and future perspectives of combined modality treatment approaches. Radiat Oncol 14(1):141
17. Tariq NU, McNamara MG, Valle JW (2019) Biliary tract cancers: current knowledge, clinical candidates and future challenges. Cancer Manag Res 11:2623–2642
18. Ferrone CR, Marchegiani G, Hong TS, Ryan DP, Deshpande V, McDonnell EI et al (2015) Radiological and surgical implications of neoadjuvant treatment with FOLFIRINOX for locally advanced and borderline resectable pancreatic cancer. Ann Surg 261(1):12–17
19. Dvorak HF (1986) Tumors: wounds that do not heal. Similarities between tumor stroma generation and wound healing. N Engl J Med 315(26):1650–1659
20. Pandolfi F, Altamura S, Frosali S, Conti P (2016) Key role of DAMP in inflammation, cancer, and tissue repair. Clin Ther 38(5):1017–1028
21. Baker KJ, Houston A, Brint E (2019) IL-1 family members in cancer; two sides to every story. Front Immunol 10:1197
22. O'Toole A, Michielsen AJ, Nolan B, Tosetto M, Sheahan K, Mulcahy HE et al (2014) Tumour microenvironment of both early- and late-stage colorectal cancer is equally immunosuppressive. Br J Cancer 111(5):927–932
23. Karamitopoulou E (2019) Tumour microenvironment of pancreatic cancer: immune landscape is dictated by molecular and histopathological features. Br J Cancer 121(1):5–14
24. Papaccio F, Paino F, Regad T, Papaccio G, Desiderio V, Tirino V (2017) Concise review: cancer cells, cancer stem cells, and mesenchymal stem cells: influence in cancer development. Stem Cells Transl Med 6(12):2115–2125

25. Pon JR, Marra MA (2015) Driver and passenger mutations in cancer. Annu Rev Pathol 10:25–50
26. Cannon A, Thompson C, Hall BR, Jain M, Kumar S, Batra SK (2018) Desmoplasia in pancreatic ductal adenocarcinoma: insight into pathological function and therapeutic potential. Genes Cancer 9(3–4):78–86
27. Apte MV, Wilson JS, Lugea A, Pandol SJ (2013) A starring role for stellate cells in the pancreatic cancer microenvironment. Gastroenterology 144(6):1210–1219
28. Lohr M, Schmidt C, Ringel J, Kluth M, Muller P, Nizze H et al (2001) Transforming growth factor-beta1 induces desmoplasia in an experimental model of human pancreatic carcinoma. Cancer Res 61(2):550–555
29. Bachem MG, Schunemann M, Ramadani M, Siech M, Beger H, Buck A et al (2005) Pancreatic carcinoma cells induce fibrosis by stimulating proliferation and matrix synthesis of stellate cells. Gastroenterology 128(4):907–921
30. Murakami T, Hiroshima Y, Matsuyama R, Homma Y, Hoffman RM, Endo I (2019) Role of the tumor microenvironment in pancreatic cancer. Ann Gastroenterol Surg 3(2): 130–137
31. Shan T, Chen S, Chen X, Lin WR, Li W, Ma J et al (2017) Cancer-associated fibroblasts enhance pancreatic cancer cell invasion by remodeling the metabolic conversion mechanism. Oncol Rep 37(4):1971–1979
32. Mace TA, Ameen Z, Collins A, Wojcik S, Mair M, Young GS et al (2013) Pancreatic cancer-associated stellate cells promote differentiation of myeloid-derived suppressor cells in a STAT3-dependent manner. Cancer Res 73(10):3007–3018
33. Halbrook CJ, Lyssiotis CA (2017) Employing metabolism to improve the diagnosis and treatment of pancreatic cancer. Cancer Cell 31(1):5–19
34. Lyssiotis CA, Kimmelman AC (2017) Metabolic interactions in the tumor microenvironment. Trends Cell Biol 27(11):863–875
35. Brabletz T, Kalluri R, Nieto MA, Weinberg RA (2018) EMT in cancer. Nat Rev Cancer 18(2):128–134
36. Jolly MK, Boareto M, Huang B, Jia D, Lu M, Ben-Jacob E et al (2015) Implications of the hybrid epithelial/mesenchymal phenotype in metastasis. Front Oncol 5:155
37. Roche J (2018) The epithelial-to-mesenchymal transition in cancer. Cancers (Basel) 10(2):52
38. Gaianigo N, Melisi D, Carbone C (2017) EMT and treatment resistance in pancreatic cancer. Cancers (Basel) 9(9):122
39. Vu T, Datta PK (2017) Regulation of EMT in colorectal cancer: a culprit in metastasis. Cancers (Basel) 9(12):171
40. Ramesh V, Brabletz T, Ceppi P (2020) Targeting EMT in cancer with repurposed metabolic inhibitors. Trends Cancer 6(11):942–950
41. Huels DJ, Sansom OJ (2015) Stem vs non-stem cell origin of colorectal cancer. Br J Cancer 113(1):1–5
42. Xu Y, Liu J, Nipper M, Wang P (2019) Ductal vs. acinar? Recent insights into identifying cell lineage of pancreatic ductal adenocarcinoma. Ann Pancreat Cancer 2:11
43. Barker N, Ridgway RA, van Es JH, van de Wetering M, Begthel H, van den Born M et al (2009) Crypt stem cells as the cells-of-origin of intestinal cancer. Nature 457(7229): 608–611
44. Powell AE, Vlacich G, Zhao ZY, McKinley ET, Washington MK, Manning HC et al (2014) Inducible loss of one Apc allele in Lrig1-expressing progenitor cells results in multiple distal colonic tumors with features of familial adenomatous polyposis. Am J Physiol Gastrointest Liver Physiol 307(1):G16–G23
45. Zhu L, Gibson P, Currle DS, Tong Y, Richardson RJ, Bayazitov IT et al (2009) Prominin 1 marks intestinal stem cells that are susceptible to neoplastic transformation. Nature 457(7229):603–607
46. Davis H, Irshad S, Bansal M, Rafferty H, Boitsova T, Bardella C et al (2015) Aberrant epithelial GREM1 expression initiates colonic tumorigenesis from cells outside the stem cell niche. Nat Med 21(1):62–70

47. Schwitalla S, Fingerle AA, Cammareri P, Nebelsiek T, Goktuna SI, Ziegler PK et al (2013) Intestinal tumorigenesis initiated by dedifferentiation and acquisition of stem-cell-like properties. Cell 152(1–2):25–38
48. Busnardo AC, DiDio LJ, Tidrick RT, Thomford NR (1983) History of the pancreas. Am J Surg 146(5):539–550
49. Brembeck FH, Schreiber FS, Deramaudt TB, Craig L, Rhoades B, Swain G et al (2003) The mutant K-ras oncogene causes pancreatic periductal lymphocytic infiltration and gastric mucous neck cell hyperplasia in transgenic mice. Cancer Res 63(9):2005–2009
50. Lee AYL, Dubois CL, Sarai K, Zarei S, Schaeffer DF, Sander M et al (2019) Cell of origin affects tumour development and phenotype in pancreatic ductal adenocarcinoma. Gut 68(3):487–498
51. Lynch MD, Watt FM (2018) Fibroblast heterogeneity: implications for human disease. J Clin Invest 128(1):26–35
52. Kalluri R (2016) The biology and function of fibroblasts in cancer. Nat Rev Cancer 16(9):582–598
53. Ohlund D, Handly-Santana A, Biffi G, Elyada E, Almeida AS, Ponz-Sarvise M et al (2017) Distinct populations of inflammatory fibroblasts and myofibroblasts in pancreatic cancer. J Exp Med 214(3):579–596
54. Koshida Y, Kuranami M, Watanabe M (2006) Interaction between stromal fibroblasts and colorectal cancer cells in the expression of vascular endothelial growth factor. J Surg Res 134(2):270–277
55. Zhu HF, Zhang XH, Gu CS, Zhong Y, Long T, Ma YD et al (2019) Cancer-associated fibroblasts promote colorectal cancer progression by secreting CLEC3B. Cancer Biol Ther 20(7):967–978
56. Rhim AD, Oberstein PE, Thomas DH, Mirek ET, Palermo CF, Sastra SA et al (2014) Stromal elements act to restrain, rather than support, pancreatic ductal adenocarcinoma. Cancer Cell 25(6):735–747
57. Ozdemir BC, Pentcheva-Hoang T, Carstens JL, Zheng X, Wu CC, Simpson TR et al (2014) Depletion of carcinoma-associated fibroblasts and fibrosis induces immunosuppression and accelerates pancreas cancer with reduced survival. Cancer Cell 25(6):719–734
58. Lee JJ, Rothenberg ME, Seeley ES, Zimdahl B, Kawano S, Lu WJ et al (2016) Control of inflammation by stromal Hedgehog pathway activation restrains colitis. Proc Natl Acad Sci U S A 113(47):E7545–E7553
59. Ohlund D, Elyada E, Tuveson D (2014) Fibroblast heterogeneity in the cancer wound. J Exp Med 211(8):1503–1523
60. Elyada E, Bolisetty M, Laise P, Flynn WF, Courtois ET, Burkhart RA et al (2019) Cross-species single-cell analysis of pancreatic ductal adenocarcinoma reveals antigen-presenting cancer-associated fibroblasts. Cancer Discov 9(8):1102–1123
61. Dominguez CX, Muller S, Keerthivasan S, Koeppen H, Hung J, Gierke S et al (2020) Single-cell RNA sequencing reveals stromal evolution into LRRC15(+) myofibroblasts as a determinant of patient response to cancer immunotherapy. Cancer Discov 10(2):232–253
62. Mace TA, Shakya R, Pitarresi JR, Swanson B, McQuinn CW, Loftus S et al (2018) IL-6 and PD-L1 antibody blockade combination therapy reduces tumour progression in murine models of pancreatic cancer. Gut 67(2):320–332
63. Zhang R, Qi F, Zhao F, Li G, Shao S, Zhang X et al (2019) Cancer-associated fibroblasts enhance tumor-associated macrophages enrichment and suppress NK cells function in colorectal cancer. Cell Death Dis 10(4):273
64. Ahmadzadeh M, Rosenberg SA (2005) TGF-beta 1 attenuates the acquisition and expression of effector function by tumor antigen-specific human memory CD8 T cells. J Immunol 174(9):5215–5223
65. Thomas DA, Massague J (2005) TGF-beta directly targets cytotoxic T cell functions during tumor evasion of immune surveillance. Cancer Cell 8(5):369–380
66. Krenkel O, Tacke F (2017) Liver macrophages in tissue homeostasis and disease. Nat Rev Immunol 17(5):306–321

67. Kuang DM, Peng C, Zhao Q, Wu Y, Chen MS, Zheng L (2010) Activated monocytes in peritumoral stroma of hepatocellular carcinoma promote expansion of memory T helper 17 cells. Hepatology 51(1):154–164
68. Zhu Y, Herndon JM, Sojka DK, Kim KW, Knolhoff BL, Zuo C et al (2017) Tissue-resident macrophages in pancreatic ductal adenocarcinoma originate from embryonic hematopoiesis and promote tumor progression. Immunity 47(2):323–38.e6
69. Nywening TM, Belt BA, Cullinan DR, Panni RZ, Han BJ, Sanford DE et al (2018) Targeting both tumour-associated CXCR2(+) neutrophils and CCR2(+) macrophages disrupts myeloid recruitment and improves chemotherapeutic responses in pancreatic ductal adenocarcinoma. Gut 67(6):1112–1123
70. Grossman JG, Nywening TM, Belt BA, Panni RZ, Krasnick BA, DeNardo DG et al (2018) Recruitment of CCR2(+) tumor associated macrophage to sites of liver metastasis confers a poor prognosis in human colorectal cancer. Oncoimmunology 7(9):e1470729
71. Mantovani A, Sozzani S, Locati M, Allavena P, Sica A (2002) Macrophage polarization: tumor-associated macrophages as a paradigm for polarized M2 mononuclear phagocytes. Trends Immunol 23(11):549–555
72. Murray PJ, Allen JE, Biswas SK, Fisher EA, Gilroy DW, Goerdt S et al (2014) Macrophage activation and polarization: nomenclature and experimental guidelines. Immunity 41(1):14–20
73. Stein M, Keshav S, Harris N, Gordon S (1992) Interleukin 4 potently enhances murine macrophage mannose receptor activity: a marker of alternative immunologic macrophage activation. J Exp Med 176(1):287–292
74. Xue J, Schmidt SV, Sander J, Draffehn A, Krebs W, Quester I et al (2014) Transcriptome-based network analysis reveals a spectrum model of human macrophage activation. Immunity 40(2):274–288
75. Mills CD, Kincaid K, Alt JM, Heilman MJ, Hill AM (2000) M-1/M-2 macrophages and the Th1/Th2 paradigm. J Immunol 164(12):6166–6173
76. Barbera-Guillem E, Nyhus JK, Wolford CC, Friece CR, Sampsel JW (2002) Vascular endothelial growth factor secretion by tumor-infiltrating macrophages essentially supports tumor angiogenesis, and IgG immune complexes potentiate the process. Cancer Res 62(23):7042–7049
77. Jedinak A, Dudhgaonkar S, Sliva D (2010) Activated macrophages induce metastatic behavior of colon cancer cells. Immunobiology 215(3):242–249
78. Cantero-Cid R, Casas-Martin J, Hernandez-Jimenez E, Cubillos-Zapata C, Varela-Serrano A, Avendano-Ortiz J et al (2018) PD-L1/PD-1 crosstalk in colorectal cancer: are we targeting the right cells? BMC Cancer 18(1):945
79. Forssell J, Oberg A, Henriksson ML, Stenling R, Jung A, Palmqvist R (2007) High macrophage infiltration along the tumor front correlates with improved survival in colon cancer. Clin Cancer Res 13(5):1472–1479
80. Edin S, Wikberg ML, Dahlin AM, Rutegard J, Oberg A, Oldenborg PA et al (2012) The distribution of macrophages with a M1 or M2 phenotype in relation to prognosis and the molecular characteristics of colorectal cancer. PLoS One 7(10):e47045
81. Narayanan S, Kawaguchi T, Peng X, Qi Q, Liu S, Yan L et al (2019) Tumor infiltrating lymphocytes and macrophages improve survival in microsatellite unstable colorectal cancer. Sci Rep 9(1):13455
82. Panni RZ, Herndon JM, Zuo C, Hegde S, Hogg GD, Knolhoff BL et al (2019) Agonism of CD11b reprograms innate immunity to sensitize pancreatic cancer to immunotherapies. Sci Transl Med 11(499):eaau9240
83. Bronte V, Wang M, Overwijk WW, Surman DR, Pericle F, Rosenberg SA et al (1998) Apoptotic death of CD8+ T lymphocytes after immunization: induction of a suppressive population of Mac-1+/Gr-1+ cells. J Immunol 161(10):5313–5320
84. Pekarek LA, Starr BA, Toledano AY, Schreiber H (1995) Inhibition of tumor growth by elimination of granulocytes. J Exp Med 181(1):435–440

85. Gabrilovich DI, Bronte V, Chen SH, Colombo MP, Ochoa A, Ostrand-Rosenberg S et al (2007) The terminology issue for myeloid-derived suppressor cells. Cancer Res 67(1):425; author reply 6
86. Movahedi K, Guilliams M, Van den Bossche J, Van den Bergh R, Gysemans C, Beschin A et al (2008) Identification of discrete tumor-induced myeloid-derived suppressor cell subpopulations with distinct T cell-suppressive activity. Blood 111(8):4233–4244
87. Youn JI, Collazo M, Shalova IN, Biswas SK, Gabrilovich DI (2012) Characterization of the nature of granulocytic myeloid-derived suppressor cells in tumor-bearing mice. J Leukoc Biol 91(1):167–181
88. Bronte V, Brandau S, Chen SH, Colombo MP, Frey AB, Greten TF et al (2016) Recommendations for myeloid-derived suppressor cell nomenclature and characterization standards. Nat Commun 7:12150
89. Li H, Han Y, Guo Q, Zhang M, Cao X (2009) Cancer-expanded myeloid-derived suppressor cells induce anergy of NK cells through membrane-bound TGF-beta 1. J Immunol 182(1):240–249
90. Elkabets M, Ribeiro VS, Dinarello CA, Ostrand-Rosenberg S, Di Santo JP, Apte RN et al (2010) IL-1beta regulates a novel myeloid-derived suppressor cell subset that impairs NK cell development and function. Eur J Immunol 40(12):3347–3357
91. Murdoch C, Giannoudis A, Lewis CE (2004) Mechanisms regulating the recruitment of macrophages into hypoxic areas of tumors and other ischemic tissues. Blood 104(8): 2224–2234
92. Allavena P, Sica A, Solinas G, Porta C, Mantovani A (2008) The inflammatory micro-environment in tumor progression: the role of tumor-associated macrophages. Crit Rev Oncol Hematol 66(1):1–9
93. Noman MZ, Desantis G, Janji B, Hasmim M, Karray S, Dessen P et al (2014) PD-L1 is a novel direct target of HIF-1alpha, and its blockade under hypoxia enhanced MDSC-mediated T cell activation. J Exp Med 211(5):781–790
94. Hossain F, Al-Khami AA, Wyczechowska D, Hernandez C, Zheng L, Reiss K et al (2015) Inhibition of fatty acid oxidation modulates immunosuppressive functions of myeloid-derived suppressor cells and enhances cancer therapies. Cancer Immunol Res 3(11):1236–1247
95. Raber PL, Thevenot P, Sierra R, Wyczechowska D, Halle D, Ramirez ME et al (2014) Subpopulations of myeloid-derived suppressor cells impair T cell responses through independent nitric oxide-related pathways. Int J Cancer 134(12):2853–2864
96. Rodriguez PC, Ochoa AC (2008) Arginine regulation by myeloid derived suppressor cells and tolerance in cancer: mechanisms and therapeutic perspectives. Immunol Rev 222:180–191
97. Srivastava MK, Sinha P, Clements VK, Rodriguez P, Ostrand-Rosenberg S (2010) Myeloid-derived suppressor cells inhibit T-cell activation by depleting cystine and cysteine. Cancer Res 70(1):68–77
98. Groth C, Hu X, Weber R, Fleming V, Altevogt P, Utikal J et al (2019) Immunosuppression mediated by myeloid-derived suppressor cells (MDSCs) during tumour progression. Br J Cancer 120(1):16–25
99. Chun E, Lavoie S, Michaud M, Gallini CA, Kim J, Soucy G et al (2015) CCL2 promotes colorectal carcinogenesis by enhancing polymorphonuclear myeloid-derived suppressor cell population and function. Cell Rep 12(2):244–257
100. Porembka MR, Mitchem JB, Belt BA, Hsieh CS, Lee HM, Herndon J et al (2012) Pancreatic adenocarcinoma induces bone marrow mobilization of myeloid-derived suppressor cells which promote primary tumor growth. Cancer Immunol Immunother 61(9):1373–1385
101. Kumar BV, Connors TJ, Farber DL (2018) Human T cell development, localization, and function throughout life. Immunity 48(2):202–213
102. Smith-Garvin JE, Koretzky GA, Jordan MS (2009) T cell activation. Annu Rev Immunol 27:591–619
103. Weiss A, Stobo JD (1984) Requirement for the coexpression of T3 and the T cell antigen receptor on a malignant human T cell line. J Exp Med 160(5):1284–1299

104. Birnbaum ME, Berry R, Hsiao YS, Chen Z, Shingu-Vazquez MA, Yu X et al (2014) Molecular architecture of the alphabeta T cell receptor-CD3 complex. Proc Natl Acad Sci U S A 111(49):17576–17581
105. Luckheeram RV, Zhou R, Verma AD, Xia B (2012) CD4(+)T cells: differentiation and functions. Clin Dev Immunol 2012:925135
106. Zhang N, Bevan MJ (2011) CD8(+) T cells: foot soldiers of the immune system. Immunity 35(2):161–168
107. Bennett SR, Carbone FR, Karamalis F, Flavell RA, Miller JF, Heath WR (1998) Help for cytotoxic-T-cell responses is mediated by CD40 signalling. Nature 393(6684):478–480
108. Schoenberger SP, Toes RE, van der Voort EI, Offringa R, Melief CJ (1998) T-cell help for cytotoxic T lymphocytes is mediated by CD40-CD40L interactions. Nature 393(6684):480–483
109. Wilson EB, Livingstone AM (2008) Cutting edge: CD4+ T cell-derived IL-2 is essential for help-dependent primary CD8+ T cell responses. J Immunol 181(11):7445–7448
110. Valitutti S (2012) The serial engagement model 17 years after: from TCR triggering to immunotherapy. Front Immunol 3:272
111. Gil D, Schrum AG, Alarcon B, Palmer E (2005) T cell receptor engagement by peptide-MHC ligands induces a conformational change in the CD3 complex of thymocytes. J Exp Med 201(4):517–522
112. Chen L, Flies DB (2013) Molecular mechanisms of T cell co-stimulation and co-inhibition. Nat Rev Immunol 13(4):227–242
113. Mueller DL, Jenkins MK, Schwartz RH (1989) Clonal expansion versus functional clonal inactivation: a costimulatory signalling pathway determines the outcome of T cell antigen receptor occupancy. Annu Rev Immunol 7:445–480
114. June CH, Ledbetter JA, Gillespie MM, Lindsten T, Thompson CB (1987) T-cell proliferation involving the CD28 pathway is associated with cyclosporine-resistant interleukin 2 gene expression. Mol Cell Biol 7(12):4472–4481
115. Ross SH, Cantrell DA (2018) Signaling and function of interleukin-2 in T lymphocytes. Annu Rev Immunol 36:411–433
116. de Goer de Herve MG, Jaafoura S, Vallee M, Taoufik Y (2012) FoxP3(+) regulatory CD4 T cells control the generation of functional CD8 memory. Nat Commun 3:986
117. McNally A, Hill GR, Sparwasser T, Thomas R, Steptoe RJ (2011) CD4+CD25+ regulatory T cells control CD8+ T-cell effector differentiation by modulating IL-2 homeostasis. Proc Natl Acad Sci U S A 108(18):7529–7534
118. Qin S, Xu L, Yi M, Yu S, Wu K, Luo S (2019) Novel immune checkpoint targets: moving beyond PD-1 and CTLA-4. Mol Cancer 18(1):155
119. Foerster F, Hess M, Gerhold-Ay A, Marquardt JU, Becker D, Galle PR et al (2018) The immune contexture of hepatocellular carcinoma predicts clinical outcome. Sci Rep 8(1):5351
120. Zheng X, Song X, Shao Y, Xu B, Chen L, Zhou Q et al (2017) Prognostic role of tumor-infiltrating lymphocytes in gastric cancer: a meta-analysis. Oncotarget 8(34):57386–57398
121. Ye L, Zhang T, Kang Z, Guo G, Sun Y, Lin K et al (2019) Tumor-infiltrating immune cells act as a marker for prognosis in colorectal cancer. Front Immunol 10:2368
122. Miksch RC, Schoenberg MB, Weniger M, Bosch F, Ormanns S, Mayer B et al (2019) Prognostic impact of tumor-infiltrating lymphocytes and neutrophils on survival of patients with upfront resection of pancreatic cancer. Cancers (Basel) 11(1):39
123. Ware MB, El-Rayes BF, Lesinski GB (2020) Mirage or long-awaited oasis: reinvigorating T-cell responses in pancreatic cancer. J Immunother Cancer 8(2):e001100
124. Chen X, Wang L, Li P, Song M, Qin G, Gao Q et al (2018) Dual TGF-beta and PD-1 blockade synergistically enhances MAGE-A3-specific CD8(+) T cell response in esophageal squamous cell carcinoma. Int J Cancer 143(10):2561–2574
125. Oshima Y, Shimada H, Yajima S, Nanami T, Matsushita K, Nomura F et al (2016) NY-ESO-1 autoantibody as a tumor-specific biomarker for esophageal cancer: screening in 1969 patients with various cancers. J Gastroenterol 51(1):30–34

126. Spear S, Candido JB, McDermott JR, Ghirelli C, Maniati E, Beers SA et al (2019) Discrepancies in the tumor microenvironment of spontaneous and orthotopic murine models of pancreatic cancer uncover a new immunostimulatory phenotype for B cells. Front Immunol 10:542
127. Roghanian A, Fraser C, Kleyman M, Chen J (2016) B cells promote pancreatic tumorigenesis. Cancer Discov 6(3):230–232
128. Edin S, Kaprio T, Hagstrom J, Larsson P, Mustonen H, Bockelman C et al (2019) The prognostic importance of CD20(+) B lymphocytes in colorectal cancer and the relation to other immune cell subsets. Sci Rep 9(1):19997
129. Brodt P, Gordon J (1978) Anti-tumor immunity in B lymphocyte-deprived mice. I. Immunity to a chemically induced tumor. J Immunol 121(1):359–362
130. Shah S, Divekar AA, Hilchey SP, Cho HM, Newman CL, Shin SU et al (2005) Increased rejection of primary tumors in mice lacking B cells: inhibition of anti-tumor CTL and TH1 cytokine responses by B cells. Int J Cancer 117(4):574–586
131. de Visser KE, Korets LV, Coussens LM (2005) De novo carcinogenesis promoted by chronic inflammation is B lymphocyte dependent. Cancer Cell 7(5):411–423
132. Fristedt R, Borg D, Hedner C, Berntsson J, Nodin B, Eberhard J et al (2016) Prognostic impact of tumour-associated B cells and plasma cells in oesophageal and gastric adenocarcinoma. J Gastrointest Oncol 7(6):848–859
133. Berntsson J, Nodin B, Eberhard J, Micke P, Jirstrom K (2016) Prognostic impact of tumour-infiltrating B cells and plasma cells in colorectal cancer. Int J Cancer 139(5):1129–1139
134. Barnett LG, Simkins HM, Barnett BE, Korn LL, Johnson AL, Wherry EJ et al (2014) B cell antigen presentation in the initiation of follicular helper T cell and germinal center differentiation. J Immunol 192(8):3607–3617
135. Crawford A, Macleod M, Schumacher T, Corlett L, Gray D (2006) Primary T cell expansion and differentiation in vivo requires antigen presentation by B cells. J Immunol 176(6):3498–3506
136. Aloisi F, Pujol-Borrell R (2006) Lymphoid neogenesis in chronic inflammatory diseases. Nat Rev Immunol 6(3):205–217
137. Carragher DM, Rangel-Moreno J, Randall TD (2008) Ectopic lymphoid tissues and local immunity. Semin Immunol 20(1):26–42
138. Moyron-Quiroz JE, Rangel-Moreno J, Hartson L, Kusser K, Tighe MP, Klonowski KD et al (2006) Persistence and responsiveness of immunologic memory in the absence of secondary lymphoid organs. Immunity 25(4):643–654
139. Di Caro G, Bergomas F, Grizzi F, Doni A, Bianchi P, Malesci A et al (2014) Occurrence of tertiary lymphoid tissue is associated with T-cell infiltration and predicts better prognosis in early-stage colorectal cancers. Clin Cancer Res 20(8):2147–2158
140. Pylayeva-Gupta Y, Das S, Handler JS, Hajdu CH, Coffre M, Koralov SB et al (2016) IL35-producing B cells promote the development of pancreatic neoplasia. Cancer Discov 6(3):247–255
141. Gunderson AJ, Kaneda MM, Tsujikawa T, Nguyen AV, Affara NI, Ruffell B et al (2016) Bruton tyrosine kinase-dependent immune cell cross-talk drives pancreas cancer. Cancer Discov 6(3):270–285
142. Huang C, Li N, Li Z, Chang A, Chen Y, Zhao T et al (2017) Tumour-derived Interleukin 35 promotes pancreatic ductal adenocarcinoma cell extravasation and metastasis by inducing ICAM1 expression. Nat Commun 8:14035
143. Caligiuri MA (2008) Human natural killer cells. Blood 112(3):461–469
144. Shimasaki N, Jain A, Campana D (2020) NK cells for cancer immunotherapy. Nat Rev Drug Discov 19(3):200–218
145. Dunn GP, Old LJ, Schreiber RD (2004) The immunobiology of cancer immunosurveillance and immunoediting. Immunity 21(2):137–148
146. Karre K, Ljunggren HG, Piontek G, Kiessling R (1986) Selective rejection of H-2-deficient lymphoma variants suggests alternative immune defence strategy. Nature 319(6055):675–678

147. Guillerey C, Huntington ND, Smyth MJ (2016) Targeting natural killer cells in cancer immunotherapy. Nat Immunol 17(9):1025–1036
148. Malmberg KJ, Carlsten M, Bjorklund A, Sohlberg E, Bryceson YT, Ljunggren HG (2017) Natural killer cell-mediated immunosurveillance of human cancer. Semin Immunol 31:20–29
149. Imai K, Matsuyama S, Miyake S, Suga K, Nakachi K (2000) Natural cytotoxic activity of peripheral-blood lymphocytes and cancer incidence: an 11-year follow-up study of a general population. Lancet 356(9244):1795–1799
150. Tang YP, Xie MZ, Li KZ, Li JL, Cai ZM, Hu BL (2020) Prognostic value of peripheral blood natural killer cells in colorectal cancer. BMC Gastroenterol 20(1):31
151. Van Audenaerde JRM, Roeyen G, Darcy PK, Kershaw MH, Peeters M, Smits ELJ (2018) Natural killer cells and their therapeutic role in pancreatic cancer: a systematic review. Pharmacol Ther 189:31–44
152. Lim SA, Kim J, Jeon S, Shin MH, Kwon J, Kim TJ et al (2019) Defective localization with impaired tumor cytotoxicity contributes to the immune escape of NK cells in pancreatic cancer patients. Front Immunol 10:496
153. Bottcher JP, Bonavita E, Chakravarty P, Blees H, Cabeza-Cabrerizo M, Sammicheli S et al (2018) NK cells stimulate recruitment of cDC1 into the tumor microenvironment promoting cancer immune control. Cell 172(5):1022–37.e14
154. Li H, Zhai N, Wang Z, Song H, Yang Y, Cui A et al (2018) Regulatory NK cells mediated between immunosuppressive monocytes and dysfunctional T cells in chronic HBV infection. Gut 67(11):2035–2044
155. Patente TA, Pinho MP, Oliveira AA, Evangelista GCM, Bergami-Santos PC, Barbuto JAM (2018) Human dendritic cells: their heterogeneity and clinical application potential in cancer immunotherapy. Front Immunol 9:3176
156. Steinman RM (1991) The dendritic cell system and its role in immunogenicity. Annu Rev Immunol 9:271–296
157. Matzinger P (1994) Tolerance, danger, and the extended family. Annu Rev Immunol 12:991–1045
158. Shortman K, Liu YJ (2002) Mouse and human dendritic cell subtypes. Nat Rev Immunol 2(3):151–161
159. Pinzon-Charry A, Maxwell T, Lopez JA (2005) Dendritic cell dysfunction in cancer: a mechanism for immunosuppression. Immunol Cell Biol 83(5):451–461
160. Almand B, Clark JI, Nikitina E, van Beynen J, English NR, Knight SC et al (2001) Increased production of immature myeloid cells in cancer patients: a mechanism of immunosuppression in cancer. J Immunol 166(1):678–689
161. Yamamoto T, Yanagimoto H, Satoi S, Toyokawa H, Yamao J, Kim S et al (2012) Circulating myeloid dendritic cells as prognostic factors in patients with pancreatic cancer who have undergone surgical resection. J Surg Res 173(2):299–308
162. Orsini G, Legitimo A, Failli A, Ferrari P, Nicolini A, Spisni R et al (2014) Quantification of blood dendritic cells in colorectal cancer patients during the course of disease. Pathol Oncol Res 20(2):267–276
163. Mazzolini G, Murillo O, Atorrasagasti C, Dubrot J, Tirapu I, Rizzo M et al (2007) Immunotherapy and immunoescape in colorectal cancer. World J Gastroenterol 13(44):5822–5831
164. van Duijneveldt G, Griffin MDW, Putoczki TL (2020) Emerging roles for the IL-6 family of cytokines in pancreatic cancer. Clin Sci (Lond) 134(16):2091–2115
165. Nagathihalli NS, Castellanos JA, VanSaun MN, Dai X, Ambrose M, Guo Q et al (2016) Pancreatic stellate cell secreted IL-6 stimulates STAT3 dependent invasiveness of pancreatic intraepithelial neoplasia and cancer cells. Oncotarget 7(40):65982–65992
166. Wormann SM, Diakopoulos KN, Lesina M, Algul H (2014) The immune network in pancreatic cancer development and progression. Oncogene 33(23):2956–2967
167. Seifert AM, List J, Heiduk M, Decker R, von Renesse J, Meinecke AC et al (2020) Gamma-delta T cells stimulate IL-6 production by pancreatic stellate cells in pancreatic ductal adenocarcinoma. J Cancer Res Clin Oncol 146(12):3233–3240

168. Holmer R, Goumas FA, Waetzig GH, Rose-John S, Kalthoff H (2014) Interleukin-6: a villain in the drama of pancreatic cancer development and progression. Hepatobiliary Pancreat Dis Int 13(4):371–380
169. Kim HW, Lee JC, Paik KH, Kang J, Kim J, Hwang JH (2017) Serum interleukin-6 is associated with pancreatic ductal adenocarcinoma progression pattern. Medicine (Baltimore) 96(5):e5926
170. Long KB, Tooker G, Tooker E, Luque SL, Lee JW, Pan X et al (2017) IL6 receptor blockade enhances chemotherapy efficacy in pancreatic ductal adenocarcinoma. Mol Cancer Ther 16(9):1898–1908
171. Iwahasi S, Rui F, Morine Y, Yamada S, Saito YU, Ikemoto T et al (2020) Hepatic stellate cells contribute to the tumor malignancy of hepatocellular carcinoma through the IL-6 pathway. Anticancer Res 40(2):743–749
172. Hsieh CC, Hung CH, Chiang M, Tsai YC, He JT (2019) Hepatic stellate cells enhance liver cancer progression by inducing myeloid-derived suppressor cells through interleukin-6 signaling. Int J Mol Sci 20(20):5079
173. Kalbasi A, Komar C, Tooker GM, Liu M, Lee JW, Gladney WL et al (2017) Tumor-derived CCL2 mediates resistance to radiotherapy in pancreatic ductal adenocarcinoma. Clin Cancer Res 23(1):137–148
174. Long KB, Gladney WL, Tooker GM, Graham K, Fraietta JA, Beatty GL (2016) IFNgamma and CCL2 cooperate to redirect tumor-infiltrating monocytes to degrade fibrosis and enhance chemotherapy efficacy in pancreatic carcinoma. Cancer Discov 6(4):400–413
175. McCarthy EF (2006) The toxins of William B. Coley and the treatment of bone and soft-tissue sarcomas. Iowa Orthop J 26:154–158
176. Ganesh K, Stadler ZK, Cercek A, Mendelsohn RB, Shia J, Segal NH et al (2019) Immunotherapy in colorectal cancer: rationale, challenges and potential. Nat Rev Gastroenterol Hepatol 16(6):361–375
177. Kelly RJ (2019) The emerging role of immunotherapy for esophageal cancer. Curr Opin Gastroenterol 35(4):337–343
178. Kelly RJ (2017) Immunotherapy for esophageal and gastric cancer. Am Soc Clin Oncol Educ Book 37:292–300
179. Smyth EC, Cervantes A (2020) Addition of nivolumab to chemotherapy in patients with advanced gastric cancer: a relevant step ahead, but still many questions to answer. ESMO Open 5(6):e001107
180. Yang L, Wang Y, Wang H (2019) Use of immunotherapy in the treatment of gastric cancer. Oncol Lett 18(6):5681–5690
181. Nomi T, Sho M, Akahori T, Hamada K, Kubo A, Kanehiro H et al (2007) Clinical significance and therapeutic potential of the programmed death-1 ligand/programmed death-1 pathway in human pancreatic cancer. Clin Cancer Res 13(7):2151–2157
182. Kamath SD, Kalyan A, Kircher S, Nimeiri H, Fought AJ, Benson A 3rd et al (2020) Ipilimumab and gemcitabine for advanced pancreatic cancer: a phase Ib study. Oncologist 25(5):e808–e815
183. Winograd R, Byrne KT, Evans RA, Odorizzi PM, Meyer AR, Bajor DL et al (2015) Induction of T-cell immunity overcomes complete resistance to PD-1 and CTLA-4 blockade and improves survival in pancreatic carcinoma. Cancer Immunol Res 3(4):399–411
184. O'Hara MH, O'Reilly EM, Varadhachary G, Wolff RA, Wainberg ZA, Ko AH et al (2021) CD40 agonistic monoclonal antibody APX005M (sotigalimab) and chemotherapy, with or without nivolumab, for the treatment of metastatic pancreatic adenocarcinoma: an open-label, multicentre, phase 1b study. Lancet Oncol 22(1):118–131
185. Sarantis P, Koustas E, Papadimitropoulou A, Papavassiliou AG, Karamouzis MV (2020) Pancreatic ductal adenocarcinoma: treatment hurdles, tumor microenvironment and immunotherapy. World J Gastrointest Oncol 12(2):173–181
186. Balachandran VP, Beatty GL, Dougan SK (2019) Broadening the impact of immunotherapy to pancreatic cancer: challenges and opportunities. Gastroenterology 156(7): 2056–2072

187. Gajiwala S, Torgeson A, Garrido-Laguna I, Kinsey C, Lloyd S (2018) Combination immunotherapy and radiation therapy strategies for pancreatic cancer-targeting multiple steps in the cancer immunity cycle. J Gastrointest Oncol. 9(6):1014–1026
188. Akce M, Zaidi MY, Waller EK, El-Rayes BF, Lesinski GB (2018) The potential of CAR T cell therapy in pancreatic cancer. Front Immunol 9:2166
189. Rahal A, Musher B (2017) Oncolytic viral therapy for pancreatic cancer. J Surg Oncol 116(1):94–103
190. Jakubowski CD, Azad NS (2020) Immune checkpoint inhibitor therapy in biliary tract cancer (cholangiocarcinoma). Chin Clin Oncol 9(1):2
191. Duffy AG, Ulahannan SV, Makorova-Rusher O, Rahma O, Wedemeyer H, Pratt D et al (2017) Tremelimumab in combination with ablation in patients with advanced hepatocellular carcinoma. J Hepatol 66(3):545–551
192. Sangro B, Gomez-Martin C, de la Mata M, Inarrairaegui M, Garralda E, Barrera P et al (2013) A clinical trial of CTLA-4 blockade with tremelimumab in patients with hepatocellular carcinoma and chronic hepatitis C. J Hepatol 59(1):81–88
193. Qin S, Finn RS, Kudo M, Meyer T, Vogel A, Ducreux M et al (2019) RATIONALE 301 study: tislelizumab versus sorafenib as first-line treatment for unresectable hepatocellular carcinoma. Future Oncol 15(16):1811–1822
194. Finn RS, Ryoo BY, Merle P, Kudo M, Bouattour M, Lim HY et al (2020) Pembrolizumab as second-line therapy in patients with advanced hepatocellular carcinoma in KEYNOTE-240: a randomized, double-blind, phase III trial. J Clin Oncol 38(3):193–202
195. Finn RS, Qin S, Ikeda M, Galle PR, Ducreux M, Kim TY et al (2020) Atezolizumab plus bevacizumab in unresectable hepatocellular carcinoma. N Engl J Med 382(20):1894–1905
196. Ghiringhelli F, Fumet JD (2019) Is there a place for immunotherapy for metastatic microsatellite stable colorectal cancer? Front Immunol 10:1816
197. Brahmer JR, Drake CG, Wollner I, Powderly JD, Picus J, Sharfman WH et al (2010) Phase I study of single-agent anti-programmed death-1 (MDX-1106) in refractory solid tumors: safety, clinical activity, pharmacodynamics, and immunologic correlates. J Clin Oncol 28(19):3167–3175
198. Topalian SL, Hodi FS, Brahmer JR, Gettinger SN, Smith DC, McDermott DF et al (2012) Safety, activity, and immune correlates of anti-PD-1 antibody in cancer. N Engl J Med 366(26):2443–2454
199. Fabrizio DA, George TJ Jr, Dunne RF, Frampton G, Sun J, Gowen K et al (2018) Beyond microsatellite testing: assessment of tumor mutational burden identifies subsets of colorectal cancer who may respond to immune checkpoint inhibition. J Gastrointest Oncol 9(4):610–617
200. Andre T, Shiu KK, Kim TW, Jensen BV, Jensen LH, Punt C et al (2020) Pembrolizumab in microsatellite-instability-high advanced colorectal cancer. N Engl J Med 383(23):2207–2218
201. Banerjea A, Bustin SA, Dorudi S (2005) The immunogenicity of colorectal cancers with high-degree microsatellite instability. World J Surg Oncol 3:26
202. Pages F, Mlecnik B, Marliot F, Bindea G, Ou FS, Bifulco C et al (2018) International validation of the consensus Immunoscore for the classification of colon cancer: a prognostic and accuracy study. Lancet 391(10135):2128–2139
203. Marcus L, Lemery SJ, Keegan P, Pazdur R (2019) FDA approval summary: pembrolizumab for the treatment of microsatellite instability-high solid tumors. Clin Cancer Res 25(13):3753–3758

Part II

Esophagus

Approach to Immunotherapy in Oesophageal Cancer

Su Li and Ian Chau

Contents

Abstract

Globally, oesophageal cancer ranks sixth highest in cancer mortality. Patients who present with metastatic disease would expect to live less than a year with chemotherapy. There have been several trials utilising anti-programmed cell death protein 1 (anti-PD-1) therapy in an attempt to improve the outcomes of oesophageal cancer. Modest activity has been demonstrated in single-agent anti-PD-1 therapy in pre-treated oesophageal squamous cell carcinoma (OSCC) and oesophageal adenocarcinoma (OAC). However, recent pivotal trials have established anti-PD-1 treatment in combination with chemotherapy as the new standard of care in the first-line advanced setting. Anti-PD-1 therapy in the form of

S. Li · I. Chau (✉)
Department of Medicine, Royal Marsden NHS Foundation Trust, London and Surrey, UK
e-mail: ian.chau@rmh.nhs.uk

Cancer Immunotherapy (2022)
https://doi.org/10.1007/13905_2021_11,
Published Online: 31 March 2022

nivolumab in combination with ipilimumab, an anti-cytotoxic T-lymphocyte-associated protein 4 (CTLA-4) antibody, also represents a chemotherapy-free treatment option in OSCC. In early disease setting, adjuvant nivolumab has also shown to benefit patients who do not achieve a pathological complete response after neoadjuvant chemoradiation, and trials are ongoing to assess immunotherapy in the setting of definitive chemoradiation. This chapter discusses the data behind these trials and addresses the importance of a distinction between OSCC and OAC as separate diseases and the role of PD-L1 expression as a key biomarker.

Keywords

Immunotherapy · PD-L1 · Oesophageal cancer · Oesophageal squamous cancer · Oesophageal adenocarcinoma · Gastro-oesophageal junction

1 Background

Globally in 2020, oesophageal cancer ranked seventh in terms of cancer incidence (604,000 new cases; 3.1% of all new cases of cancer) and is associated with a high disease-related mortality, resulting to be the sixth highest in cancer mortality overall (544,000 deaths; 5.5% of all cancer deaths) [1]. Approximately 70% of cases occur in men. The highest regional incidence is found in Eastern Asia mainly due to the large burden of disease in China, with the Asian continent making up a total of 79.7% of global cases in 2020, which is markedly higher than other regions (Europe 8.8%, Africa 4.6%, North America 3.4%, Latin America and Caribbean 3.1%).

The two most common histological subtypes account for almost all of the global cases as squamous cell carcinoma (SCC) composing of 84% of the cases and adenocarcinoma (AC) composing of 15% of the cases [2]. Oesophageal SCC (OSCC) mostly occurs in the stratified squamous epithelium lining the upper two-thirds of the oesophagus, whereas oesophageal AC (OAC) typically develops in the lower third of the oesophagus and originates from Barrett's mucosa. Smoking and heavy alcohol consumption have been linked to OSCC in Western populations; however, in non-Western countries the risk factors have been less established. There has been a rising incidence of OAC in high-income countries, which has been mainly attributed to increasing body weight and gastro-oesophageal reflux disease and possibly associated with a decrease of chronic infection with *H. pylori* which has been postulated to protect from OAC through the development of atrophic gastritis [3].

Although OSCC and OAC are both cancers of the oesophagus, there is evidence to suggest that they are molecularly distinct entities. The Cancer Genome Atlas performed a comprehensive molecular analysis of 164 carcinomas of the oesophagus (90 SCC, 72 AC, 2 undifferentiated carcinomas) and it is suggested that OSCC resembles SCC of other organs more than OAC, whereas OAC resembles the chromosomally unstable variant of gastric adenocarcinoma, which is the most frequently occurring subtype [4]. This chromosome instability (CIN) subtype is thought to be distinct from the microsatellite instability high (MSI-H) subtype and Epstein–Barr virus (EBV) subtype found in gastric cancer; EBV and MSI-H subtype are thought to be predictive of a response to immunotherapy in the form of immune checkpoint inhibitors (ICIs) such as anti-programmed death 1 (PD-1)/programmed death ligand-1 (PD-L1) antibodies [5, 6].

This lack of EBV and MSI-H/mismatch repair-deficient (MMRd) oesophageal cancers is further supported in a large multicentre study of gastric and oesophageal cancers where it was found that only 7 (0.8%) out of 916 oesophageal cancer samples (764 AC, 138 SCC, 14 other histologies) could be classified as MMRd and all were EBV negative [7] and therefore this is likely to be a less relevant biomarker in oesophageal cancer due to its rarity.

Several oesophageal clinical trials enrolling patients to receive ICIs have evaluated the predictive value of PD-L1 expression on the tumour cells and/or on the surrounding macrophages and lymphocytes. Frequently, PD-L1 expression scores have been expressed as a combined positive score (CPS) where it is defined as the number of PD-L1-positive cells (tumour cells, macrophages and lymphocytes) divided by the total number of tumour cells, multiplied by 100. An alternative method is to assess PD-L1 positivity by the expression on tumour cells only; however, this may not reflect the impact of the tumour microenvironment on the biological mechanisms of immune suppression. Other potential biomarkers such as tumour mutational burden have been assessed in other cancers [8] but have not been prospectively evaluated in oesophageal cancer ICI trials; however, the prevalence of high tumour mutational burden is estimated to be low in oesophageal cancers [9].

2 Oesophageal Squamous Cell Cancer

2.1 Single-Agent Anti-PD-1 Antibodies

First-line doublet platinum-based chemotherapy for advanced OSCC cancer has been the standard of care; however, after first-line therapy there has been no accepted standard of care; taxanes and irinotecan can be used, although the benefit compared to the best supportive care is incremental. In an attempt to improve outcomes for patients on progression of first-line therapy, single-agent PD-1/PD-L1 therapies have been explored as an alternative to second-line chemotherapy as single-arm studies.

ATTRACTION-01 [10] and KEYNOTE-180 [11] were single-arm studies investigating single-agent anti-PD-1 antibodies nivolumab and pembrolizumab, respectively, in patients with previously treated oesophageal cancer although ATTRACTION-01 only had OSCC patients whereas KEYNOTE-180 had a mix of both OAC and OSCC patients (52.1% OSCC and 47.9% OAC). An objective response rate (ORR) of 17% (95% confidential interval, CI 10–28) was achieved in ATTRACTION-1 and ORR of 14.3% (95% CI, 6.7–25.4%) was achieved in the OSCC group in KEYNOTE-180.

These studies informed the development of phase 3 studies ATTRACTION-03 [12] and KEYNOTE-181 [13] which assessed whether single-agent PD-1 inhibitors could pose as a feasible alternative to chemotherapy.

KEYNOTE-181 was a global phase III trial investigating second-line pembrolizumab vs. physician's-choice chemotherapy in patients with advanced oesophageal cancer. As with KEYNOTE-180, this trial again included both squamous and adenocarcinoma histology; however, a subgroup analysis of OSCC outcomes was prespecified along with a separate subgroup analysis of PD-L1-positive (defined as CPS $\geq$ 10) patients. 628 patients enrolled in this study, out of which 401 had OSCC and remaining 227 had OAC. The overall survival (OS) benefit for pembrolizumab vs. chemotherapy was not significant in the intention to treat group (HR 0.89, 95% CI 0.75–1.05); however, a significant benefit was seen in the OSCC group (HR 0.77, 95% CI 0.63–0.96). Within the OSCC cohort, PD-L1 positivity was also predictive of benefit as OSCC CPS $\geq$10 had a greater benefit (HR 0.64, 95% CI 0.46–0.90).

ATTRACTION-03 was a global phase III study investigating nivolumab vs. paclitaxel in the second-line setting for advanced OSCC; however, it is noted that 96% of the patients were of Asian ethnicity. This study met its primary end point for overall survival (HR 0.77, 95% CI 0.62–0.96). Biomarker analysis for PD-L1 expression was also performed; however, PD-L1 positivity was defined by tumour cell positivity for PD-L1 staining instead of CPS. In the subgroup analysis, it can be inferred that PD-L1-positive patients may benefit more from nivolumab (PD-L1 $\geq$1% HR for death 0.69, 95% CI 0.51–0.94; PD-L1 $<$1% HR for death 0.84, 95% CI 0.62–1.14).

Further data for use of a single-agent anti-PD-1 therapy can be found from ESCORT [14], a Chinese phase 3 study evaluating an anti-PD-1 antibody camrelizumab in second-line advanced OSCC compared to investigator-choice chemotherapy. This also showed benefit in the overall survival of camrelizumab vs. chemotherapy (HR 0.71, 95% CI 0.57–0.87) with more benefit seen in PD-L1-positive patients (PD-L1 $<$1% HR 0.82, 95% CI 0.62–1.09 vs. PD-L1 $\geq$1% HR 0.58, 95% CI 0.42–0.81). RATIONALE-302 [15] has also reported positive outcomes with an anti-PD-1 antibody, tislelizumab, compared to investigator-choice chemotherapy. 79% of patients were from Asia and 21% of patients were from Europe and North America. The study met its primary end point for OS in the ITT population (HR 0.70 95%, CI 0.57–0.85) with enrichment of benefit in the PD-L1-positive patients (CPS $\geq$10 HR 0.54, 95% CI 0.36–0.79).

2.2 Anti-PD-1 Antibodies in Combination with Other Systemic Therapies

In first-line advanced OSCC, single-agent anti-PD-1 antibodies have not been assessed in a phase 3 trial; however, recently there have been phase 3 data to support its use in combination with doublet platinum-based chemotherapy and in combination with ipilimumab, an inhibitor of cytotoxic T-lymphocyte-associated protein 4 (CTLA-4), which is another immune checkpoint.

KEYNOTE-590 [16] was a phase 3 study evaluating pembrolizumab plus cisplatin 5FU vs. placebo plus cisplatin 5FU in advanced oesophageal cancer in the first-line setting. 749 patients enrolled, of which 73% had OSCC, with the remainder being OAC. A benefit in the overall survival was seen with the addition of pembrolizumab in both the OSCC and intention-to-treat (ITT) group, although OSCC did make up the majority of the ITT (HR for death, OSCC, 0.72, 95% CI 0.60–0.88, HR for death, ITT, 0.73, 95% CI 0.62–0.86). OSCC patients that were PD-L1 CPS ≥10 had a more marked improvement in the overall survival with the addition of pembrolizumab (HR 0.57, 95% CI 0.43–0.75). Therefore, pembrolizumab can be considered with chemotherapy in OSCC patients and particularly in OSCC patients with CPS ≥10. However, it is noted that CPS <10 patients in the ITT appeared to benefit less than CPS ≥10 (CPS <10 HR 0.86, 95% CI 0.68–1.10; CPS ≥10 HR 0.62, 95% CI) and therefore it would be of interest to know the impact of pembrolizumab in patients with CPS <1.

CheckMate 648 [17] was a phase 3 study evaluating first-line chemotherapy (cisplatin 5FU) in advanced OSCC vs. chemotherapy plus nivolumab and also vs. nivolumab with ipilimumab. Again, this showed an improvement in OS with chemotherapy plus nivolumab vs. chemotherapy alone (HR 0.74, 95% CI 0.58–0.96) with a larger effect on the tumour cell PD-L1 ≥1% group (HR 0.54, 95% CI 0.37–0.80). OS is also improved in nivolumab plus ipilimumab vs. chemotherapy (HR for death 0.78, 95% CI 0.62–0.98) with further improvement in PD-L1 ≥1% group (HR for death 0.64, 95% CI 0.46–0.90). The HR for progression with nivolumab and ipilimumab vs. chemotherapy however appeared to favour chemotherapy in the ITT group (HR 1.26, 95% CI 1.04–1.52) and also in the PD-L1 ≥1% group (HR 1.02, 95% CI 0.73–1.43). Despite the lack of PFS benefit, the nivolumab and ipilimumab group achieved a longer OS compared to chemotherapy alone due to the longer median duration of response to nivolumab plus ipilimumab (11.1 months) compared to chemotherapy (7.1 months). Although the chances of progression may be higher in the nivolumab and ipilimumab group, as there was a benefit to overall survival it may still be an attractive option to patients where chemotherapy is undesirable and achieving a response quickly is not critical, e.g., patients with low disease burden.

This study was not designed to compare the nivolumab-containing arms against each other; however, the ORR of the nivolumab plus chemotherapy arm was higher at 47% compared to ORR of 28% with nivolumab plus ipilimumab although OS was similar (chemotherapy plus nivolumab arm 13.2m and nivolumab plus ipilimumab 12.8m). PD-L1 positivity did not appear to be a discriminating factor as to whether one should receive nivolumab plus ipilimumab rather than chemotherapy plus nivolumab, as the mOS and ORR in PD-L1 ≥1% patients were 15.4m and 53% with chemotherapy plus nivolumab and 13.7m and 35% with nivolumab plus ipilimumab, respectively. The HR for death in the PD-L1 negative group was 0.98 for chemotherapy plus nivolumab vs. chemotherapy and 0.96 for nivolumab plus ipililumab vs. chemotherapy and therefore it is uncertain as to how mcuh benefit PD-L1 negative patients will receive from nivolumab. However, the study was not powered to assess the outcomes of the PD-L1-negative patients in isolation from the ITT. Of note, the PD-L1 expression in this study was assessed by tumour cell PD-L1; however, it would be interesting to know the outcome of patients according to PD-L1 CPS.

ESCORT-1st [18] was a Chinese study looking at chemotherapy plus camrelizumab vs. chemotherapy plus placebo in first-line advanced OSCC. The chemotherapy used in this study was cisplatin and paclitaxel, which differs to the platinum-fluoropyrimidine doublet used in KEYNOTE-590 and CheckMate 648. This trial also showed an overall survival advantage with the addition of camrelizumab (HR for death 0.70, 95% CI 0.56–0.88). The subgroup analysis suggests that PD-L1 positive patients may benefit more this (PD-L1 ≥1% HR for death 0.59, 95% CI 0.43–0.80; PD-L1 <1% HR for death 0.79, 95% CI 0.57–1.11).

2.3 Early Disease

Early OSCC can be treated with definitive chemoradiation or with neoadjuvant chemoradiation (CRT) followed by radical oesophagectomy. CheckMate 577 [19] investigated the role of adjuvant nivolumab vs. placebo in patients who did not have a complete pathological response (pCR) to neoadjuvant chemoradiotherapy. In CheckMate 577, both squamous cell (29%) and adenocarcinoma (71%) patients were accrued. There was a statistically significant improvement in disease-free survival (HR 0.70, 95% CI 0.58–0.86) in the overall cohort. Although the SCC subgroup was less represented, it can be estimated that this group also benefited, perhaps to a greater degree, as the HR for progression in OSCC group was more favourable than the ITT (HR 0.61, 95% CI 0.42–0.88). This study will likely lead to the use of adjuvant nivolumab in OSCC patients who do not achieve a pCR after completion of neoadjuvant CRT; however, in patients who have definitive CRT instead the role of immunotherapy is yet to be addressed. In ongoing phase 3 trials, KEYNOTE-975 [20] is assessing the role of pembrolizumab with definitive CRT followed by adjuvant pembrolizumab whereas SKYSCRAPER-07 (NCT04543617) is assessing adjuvant PD-L1 inhibitor atezolizumab with or without tiragolumab, an immune checkpoint inhibitor of T-cell immunoreceptor with immunoglobulin and ITIM domain (TIGIT), after completion of definitive CRT.

3 Oesophageal Adenocarcinoma

3.1 Single-Agent Anti-PD-1 Antibodies

Advanced OAC shares a similar treatment paradigm to OSCC as these cancers have also been treated with platinum doublet in first line with poor outcomes in the second-line setting. However, as described in the Cancer Genome Atlas, OAC is molecularly more similar to CIN gastric cancer than to OSCC and therefore the responses to immunotherapy in OSCC may be different.

KEYNOTE-180 was an oesophageal trial as previously discussed, where approximately half of the patients were of OAC and half of OSCC. It was noted in this study that the ORR of the OAC was 5.2% whereas it was 14.3% in OSCC, which suggested that OSCC may be more responsive to pembrolizumab than OAC. This was further explored in the phase 3 study KEYNOTE-181 where 227 out of the 628 patients with oesophageal cancer were of adenocarcinoma histology. The overall ITT was not deemed to have a significant benefit of pembrolizumab over chemotherapy; however, there was significant benefit for OSCC. Although the study was not powered to look at OAC outcomes separately, HR for death in OAC was 1.12 (95% CI 0.85–1.47) favouring chemotherapy which again suggested that OSCC may respond better to pembrolizumab than OAC. Furthermore, in CPS ≥10 OAC group, there was no benefit in survival with pembrolizumab over chemotherapy (mOS pembrolizumab 6.3m vs. chemotherapy 6.9).

Due to the molecular similarities of OAC to CIN gastric cancer, gastric cancer studies may inform on the possible effect of immunotherapy on OAC. To discuss the gastric studies in detail would be beyond the scope of this chapter and this data can be found in the gastric chapter of this book. In summary, single-agent anti-PD-1 therapy has failed to show superiority to chemotherapy in randomised control studies [21–24]; however, its use may be considered in the third line if no other suitable options are available [25, 26]. In light of these studies, single-agent anti-PD-1 therapy is not superior to chemotherapy in the treatment of OAC.

3.2 Anti-PD-1 Antibodies in Combination with Other Systemic Antibodies

Single-agent anti-PD-1 therapy does not demonstrate superiority to chemotherapy in OAC; however, the combination of anti-PD-1 antibodies with chemotherapy has shown promising outcomes.

KEYNOTE-590, as discussed previously, was a first-line phase 3 advanced oesophageal study investigating chemotherapy plus pembrolizumab vs. chemotherapy plus placebo. 201 out of the 749 (21%) patients enrolled were of adenocarcinoma histology (91 GOJ, 110 oesophageal) with the remainder being OSCC. This was a positive trial for the ITT and the OSCC population; however, it was not powered to look at the adenocarcinoma outcomes separately. Due to the molecular differences identified in the Cancer Genome Atlas between OAC and OSCC [4] and the smaller proportion of OAC patients in the ITT, the impact on oesophageal adenocarcinoma from KEYNOTE-590 may be contentious. In the subgroup analysis there did also appear to be a trend towards benefit of the addition of pembrolizumab in the adenocarcinoma cohort (HR for death 0.74, 95% CI 0.54–1.02); however, the outcomes according to CPS in the adenocarcinoma group are yet to be published. Although outcomes stratified by CPS <10 and ≥10 have been reported, it is not possible to extrapolate the outcomes from the ITT onto OAC subgroup as OAC only represents 21% of the ITT.

However, support for chemotherapy plus anti-PD-1 in oesophageal adenocarcinoma can also be found in CheckMate 649 [27] and ATTRACTION-04 [28], which were positive phase 3 first-line advanced gastric/GOJ/OAC studies. CheckMate 649 was a global study recruiting 70% gastric and 30% GOJ/OAC. ATTRACTION-04 differs more as this was an Asian study with 89% gastric and 11% GOJ patients. Further discussion of these studies in detail will be found in the gastric chapter of this book; however, in summary a significant OS and PFS benefit was seen in CheckMate 649 and a significant PFS benefit was seen in ATTRACTION-04 in the

ITT. An OS benefit was not seen in ATTRACTION-04; however, it can be speculated that patients who progressed on the chemotherapy arm may have benefited from subsequent nivolumab as this was approved in the participating countries of ATTRACTION-04 (Japan, Korea and Taiwan).

Although the GOJ and oesophageal group is not powered to be assessed in isolation from the gastric patients who made up the majority in CheckMate 649 and ATTRACTION-04, it may be acceptable to apply the benefit of the ITT to OAC patients as molecular data suggests that oesophageal adenocarcinomas are similar to CIN gastric adenocarcinomas which make up the majority of gastric cancers. However, a difference in response to immunotherapy may exist between gastric and GOJ, as in the subgroup analysis of CheckMate 649, patients who had GOJ cancer may have benefited less from the addition of nivolumab compared to patients with gastric cancer (HR for death in chemotherapy and nivolumab vs. chemotherapy: gastric 0.76, GOJ 0.90, oesophageal 0.82. HR for death in CPS ≥5 chemotherapy plus nivolumab vs. chemotherapy: gastric 0.65, GOJ 0.84, oesophageal 0.78). Differences in response to immunotherapy between the gastric and OAC groups may occur as MSI high and EBV gastric cancers do not overlap with OAC; however, these subtypes are in the minority. For example, in CheckMate 649, although MSI-H patients greatly benefited from the addition of nivolumab (HR for death 0.37) this group only made up 44 out of the 1421 patients with an evaluable MSI status.

3.3 Early Disease

As discussed before, CheckMate 577 assessed adjuvant nivolumab after neoadjuvant CRT in oesophageal cancer patients who did not achieve a pCR. The majority of patients were of adenocarcinoma histology (71%) with the remainder being SCC. The SCC patients, as discussed above, achieved a HR of 0.61 for mDFS benefit for the addition of nivolumab; however, the HR for adenocarcinoma was 0.75 (95% CI 0.59–0.96) and therefore it is possible that the benefit of adjuvant nivolumab is greater in OSCC than OAC. Furthermore, it is unclear as to what the benefit of adjuvant nivolumab is in CPS-negative patients as it appears that CPS <5 patients may benefit less than CPS ≥5 (HR for progression in CPS <5 0.89, 95% CI 0.65–1.22; CPS ≥5 0.62, 95% CI 0.46–0.83). Nevertheless, the results of CheckMate 577 are likely to change the standard of care for patients after neoadjuvant CRT although overall survival data is awaited and will be of relevance especially as the role of immunotherapy evolves in the advanced setting. The results of CheckMate 577 may also have a limited impact in centres where perioperative chemotherapy is preferred over neoadjuvant CRT for GOJ adenocarcinoma.

4 Concluding Remarks

Combination of chemotherapy and nivolumab [17], pembrolizumab [16] or camrelizumab [18] will become first-line standard of care in patients with advanced OSCC. Nivolumab plus ipilimumab [17] also represents an option associated with durable disease responses in first-line advanced OSCC in patients where chemotherapy is undesirable or in patients who do not have an urgent requirement for a reduction of tumour disease burden. Studies have suggested a role of single-agent nivolumab [12], pembrolizumab [13], camrelizumab [14] or tislelizumab [15] in the second-line setting in OSCC; however, this is likely to be replaced with front-line immunotherapy with chemotherapy especially as many patients with oesophageal cancer are not fit enough for second-line treatment when they progress. If checkpoint inhibitors are used upfront, then second-line PD-1 antibodies are likely to be replaced with cytotoxic drugs such as irinotecan and taxanes. There is less evidence for single-agent anti-PD-1 therapy in OAC; however, this may be considered in the third-line advanced setting if there are no suitable alternatives. However, there is now a possibility in OAC to offer nivolumab [27] or pembrolizumab [16] in combination with chemotherapy in the first-line advanced setting. So far in the early disease setting, adjuvant nivolumab [29] can be considered for patients who have had neoadjuvant chemoradiotherapy and do not achieve a pCR; however, the smaller OSCC subgroup appeared to benefit more than the adenocarcinoma group. There may be a greater benefit to ICI with OSCC compared to OAC indicating that OSCC and OAC may be very different diseases as molecular data [4] has already suggested. Therefore, combining the two histologies in studies should be discouraged as this may provide confusing results and going forward, studies recruiting each histology exclusively are recommended. PD-L1 expression is a relevant biomarker for response to ICI in both OSCC and OAC as several trials demonstrate favourable outcomes to ICI in PD-L1-positive tumours whereas controversy exists over its impact in PD-L1-negative tumours. Nevertheless, despite these uncertainties, there is sufficient evidence to support ICI as a standard of care in oesophageal cancer.

Compliance with Ethical Standards

Disclosure of Interests Ian Chau is on the advisory board at Eli Lilly, Bristol Myers Squibb, MSD, Bayer, Roche, Merck Serono, Five Prime Therapeutics, AstraZeneca, OncXerna, Pierre Fabre, Boehringer Ingelheim, Incyte, Astella, GSK, Sotio and Eisai. He has received research funding from Eli Lilly and Janssen-Cilag and honorarium from Eli Lilly, Eisai and Servier.

Su Li has no competing interests.

References

1. Sung H, Ferlay J, Siegel RL, Laversanne M, Soerjomataram I et al (2021) Global Cancer Statistics 2020: GLOBOCAN estimates of incidence and mortality worldwide for 36 cancers in 185 countries. CA: Cancer J Clin 71:209–249
2. Arnold M, Ferlay J, van Berge Henegouwen MI, Soerjomataram I (2020) Global burden of oesophageal and gastric cancer by histology and subsite in 2018. Gut 69:1564
3. de Martel C, Georges D, Bray F, Ferlay J, Clifford GM (2020) Global burden of cancer attributable to infections in 2018: a worldwide incidence analysis. Lancet Global Health 8:e180–ee90
4. Kim J, Bowlby R, Mungall AJ, Robertson AG, Odze RD et al (2017) Integrated genomic characterization of oesophageal carcinoma. Nature 541:169–175
5. Le DA-O, Durham JA-O, Smith KA-O, Wang H, Bartlett BA-O et al Mismatch repair deficiency predicts response of solid tumors to PD-1 blockade. Science 357(6349):409–413

6. Kim ST, Cristescu R, Bass AJ, Kim K-M, Odegaard JI et al (2018) Comprehensive molecular characterization of clinical responses to PD-1 inhibition in metastatic gastric cancer. Nat Med 24:1449–1458
7. Hewitt LC, Inam IZ, Saito Y, Yoshikawa T, Quaas A et al (2018) Epstein-Barr virus and mismatch repair deficiency status differ between oesophageal and gastric cancer: a large multicentre study. Eur J Cancer 94:104–114
8. Marabelle A, Fakih M, Lopez J, Shah M, Shapira-Frommer R et al (2020) Association of tumour mutational burden with outcomes in patients with advanced solid tumours treated with pembrolizumab: prospective biomarker analysis of the multicohort, open-label, phase 2 KEYNOTE-158 study. Lancet Oncol 21:1353–1365
9. Cui Y, Chen H, Xi R, Cui H, Zhao Y et al (2020) Whole-genome sequencing of 508 patients identifies key molecular features associated with poor prognosis in esophageal squamous cell carcinoma. Cell Res 30:902–913
10. Kudo T, Hamamoto Y, Kato K, Ura T, Kojima T et al (2017) Nivolumab treatment for oesophageal squamous-cell carcinoma: an open-label, multicentre, phase 2 trial. Lancet Oncol 18:631–639
11. Shah MA, Kojima T, Hochhauser D, Enzinger P, Raimbourg J et al (2019) Efficacy and safety of pembrolizumab for heavily pretreated patients with advanced, metastatic adenocarcinoma or squamous cell carcinoma of the esophagus: the phase 2 KEYNOTE-180 Study. JAMA Oncol 5(4):546–550
12. Kato K, Cho BC, Takahashi M, Okada M, Lin C-Y et al (2019) Nivolumab versus chemotherapy in patients with advanced oesophageal squamous cell carcinoma refractory or intolerant to previous chemotherapy (ATTRACTION-3): a multicentre, randomised, open-label, phase 3 trial. Lancet Oncol 20:1506–1517
13. Kojima TA-O, Shah MA-O, Muro K, Francois E, Adenis A et al (2020) Randomized phase III KEYNOTE-181 study of pembrolizumab versus chemotherapy in advanced esophageal cancer. J Clin Oncol 38(35):4138–4148
14. Huang J, Xu J, Chen Y, Zhuang W, Zhang Y et al (2020) Camrelizumab versus investigator's choice of chemotherapy as second-line therapy for advanced or metastatic oesophageal squamous cell carcinoma (ESCORT): a multicentre, randomised, open-label, phase 3 study. Lancet Oncol 21:832–842
15. Shen L, Kato K, Kim S-B, Ajani JA, Zhao K et al (2021) RATIONALE 302: randomized, phase 3 study of tislelizumab versus chemotherapy as second-line treatment for advanced unresectable/metastatic esophageal squamous cell carcinoma. J Clin Oncol 39:4012
16. Kato K, Sun J, Shah MA, Enzinger PC, Adenis A et al (2020) Pembrolizumab plus chemotherapy versus chemotherapy as first-line therapy in patients with advanced esophageal cancer: the phase 3 KEYNOTE-590 study. Ann Oncol 31(Suppl. 4):S1142–S1215. https://doi.org/10.1016/annonc/annonc325
17. Chau IDY, Ajani JA, Xu J, Wyrwicz L, Motoyama S, Ogata T, Kawakami H, Hsu CH, Adenis A, Hajbi E, Di Bartolomeo M, Braghiroli MIFM, Holtved E, Xynos I, Liu X, Lei M, Kondo K, Kato K, Kitagawa Y (2021) Nivolumab (NIVO) plus ipilimumab (IPI) or NIVO plus chemotherapy (chemo) versus chemo as first-line (1L) treatment for advanced esophageal squamous cell carcinoma (ESCC): First results of the CheckMate 648 study. J Clin Oncol 39(Suppl. 18):LBA4001
18. Xu R-h, Luo H, Lu J, Bai Y, Mao T et al (2021) ESCORT-1st: a randomized, double-blind, placebo-controlled, phase 3 trial of camrelizumab plus chemotherapy versus chemotherapy in patients with untreated advanced or metastatic esophageal squamous cell carcinoma (ESCC). J Clin Oncol 39:4000
19. Kelly RJ, Ajani JA, Kuzdzal J, Zander T, Van Cutsem E et al (2021) Adjuvant nivolumab in resected esophageal or gastroesophageal junction cancer. N Engl J Med 384:1191–1203
20. Shah MA, Bennouna J, Doi T, Shen L, Kato K et al (2021) KEYNOTE-975 study design: a Phase III study of definitive chemoradiotherapy plus pembrolizumab in patients with esophageal carcinoma. Future Oncol 17:1143–1153

21. Shitara K, Özgüroğlu M, Bang Y-J, Di Bartolomeo M, Mandalà M et al (2018) Pembrolizumab versus paclitaxel for previously treated, advanced gastric or gastro-oesophageal junction cancer (KEYNOTE-061): a randomised, open-label, controlled, phase 3 trial. Lancet 392:123–133
22. Bang YJ, Ruiz EY, Van Cutsem E, Lee KW, Wyrwicz L et al (2018) Phase III, randomised trial of avelumab versus physician's choice of chemotherapy as third-line treatment of patients with advanced gastric or gastro-oesophageal junction cancer: primary analysis of JAVELIN Gastric 300. Ann Oncol 29:2052–2060
23. Tabernero J, Van Cutsem E, Bang Y-J, Fuchs CS, Wyrwicz L et al (2019) Pembrolizumab with or without chemotherapy versus chemotherapy for advanced gastric or gastroesophageal junction (G/GEJ) adenocarcinoma: the phase III KEYNOTE-062 study. J Clin Oncol 37:LBA4007
24. Moehler M, Dvorkin M, Boku N, Özgüroğlu M, Ryu M-H et al (2020) Phase III trial of avelumab maintenance after first-line induction chemotherapy versus continuation of chemotherapy in patients with gastric cancers: results from JAVELIN gastric 100. J Clin Oncol 39:966–977
25. Kang Y-K, Boku N, Satoh T, Ryu M-H, Chao Y et al (2017) Nivolumab in patients with advanced gastric or gastro-oesophageal junction cancer refractory to, or intolerant of, at least two previous chemotherapy regimens (ONO-4538-12, ATTRACTION-2): a randomised, double-blind, placebo-controlled, phase 3 trial. Lancet 390:2461–2471
26. Fuchs CS, Doi T, Jang RW, Muro K, Satoh T et al (2018) Safety and efficacy of pembrolizumab monotherapy in patients with previously treated advanced gastric and gastroesophageal junction cancer: phase 2 clinical KEYNOTE-059 trial. JAMA Oncol 4:e180013
27. Janjigian YY, Shitara K, Moehler M, Garrido M, Salman P et al (2021) First-line nivolumab plus chemotherapy versus chemotherapy alone for advanced gastric, gastro-oesophageal junction, and oesophageal adenocarcinoma (CheckMate 649): a randomised, open-label, phase 3 trial. Lancet
28. Boku N, Ryu MH, Oh DY, Oh SC, Chung HC et al (2020) LBA7_PR Nivolumab plus chemotherapy versus chemotherapy alone in patients with previously untreated advanced or recurrent gastric/gastroesophageal junction (G/GEJ) cancer: ATTRACTION-4 (ONO-4538-37) study. Ann Oncol 31:S1192
29. Kelly RJ, Ajani JA, Kuzdzal J, Zander T, Cutsem EV et al (2020) LBA9_PR - Adjuvant nivolumab in resected esophageal or gastroesophageal junction cancer (EC/GEJC) following neoadjuvant chemoradiation therapy (CRT): First results of the CheckMate 577 study. Ann Oncol 31(Suppl. 4):S1142–S1215. https://doi.org/10.1016/annonc/annonc325

Perspective on the Immunotherapy of Esophageal Cancer

Sarah Derks and Hanneke W. M. van Laarhoven

Contents

Abstract

While immune checkpoint inhibitors have revolutionized cancer treatment, in esophageal cancer, response rates are only modest. One potential explanation can be found in the composition of the tumor immune microenvironment, which is characterized by immune cell exclusion, infiltration of immune suppressive macrophages, epithelial-to-mesenchymal transition, and stromal factors that suppress local immunity. Improving success of immune checkpoint inhibitor will likely need targeting of these factors as well. Furthermore, determining the best timing of immunotherapy relative to conventional therapies such as

S. Derks
Department of Medical Oncology, Amsterdam University Medical Centers, Cancer Center Amsterdam, Free University, Amsterdam, The Netherlands
e-mail: s.derks@amsterdamumc.nl

H. W. M. van Laarhoven (✉)
Department of Medical Oncology, Amsterdam University Medical Centers, Cancer Center Amsterdam, University of Amsterdam, Amsterdam, The Netherlands
e-mail: h.vanlaarhoven@amsterdamumc.nl

Cancer Immunotherapy (2021)
https://doi.org/10.1007/13905_2021_2,
Published Online: 02 September 2021

chemotherapy and radiotherapy needs to be studied in more detail and likely influences it success. Based on this knowledge alternative immunomodulatory strategies can be developed using a precision oncology approach.

Keywords

Esophageal adenocarcinoma · Esophageal squamous cell carcinoma · Fibroblasts · Tumor associated macrophages · Tumor immune microenvironment

1 Introduction

While immune checkpoint inhibitors (ICI) have shown clear signal in patients with esophageal cancer (EC), they only benefit for a subset of patient and the fast majority of patients still fails to respond. In order to increase immunotherapy efficacy, it is crucial to identify the characteristics of responsive tumors as well as the underlying mechanism(s) of immunotherapy's failure (Fig. 1). Lack of response often occurs in tumors with few tumor infiltrating T cells, referred to as immunologically "cold" tumors, which can likely be explained by a lack of tumor cell recognition or activation of immune suppressive mechanisms within the tumor microenvironment. In addition to tumor-specific factors modulating the tumor immune microenvironment of esophageal cancer, systemic host-related factors should also be considered. For example, there is growing evidence that the human microbiome is one of the determinant factors of an individual's immune profile. Microbes identified in feces or tumors have been associated with the response to chemotherapy as well as immune checkpoint inhibitors (ICIs) [1].

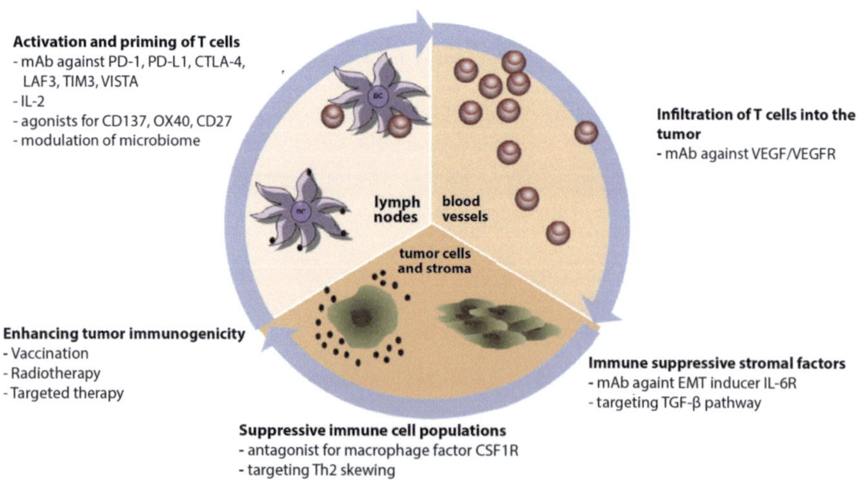

Fig. 1 Leads to increase efficacy of immunotherapy. (With permission adapted from Moehler [2])

2 The Suppressed Immune Microenvironment of ESCC and EAC and Response to Immunotherapy

In the last two decades accumulating data has shown that anti-tumor immunity in esophageal adenocarcinomas and squamous cell carcinomas is often heavily suppressed by multiple immune suppressive mechanisms. This is rather contraintuitive, as ECs harbor a high somatic mutation burden [3]. In their development at a background of chronic inflammation, ECs must have developed these suppressive mechanisms to regulate an anti-tumor immunity and become clinically apparent.

The development of esophageal adenocarcinomas (EACs) starts with exposure to gastric and bile acids which stimulates the lower esophagus to undergo metaplasia to an intestinalized epithelium, Barrett's esophagus (BE). Barrett's metaplasia is associated with a change from an acute (Th1 type) proinflammatory immune response accompanied with IFN-γ expression to a Th2 type chronic inflammatory tumor permissive microenvironment accompanied by the production of IL-4 and IL-13 [4, 5]. The Th1 to Th2 transition is associated with the infiltration of myeloid-derived suppressor cells (MDSCs) and M2-polarized macrophages [6]. MDSCs are known to suppress the anti-tumor immune response by inhibiting T cell activation and NK cell cytotoxicity and induction of regulatory T cells (Tregs). Recruitment of Tregs is also mediated by chemokine CCL17 and CCL22 which are secreted by tumor cells and macrophages in EAC [7].

In esophageal squamous cell carcinomas (ESCC) well-known risk factors such as smoking and alcohol also cause chronic irritation and inflammation. This subsequently leads to the production of reactive oxygen species (ROS) [8]. ROS production causes DNA damage and activation of multiple cancer-associated pathways. In both ESCC and EAC chronic inflammation further stimulates expression of cytokines such as IL-6 and TNFalpha which have anti-apoptotic but also immune suppressive properties. Activation of IL-6 and downstream transcription factor STAT3, for instance, allow cells to survive in inflamed areas by stimulating proliferation as well as expansion of pro-tumorigenic MDSCs. Within this chronic inflammatory state also nuclear factor-kappaB (NF-κB) pathways are activated (reviewed in [8]). NF-κB signaling stimulates CXCL8 expression which has neutrophil attractive properties but also helps tumor cell to escape from immunity.

The Th2 skewed immune microenvironment in EAC is also reflected in PD-L2 dominancy over PD-L1. Although in ESCC both the immunosuppressive checkpoints PD-L1 and PD-L2 are expressed in 48%, epithelial PD-L1 expression occurs in only 23% of EAC [9, 10]. In contrast, epithelial expression of the alternative PD-1 ligand PD-L2 was observed in ~50% of EACs. This can be explained by Th2 cytokines Il4 and Il-13, which are not only involved in the recruitment and stimulation of M2 macrophages and MDSCs, but also drive PD-L2 expression. This underscores that solely targeting the PD-1 pathway may not be sufficient to activate an anti-tumor immune response in EAC.

Besides PD-L1 and PD-L2 also expression of additional inhibitory checkpoints such as CTLA4, TIM-3, LAG3 and VISTA has been well described (recently reviewed in [11]). It is not immediately clear how the expression of these checkpoints correlates to the inflammatory state of the tumor immune microenvironment nor to response to immune checkpoint blockade. This required further exploration in future (clinical) studies.

3 Stromal Derived Immune Modulation

Intriguingly, in addition to cells usually associated with the immune microenvironment, such as T cells and macrophages, yet another cell type may be involved in the shaping of this environment, namely cancer-associated fibroblasts (CAFs). Many gastrointestinal cancers, including esophageal cancer, non-tumor cells such as fibroblasts and extracellular matrix, so-called tumor stroma, often constitute the bulk of tumor tissue. A high tumor stroma ratio is prognostic for poor outcome in esophageal cancer [12], which is attributed to its tumor-promoting properties. These properties are most predominantly related to the physical barrier it creates for systemic therapy, while at the same time causing hypoxia and hypoxia-induced cell survival, invasion, and stemness [13]. Recently, it was also shown that cancer-associated fibroblasts in esophageal adenocarcinoma (EAC) can produce the pro-inflammatory cytokine IL-6 which is commonly secreted by inflammatory cells such as B-cells and T cells [14]. In addition to the known involvement of IL-6 in immune responses, acute phase reaction, and stimulation of hemopoeisis, in EAC stromal derived IL-6 was shown to drive epithelial-to-mesenchymal transition (EMT) in tumor cells.

EMT encompasses a molecular dedifferentiation program similar to wound healing and tissue degeneration associated with soluble factors such as TGF-β and IL-8 and transcription factors snail, slug, twist, zeb1, zeb2, brachyury, and foxc2 among others. These factors jointly drive tumor cells into motile and invasive mesenchymal-like cells and also induce resistance to therapy such as neoadjuvant chemoradiation [14]. Recently it has become increasingly apparent that a mesenchymal cell state enhances resistance to cytotoxic T cell and NK cell-mediated lysis and resistance to immunotherapy [15]. In a diversity of tumor types it is has been shown that the EMT process is associated with a change from a neutrophil-rich TME to an increased number of immune suppressive M2-like macrophages. Large transcriptome studies have also identified that EMT expression signatures are associated with a decreased number of tumor infiltrating lymphocytes (TILs) and an increased expression of immunosuppressive cytokines, immune checkpoint molecules such as PD-L1 [16] and markers of T cell exhaustion [17]. Giving the immune suppressive effect of mesenchymal cells, tumors with EMT are likely to respond to immunotherapy which has indeed been shown for non-small cell lung cancer [18]. As both EMT and immune cell exclusion are central features of esophageal cancers, targeting factors that drive EMT and stroma-immune interactions such as TGF-β, IL-6, or macrophages, might be a promising strategy (recently reviewed in [19]) and is currently being explored in clinical studies (e.g., NCT04595149, NCT04554771).

4 Checkpoint Inhibition and Conventional Anti-Cancer Treatments in Esophagogastric Cancer: New Roads Ahead?

For long, chemotherapy has been one of the cornerstones of esophagogastric cancer treatment [20–22]. With the advent of checkpoint inhibitors—more specifically PD-1 and PD-L1 inhibitors—hopes were high to improve outcome in patients with esophagogastric cancer. Unfortunately, thus far, in biomarker unselected patient populations, results have been limited [23, 24]. In PD-L1 positive patients, significant improvement in outcomes has been observed with pembrolizumab [25], however, this positive effect only became apparent 6 months after start of treatment. These results raise the question whether a short course of chemotherapy followed by checkpoint inhibition might be the optimal approach. Theoretically, this would combine the best of both worlds: compared to PD-(L)-1 inhibitors alone possible negative effects in patients with fast growing tumors would be avoided, while compared to combination therapies PD-(L)-1 inhibitors and chemotherapy, patients would be saved from long-term chemotherapy induced toxicity, especially neurotoxicity [26]. The latter would not only positively impact quality of life, but also leave room for the administration of second line treatments [27]. Furthermore, chemotherapy might "prime" tumors for subsequent PD-(L)1 inhibition [28].

Following this concept, the JAVELIN GASTRIC-100 study investigated maintenance therapy with avelumab compared to continuation of chemotherapy in patients with locally advanced/metastatic HER2− gastric/gastroesophageal junction cancer adenocarcinoma, who have achieved at least stable disease following 12 weeks of first-line oxaliplatin/fluoropyrimidine chemotherapy [29]. First results presented at ASCO-GI 2020 showed that avelumab maintenance had clinical activity and favorable safety versus continued chemotherapy [30]. Unfortunately, JAVELIN Gastric 100 did not meet its primary objective of demonstrating superior overall survival in the randomized or PD-L1+ population. Results of JAVELIN Gastric 100, however, do not exclude the potential of sequential treatment with chemotherapy followed by PD-(L)1 inhibition in certain subgroups of patients, such as MSI-high cancers and gastric cancers with Epstein–Barr Virus (EBV) positivity.

In addition to chemotherapy, radiation plays a crucial role in the treatment of esophageal cancer for both the adenocarcinoma and squamous cell carcinoma subtypes [31, 32]. Several mechanisms have been identified through which radiotherapy may increase efficacy of immunotherapy (Fig. 2). For instance, radiotherapy induces immunogenic cell death which enhances specific T cell priming. Also, the expression of adhesion molecules on endothelial cell and chemokines by cancer cells can be induced, improving the extravasation of immune cells into the tumor tissue.

However, unfortunately, the combination of radiation with checkpoint inhibition does not result in improved outcomes as a matter of course. In a recent study combining neoadjuvant chemoradiation according to the CROSS regimen with atezolizumab, pathological response rates and survival were similar compared to a historic

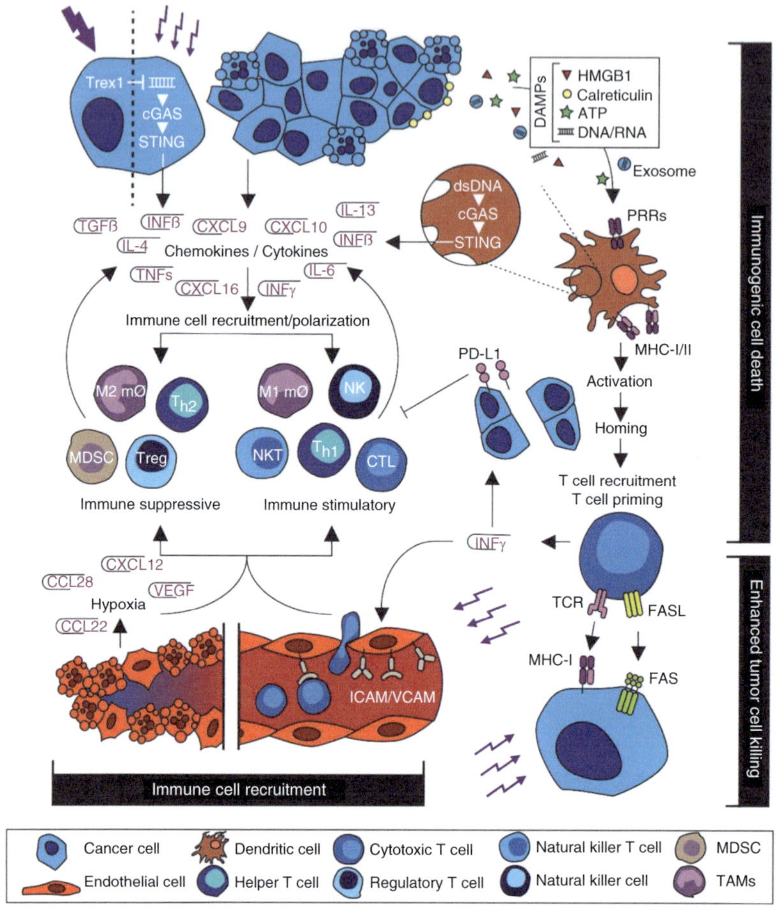

Fig. 2 Schematic overview of the main effects that occur in the immune microenvironment in response to radiotherapy. Irradiation of tumor cells can induce expression of interferon beta (IFNβ) through cytosolic dsDNA/cGAS/STING signaling. This is dependent on dosing, as high dose irradiation induces Trex1 which causes clearance of cytosolic dsDNA. Apart from IFNβ, radiotherapy induces the expression and release of several chemokines, cytokines, and growth factors that promote the recruitment of immune cells. This includes both suppressive and stimulatory immune cell subsets. At the same time, irradiation promotes an immune response via the induction of immunogenic cell death. The release of damage-associated molecular patterns (DAMPs) upon radiotherapy-induced cell death cause the activation of antigen presenting cells like dendritic cells through pattern recognition receptors (PPR). This eventually results in the recruitment and priming of cytotoxic T cells. This is accompanied by the release of cytokines like interferon gamma (IFNγ) which exerts diverging effects on the immune response. At the one hand, IFNγ induces PD-L1 expression on tumor cells which is immunosuppressive. At the other hand, it stimulates the expression of leukocyte adhesion molecules in the vessel wall which contributes to increased immune cell recruitment. Vessel regression induces hypoxia which increases expression of growth factors and chemokines that affect immune cell recruitment and polarization. Finally, radiotherapy induces the expression of molecules on the tumor cell surface like MHC-I and Fas, which increases tumor cell killing by immune cells. Targeting the immune suppressive mechanisms provides opportunities for therapeutic intervention in combination with radiotherapy. (Adapted from the open access publication by Goedegebuure et al. [33])

comparison with the CROSS trial as well as a propensity matched cohort [34]. Nevertheless, responders to this short-term neoadjuvant treatment seemed to derive survival benefit. In contrast, a recent adjuvant trial has established the benefit of long-term adjuvant nivolumab in non-responders after neoadjuvant chemoradiation (CheckMate-577) [35]. The immunoregulatory response to irradiation appears to be dose and schedule dependent, as well as determined by tumor type and the (pre-treatment) tumor microenvironment [28, 33].

Although targeted treatment of esophagogastric cancer is lagging behind compared to other tumor types, anti-HER2 treatment with trastuzumab and anti-angiogenic treatment with ramucirumab have become standard of care in the first-line metastatic setting for HER2 overexpressing adenocarcinomas of the stomach and gastroesophageal junction, and in the second line for biomarker unselected adenocarcinomas of the stomach and gastroesophageal junction, respectively [27, 36]. In both settings, outcomes may be improved by combination with immunomodulating treatment and more specifically checkpoint inhibition.

In the first-line treatment setting of HER2-positive metastatic esophagogastric cancer, promising activity of pembrolizumab in combination with trastuzumab and chemotherapy has been observed in a single-arm phase 2 study with 70% of patients being free of progression at 6 months [37]. However, the mechanism behind the positive interaction between trastuzumab and pembrolizumab remains to be elucidated. Upregulation of PD-1 and PD-L1, trastuzumab related antibody-dependent cell-mediated cytotoxicity enhancing presentation of tumor antigens, enhanced immune infiltration, augmentation of HER2-specific T-cell responses, promotion of T cell and dendritic cell trafficking, and induced expansion of peripheral memory T cells have all been suggested as potential players [38–43]. Further correlative studies should pinpoint the relevance of these pathways to find further leads to improve treatment efficacy. This is especially relevant for those 30% of patients benefiting only for a relatively short period of time from the combination of pembrolizumab, trastuzumab, and chemotherapy.

Targeting the VEGF/VEGF receptor 2 (VEGFR2) pathway may improve the efficacy of checkpoint inhibitors by reprogramming the tumor microenvironment to be more immune supportive or inflammatory, and promising results of the phase IB study combining ramucirumab and pembrolizumab in advanced gastric cancer underscore this hypothesis [44]. Also here, the exact mechanism through which targeting of the VEGF/VEGFR2 pathway improves efficacy of checkpoint inhibition has not been fully elucidated. Generally speaking, anti-angiogenic drugs have been shown to increase effector immune cell infiltration in tumors by vascular remodeling and/or relieving immunosuppression. In turn, activated immune effector cells—which can be further stimulated by checkpoint inhibitors—can secrete IFNγ, which promotes vascular remodeling, thus leading to a synergy between anti-angiogenic drugs and checkpoint inhibitors [45]. Especially in view of the development of resistance to anti-angiogenic or immune checkpoint inhibition, in depth studies on the molecular pathways affected by (the combined) use of these drugs are fundamental to further improve treatment outcomes [45]. For example, upregulation of HGF-mediated angiogenesis in response to anti-VEGF treatment may result in other molecules eliciting tumor immunosuppression than during VEGF-mediated angiogenesis, thus necessitating not only a switch in anti-angiogenic treatment, but possibly also in immunostimulatory treatment. Of note, the presumed increase in tumor uptake of checkpoint inhibitors due to vascular normalization induced by anti-angiogenic drugs may, in fact, be a marginal mechanism of action, as several reports have shown that anti-angiogenic drugs can significantly *reduce* tumor uptake of drugs [45–48]. Smart sequencing of the different drugs and/or introduction of drug holidays may circumvent this problem, but hitherto has not been implemented in clinical practice.

5 Immunotherapy Beyond Checkpoint Inhibitors

As tumor associated macrophages (TAMs) seem to play such a dominant role in the suppressed immune microenvironment of esophageal cancers, targeting TAMs is a potential alternative strategy to reactivate anti-tumor immunity (Fig. 3). It is not immediately clear how TAMs suppress T cells, but expression of arginase-1 (ARG1), IL-10, and TGF-β can have T cell suppressive effects [49]. In recent years multiple therapies to target TAMs such as colony stimulatory factor 1 receptor (CSF1R) antagonists have shown promising results in in vivo mouse studies using a diversity of tumor models [50]. Depletion of macrophages resulted in infiltration of CD8+ T cells, delay of tumor progression, and increased effectivity of PD-1 checkpoint inhibitors. Alternatively, targeting regulators of macrophages differentiation (MARCO, PI3Kγ and histone deacetylase) also reduces the T cell suppressive effects of TAMs and thereby increases the effectivity of T cell directed therapies in HNSCC and other cancers [51].

Given the role of cancer-associated fibroblasts in the production of anti-IL6, causing a treatment resistant phenotype [14], the BASALT study is currently investigating whether stroma-targeting by tocilizumab in esophageal adenocarcinoma patients with highly activated stroma increases efficacy of chemoradiotherapy (clinicaltrials.gov NCT04554771). Patients will be stratified for ADAM12, a non-invasive blood-borne marker of stromal activation [53, 54]. Also, rather than targeting of cytokines produced by CAFs, direct targeting of CAFs may be considered. However, caution should be taken with global anti-CAF treatments, since evidence is emerging on the existence of different subtypes of CAFs within tumor tissues that exert fundamentally different effects on the tumor as a whole, and clinical outcome as a result [55–59]. Indeed, also in EAC stromal activation does not always result in a treatment resistant phenotype, and activation of the tumor stroma may result in a tumor microenvironment that, in fact, supports treatment efficacy [47]. Thus, depending on specific cues that activate CAFs, a treatment resistant or treatment-facilitating tumor (immune) microenvironment may arise. Therefore, future research should aim at the development of biomarkers to distinguish subpopulations of CAFs and efforts should be undertaken to targeted the tumor stroma in a subpopulation specific way.

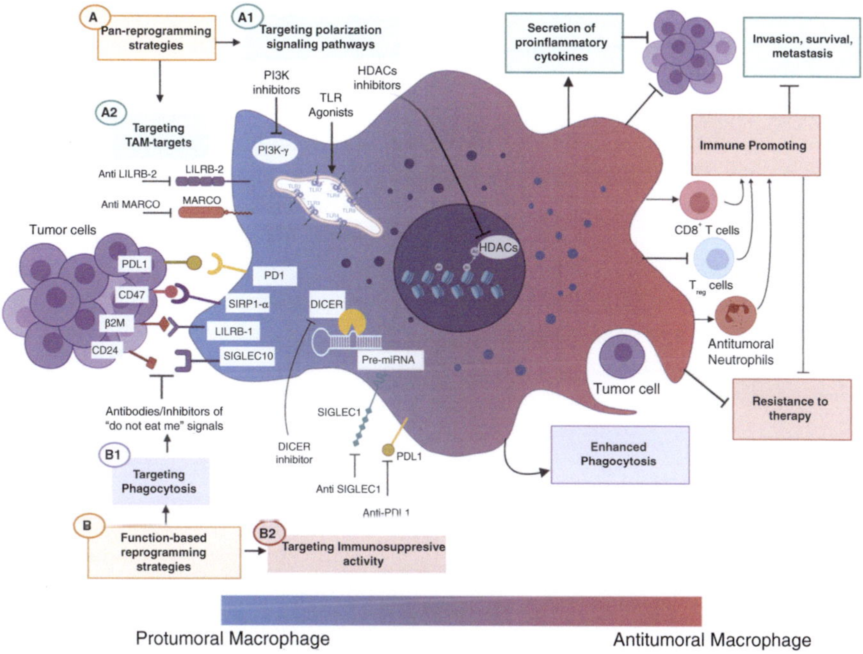

Fig. 3 Therapeutic strategies aimed at changing the phenotype of TAMs from a protumoral to an anti-tumoral state (macrophage reprogramming). TAM reprogramming strategies fall into two main categories: pan-reprogramming (A) and function-based reprogramming of TAMs (B). Pan-reprogramming includes strategies that target macrophage polarization signaling pathways (A1), such as using PI3Kγ inhibitors, TLR agonists, and HDAC inhibitors; and TAM-preferentially expressed targets (A2) such as MARCO and LILRB2. Function-based reprogramming of TAMs (B) includes targeting specific TAM functions, such as phagocytosis (B1), by targeting the macrophage tumor cell "do not eat me" signals SIRP1α–CD47, LILRB1–β2M, SIGLEC10–CD24, and PD1–PDL1, and macrophage immunosuppressive activities (B2) by inhibiting macrophage SIGLEC1, PDL1, or abrogating micro-RNA activity through DICER inhibition. Macrophage reprogramming leads to the secretion of proinflammatory cytokines, an enhancement of phagocytic ability, and macrophage-mediated immune promotion. These activities inhibit tumor progression, metastasis, and/or resistance to therapy. *HDACs* histone deacetylases, *TLRs* Toll-like receptors, *PI3Kγ* phosphoinositide 3-kinase-γ, *LILRB2* leukocyte immunoglobulin-like receptor-B2, *MARCO* macrophage receptor with collagenous structure, *PD1* programmed cell death 1, *PDL1* PD1 ligand 1, *SIRP1α* signal regulatory protein-α, *LILRB1* leukocyte immunoglobulin-like receptor-B1, *β2M* β2-microglobulin, *SIGLEC10* sialic acid–binding Ig-like lectin-10, *SIGLEC1* sialic acid–binding Ig-like lectin-1, *pre-miRNA* pre-micro-RNA, *Treg cells* regulatory T cells. (Reproduced from the open access publication by Lopez-Yrigoyen et al. [52])

6 Microbiome

In view of systemic host-related factors contributing to anti-tumor immunity and the role that is played by microbiota, and more specifically gut microbiota, modulation of this system may be used to enhance (immune)therapy efficacy. In mice, it has been shown that manipulation of the gut microbiota can improve anti-tumor response through enhancing host immune response [60–62]. In a small, proof-of-principle randomized controlled trial an improvement in disease control rate and a prolongation in median progression free and overall survival were observed after donor fecal microbiota transplantation derived from healthy obese donors compared to autologous fecal microbiota transplantation prior to first-line palliative chemotherapy in patients with advanced gastroesophageal adenocarcinoma.(manuscript submitted) However, despite these intriguing results, there is no consensus on how the "ideal" or "most beneficial" gut microbiota composition should look like to enhance anti-tumor immunity. Importantly, research thus far has mainly focused on fecal and tumor microbiota composition, while the duodenal microbiome, and the metabolites they produce, may also play a crucial role in regulation of the immune system [63, 64].

7 Concluding Remarks

Improvement of response to immunotherapy requires a deep understanding of the activation status and the key players in the pre-existing immune microenvironment. Based on this knowledge alternative immunomodulatory strategies can be developed using a precision oncology approach.

Compliance with Ethical Standards

Disclosure of interests Hanneke van Laarhoven reports a consultant or advisory role for: BMS, Lilly, Merck, Nordic Pharma, Servier and research funding and/or medication supply for: Bayer, BMS, Celgene, Janssen, Lilly, Merck, Nordic Pharma, Philips, Roche, Servier, as well as from the Dutch Cancer Society, EU, MLDS, the Netherlands Organisation for Scientific Research, and Oncode Institute.

Sarah Derks reports research funding from the Dutch Cancer Society, the Netherlands Organisation for Scientific Research, and Oncode Institute.

References

1. Gori S, Inno A, Belluomini L, Bocus P, Bisoffi Z, Russo A et al (2019) Gut microbiota and cancer: how gut microbiota modulates activity, efficacy and toxicity of antitumoral therapy. Crit Rev Oncol Hematol 143:139–147. https://doi.org/10.1016/j.critrevonc.2019.09.003
2. Moehler M (2019) Checkpoint-Inhibitoren bei fortgeschrittenen ösophagogastralen Karzinomen Ist die Immuntherapie bereits kurz vor der Zulassung? Onkologie Heute 6:10–18
3. Dulak AM, Stojanov P, Peng S, Lawrence MS, Fox C, Stewart C et al (2013) Exome and whole-genome sequencing of esophageal adenocarcinoma identifies recurrent driver events and mutational complexity. Nat Genet 45(5):478
4. Fitzgerald RC, Abdalla S, Onwuegbusi BA, Sirieix P, Saeed IT, Burnham WR et al (2002) Inflammatory gradient in Barrett's oesophagus: implications for disease complications. Gut 51(3):316–322
5. Moons LM, Kusters JG, Bultman E, Kuipers EJ, van Dekken H, Tra WM et al (2005) Barrett's oesophagus is characterized by a predominantly humoral inflammatory response. J Pathol 207(3):269–276. https://doi.org/10.1002/path.1847

6. Loke P, Allison JP (2003) PD-L1 and PD-L2 are differentially regulated by Th1 and Th2 cells. Proc Natl Acad Sci U S A 100(9):5336–5341. https://doi.org/10.1073/pnas.0931259100
7. Ichihara F, Kono K, Takahashi A, Kawaida H, Sugai H, Fujii H (2003) Increased populations of regulatory T cells in peripheral blood and tumor-infiltrating lymphocytes in patients with gastric and esophageal cancers. Clin Cancer Res 9(12):4404–4408
8. Lin EW, Karakasheva TA, Hicks PD, Bass AJ, Rustgi AK (2016) The tumor microenvironment in esophageal cancer. Oncogene 35(41):5337–5349. https://doi.org/10.1038/onc.2016.34
9. Improving End-of-Life Care (2005) National Institutes of Health statement on the state of science. AWHONN Lifelines 9(1):15–22
10. Svensson MC, Borg D, Zhang C, Hedner C, Nodin B, Uhlén M et al (2019) Expression of PD-L1 and PD-1 in chemoradiotherapy-naïve esophageal and gastric adenocarcinoma: relationship with mismatch repair status and survival. Front Oncol 9:136. https://doi.org/10.3389/fonc.2019.00136
11. Huang TX, Fu L (2019) The immune landscape of esophageal cancer. Cancer Commun (Lond) 39(1):79. https://doi.org/10.1186/s40880-019-0427-z
12. Courrech Staal EF, Wouters MW, van Sandick JW, Takkenberg MM, Smit VT, Junggeburt JM et al (2010) The stromal part of adenocarcinomas of the oesophagus: does it conceal targets for therapy? Eur J Cancer 46(4):720–728. https://doi.org/10.1016/j.ejca.2009.12.006
13. Bijlsma MF, van Laarhoven HW (2015) The conflicting roles of tumor stroma in pancreatic cancer and their contribution to the failure of clinical trials: a systematic review and critical appraisal. Cancer Metastasis Rev 34(1):97–114
14. Ebbing EA, van der Zalm AP, Steins A, Creemers A, Hermsen S, Rentenaar R et al (2019) Stromal-derived interleukin 6 drives epithelial-to-mesenchymal transition and therapy resistance in esophageal adenocarcinoma. Proc Natl Acad Sci USA 116(6):2237–2242
15. Akalay I, Janji B, Hasmim M, Noman MZ, André F, De Cremoux P et al (2013) Epithelial-to-mesenchymal transition and autophagy induction in breast carcinoma promote escape from T-cell–mediated lysis. Cancer Res 73(8):2418–2427
16. Chen J, Jiang C, Jin L, Zhang X (2016) Regulation of PD-L1: a novel role of pro-survival signalling in cancer. Ann Oncol 27(3):409–416
17. Mak MP, Tong P, Diao L, Cardnell RJ, Gibbons DL, William WN et al (2016) A patient-derived, pan-cancer EMT signature identifies global molecular alterations and immune target enrichment following epithelial-to-mesenchymal transition. Clin Cancer Res 22(3):609–620
18. Thompson JC, Hwang W-T, Davis C, Deshpande C, Jeffries S, Rajpurohit Y et al (2020) Gene signatures of tumor inflammation and epithelial-to-mesenchymal transition (EMT) predict responses to immune checkpoint blockade in lung cancer with high accuracy. Lung Cancer 139:1–8
19. Horn LA, Fousek K, Palena C (2020) Tumor plasticity and resistance to immunotherapy. Trends Cancer 6:432–441
20. van den Ende T, Ter Veer E, Machiels M, Mali RMA, Abe Nijenhuis FA, de Waal L et al (2019) The efficacy and safety of (neo)adjuvant therapy for gastric cancer: a network meta-analysis. Cancers (Basel) 11(1). https://doi.org/10.3390/cancers11010080
21. Ter Veer E, Haj MN, van Valkenhoef G, Ngai LL, Mali RMA, Anderegg MC et al (2016) The efficacy and safety of first-line chemotherapy in advanced esophagogastric cancer: a network meta-analysis. J Natl Cancer Inst 108(10). https://doi.org/10.1093/jnci/djw166
22. Ter Veer E, Mohammad NH, van Valkenhoef G, Ngai LL, Mali RM, van Oijen MG et al (2016) Second- and third-line systemic therapy in patients with advanced esophagogastric cancer: a systematic review of the literature. Cancer Metastasis Rev 35(3):439–456
23. Kang YK, Boku N, Satoh T, Ryu MH, Chao Y, Kato K et al (2017) Nivolumab in patients with advanced gastric or gastro-oesophageal junction cancer refractory to, or intolerant of, at least two previous chemotherapy regimens (ONO-4538-12, ATTRACTION-2): a randomised, double-blind, placebo-controlled, phase 3 trial. Lancet 390(10111):2461–2471. https://doi.org/10.1016/s0140-6736(17)31827-5
24. Shitara K, Ozguroglu M, Bang YJ, Di Bartolomeo M, Mandala M, Ryu MH et al (2018) Pembrolizumab versus paclitaxel for previously treated, advanced gastric or gastro-

oesophageal junction cancer (KEYNOTE-061): a randomised, open-label, controlled, phase 3 trial. Lancet 392(10142):123–133. https://doi.org/10.1016/s0140-6736(18)31257-1
25. Shitara K, Van Cutsem E, Bang YJ, Fuchs C, Wyrwicz L, Lee KW et al (2020) Efficacy and safety of pembrolizumab or pembrolizumab plus chemotherapy vs chemotherapy alone for patients with first-line, advanced gastric cancer: the KEYNOTE-062 phase 3 randomized clinical trial. JAMA Oncol 6(10):1–10. https://doi.org/10.1001/jamaoncol.2020.3370
26. Hochster HS, Grothey A, Hart L, Rowland K, Ansari R, Alberts S et al (2014) Improved time to treatment failure with an intermittent oxaliplatin strategy: results of CONcePT. Ann Oncol 25(6):1172–1178. https://doi.org/10.1093/annonc/mdu107
27. Wilke H, Muro K, Van CE, Oh SC, Bodoky G, Shimada Y et al (2014) Ramucirumab plus paclitaxel versus placebo plus paclitaxel in patients with previously treated advanced gastric or gastro-oesophageal junction adenocarcinoma (RAINBOW): a double-blind, randomised phase 3 trial. Lancet Oncol 15(11):1224–1235
28. van den Ende T, van den Boorn HG, Hoonhout NM, van Etten-Jamaludin FS, Meijer SL, Derks S et al (1874) Priming the tumor immune microenvironment with chemo(radio)therapy: a systematic review across tumor types. Biochim Biophys Acta Rev Cancer 2020(1):188386. https://doi.org/10.1016/j.bbcan.2020.188386
29. Moehler M, Ryu MH, Dvorkin M, Lee KW, Coskun HS, Wong R et al (2019) Maintenance avelumab versus continuation of first-line chemotherapy in gastric cancer: JAVELIN Gastric 100 study design. Future Oncol 15(6):567–577. https://doi.org/10.2217/fon-2018-0668
30. Moehler MH, Dvorkin M, Ozguroglu M, Ryu M-H, Muntean AS, Lonardi S et al (2020) Results of the JAVELIN Gastric 100 phase 3 trial: avelumab maintenance following first-line (1L) chemotherapy (CTx) vs continuation of CTx for HER2− advanced gastric or gastroesophageal junction cancer (GC/GEJC). J Clin Oncol. https://doi.org/10.1200/jco.2020.38.4_suppl.278
31. Shapiro J, Van Lanschot JJB, Hulshof MC, van Hagen P, van Berge Henegouwen MI, Wijnhoven BP et al (2015) Neoadjuvant chemoradiotherapy plus surgery versus surgery alone for oesophageal or junctional cancer (CROSS): long-term results of a randomised controlled trial. Lancet Oncol 16(9):1090–1098
32. Hulshof MCCM, Geijsen D, Rozema T, Oppedijk V, Buijsen J, Neelis KJ et al (2020) A randomized controlled phase III multicenter study on dose escalation in definitive chemoradiation for patients with locally advanced esophageal cancer: ARTDECO study. J Clin Oncol 38(4_Suppl):281. https://doi.org/10.1200/JCO.2020.38.4_suppl.281
33. Goedegebuure RSA, de Klerk LK, Bass AJ, Derks S, Thijssen V (2018) Combining radiotherapy with anti-angiogenic therapy and immunotherapy; a therapeutic triad for cancer? Front Immunol 9:3107. https://doi.org/10.3389/fimmu.2018.03107
34. van den Ende T, de Clercq NC, van Berge Henegouwen MI, Gisbertz SS, Meijer SL, Schokker S et al (2019) A phase II feasibility trial of neoadjuvant chemoradiotherapy combined with atezolizumab for resectable esophageal adenocarcinoma: the PERFECT trial. J Clin Oncol 37(15_Suppl):4045
35. Kelly RJ, Ajani JA, Kuzdzal J, Zander T, Van Cutsem E, Piessen G et al (2020) LBA9_PR adjuvant nivolumab in resected esophageal or gastroesophageal junction cancer (EC/GEJC) following neoadjuvant chemoradiation therapy (CRT): first results of the CheckMate 577 study. Ann Oncol 31:S1193–S1194. https://doi.org/10.1016/j.annonc.2020.08.2299
36. Bang YJ, Van CE, Feyereislova A, Chung HC, Shen L, Sawaki A et al (2010) Trastuzumab in combination with chemotherapy versus chemotherapy alone for treatment of HER2-positive advanced gastric or gastro-oesophageal junction cancer (ToGA): a phase 3, open-label, randomised controlled trial. Lancet 376(9742):687–697
37. Janjigian YY, Maron SB, Chatila WK, Millang B, Chavan SS, Alterman C et al (2020) First-line pembrolizumab and trastuzumab in HER2-positive oesophageal, gastric, or gastro-oesophageal junction cancer: an open-label, single-arm, phase 2 trial. Lancet Oncol 21(6):821–831. https://doi.org/10.1016/s1470-2045(20)30169-8
38. Melero I, Berman DM, Aznar MA, Korman AJ, Pérez Gracia JL, Haanen J (2015) Evolving synergistic combinations of targeted immunotherapies to combat cancer. Nat Rev Cancer 15(8):457–472. https://doi.org/10.1038/nrc3973

39. Varadan V, Gilmore H, Miskimen KL, Tuck D, Parsai S, Awadallah A et al (2016) Immune signatures following single dose trastuzumab predict pathologic response to preoperative trastuzumab and chemotherapy in HER2-positive early breast cancer. Clin Cancer Res 22(13):3249–3259. https://doi.org/10.1158/1078-0432.Ccr-15-2021
40. Chaganty BKR, Qiu S, Gest A, Lu Y, Ivan C, Calin GA et al (2018) Trastuzumab upregulates PD-L1 as a potential mechanism of trastuzumab resistance through engagement of immune effector cells and stimulation of IFNγ secretion. Cancer Lett 430:47–56. https://doi.org/10.1016/j.canlet.2018.05.009
41. Taylor C, Hershman D, Shah N, Suciu-Foca N, Petrylak DP, Taub R et al (2007) Augmented HER-2 specific immunity during treatment with trastuzumab and chemotherapy. Clin Cancer Res 13(17):5133–5143. https://doi.org/10.1158/1078-0432.Ccr-07-0507
42. Mortenson ED, Park S, Jiang Z, Wang S, Fu YX (2013) Effective anti-neu-initiated antitumor responses require the complex role of CD4+ T cells. Clin Cancer Res 19(6):1476–1486. https://doi.org/10.1158/1078-0432.Ccr-12-2522
43. Park S, Jiang Z, Mortenson ED, Deng L, Radkevich-Brown O, Yang X et al (2010) The therapeutic effect of anti-HER2/neu antibody depends on both innate and adaptive immunity. Cancer Cell 18(2):160–170. https://doi.org/10.1016/j.ccr.2010.06.014
44. Chau I, Penel N, Soriano AO, Arkenau HT, Cultrera J, Santana-Davila R et al (2020) Ramucirumab in combination with pembrolizumab in treatment-naïve advanced gastric or GEJ adenocarcinoma: safety and antitumor activity from the phase 1a/b JVDF trial. Cancers (Basel) 12(10). https://doi.org/10.3390/cancers12102985
45. Khan KA, Kerbel RS (2018) Improving immunotherapy outcomes with anti-angiogenic treatments and vice versa. Nat Rev Clin Oncol 15(5):310–324. https://doi.org/10.1038/nrclinonc.2018.9
46. Heskamp S, Boerman OC, Molkenboer-Kuenen JD, Oyen WJ, van der Graaf WT, van Laarhoven HW (2013) Bevacizumab reduces tumor targeting of antiepidermal growth factor and anti-insulin-like growth factor 1 receptor antibodies. Int J Cancer 133(2):307–314
47. Steins A, Klaassen R, Jacobs I, Schabel MC, van Lier MG, Ebbing EA et al (2020) Rapid stromal remodeling by short-term VEGFR2 inhibition increases chemotherapy delivery in esophagogastric adenocarcinoma. Mol Oncol 14:704–720
48. Van der Veldt AA, Lubberink M, Bahce I, Walraven M, de Boer MP, Greuter HN et al (2012) Rapid decrease in delivery of chemotherapy to tumors after anti-VEGF therapy: implications for scheduling of anti-angiogenic drugs. Cancer Cell 21(1):82–91
49. Noy R, Pollard JW (2014) Tumor-associated macrophages: from mechanisms to therapy. Immunity 41(1):49–61
50. Cassetta L, Kitamura T (2018) Macrophage targeting: opening new possibilities for cancer immunotherapy. Immunology 155(3):285–293
51. Kaneda MM, Messer KS, Ralainirina N, Li H, Leem CJ, Gorjestani S et al (2016) PI3Kγ is a molecular switch that controls immune suppression. Nature 539(7629):437–442
52. Lopez-Yrigoyen M, Cassetta L, Pollard JW Macrophage targeting in cancer. Ann N Y Acad Sci. https://doi.org/10.1111/nyas.14377
53. Schokker S, van der Woude SO, van Kleef JJ, van Zoen DJ, van Oijen MGH, Mearadji B et al (2019) Phase I dose escalation study with expansion cohort of the addition of nab-paclitaxel to capecitabine and oxaliplatin (CapOx) as first-line treatment of metastatic esophagogastric adenocarcinoma (ACTION Study). Cancers (Basel) 11(6). https://doi.org/10.3390/cancers11060827
54. Veenstra VL, Damhofer H, Waasdorp C, van Rijssen LB, van de Vijver MJ, Dijk F et al (2018) ADAM12 is a circulating marker for stromal activation in pancreatic cancer and predicts response to chemotherapy. Oncogenesis 7(11):87. https://doi.org/10.1038/s41389-018-0096-9
55. Kalluri R (2016) The biology and function of fibroblasts in cancer. Nat Rev Cancer 16(9):582
56. Sugimoto H, Mundel TM, Kieran MW, Kalluri R (2006) Identification of fibroblast heterogeneity in the tumor microenvironment. Cancer Biol Ther 5(12):1640–1646

57. Öhlund D, Elyada E, Tuveson D (2014) Fibroblast heterogeneity in the cancer wound. J Exp Med 211(8):1503–1523
58. Öhlund D, Handly-Santana A, Biffi G, Elyada E, Almeida AS, Ponz-Sarvise M et al (2017) Distinct populations of inflammatory fibroblasts and myofibroblasts in pancreatic cancer. J Exp Med 214(3):579–596
59. Su S, Chen J, Yao H, Liu J, Yu S, Lao L et al (2018) CD10+ GPR77+ cancer-associated fibroblasts promote cancer formation and chemoresistance by sustaining cancer stemness. Cell 172(4):841–56.e16
60. Sivan A, Corrales L, Hubert N, Williams JB, Aquino-Michaels K, Earley ZM et al (2015) Commensal bifidobacterium promotes antitumor immunity and facilitates anti-PD-L1 efficacy. Science 350(6264):1084–1089
61. Gopalakrishnan V, Spencer C, Nezi L, Reuben A, Andrews M, Karpinets T et al (2018) Gut microbiome modulates response to anti–PD-1 immunotherapy in melanoma patients. Science 359(6371):97–103
62. Routy B, Le Chatelier E, Derosa L, Duong CPM, Alou MT, Daillere R et al (2018) Gut microbiome influences efficacy of PD-1-based immunotherapy against epithelial tumors. Science 359(6371):91–97. https://doi.org/10.1126/science.aan3706
63. Santaolalla R, Fukata M, Abreu MT (2011) Innate immunity in the small intestine. Curr Opin Gastroenterol 27(2):125–131. https://doi.org/10.1097/MOG.0b013e3283438dea
64. de Clercq NC, van den Ende T, Prodan A, van Berge Henegouwen MI, Gisbertz SS, Meijer SL et al (2020) Intestinal and tumor microbiome analysis combined with metabolomics of the anti-PD-L1 phase II PERFECT trial for resectable esophageal adenocarcinoma. J Clin Oncol 38(15_Suppl):4556. https://doi.org/10.1200/JCO.2020.38.15_suppl.4556

Part III

Stomach

Immunotherapy of Gastric Cancer: Focus on Perioperative Strategies

Virginia Arrazubi and Maria Alsina

Contents

Abstract

Gastric and gastro-oesophageal junction cancer (GC) remains a world-wide problem. When diagnosis occur with a locally advanced disease (stages Ib-III), perioperative treatment with chemotherapy a surgery is mandatory. However, 50% of these patients will recur. In this context, novel strategies should improve their prognosis, and immune combinations are emerging as the most interesting one.

V. Arrazubi
Medical Oncology Department, Complejo Hospitalario de Navarra (CHN), Pamplona, Spain
e-mail: virginia.arrazubi.arrula@navarra.es

M. Alsina (✉)
Medical Oncology Department, Complejo Hospitalario de Navarra (CHN), Pamplona, Spain

Vall d'Hebron Institute of Oncology (VHIO), Barcelona, Spain
e-mail: malsinamaqued@gmail.com

Cancer Immunotherapy (2021)
https://doi.org/10.1007/13905_2021_3,

Published Online: 17 August 2021

Considering the recognized link with a precursor chronic inflammatory lesion and the high mutational rate of GC, enough rational supports the treatment with immunotherapy. Whether combinations of immune checkpoints (ICIs) with chemotherapy have demonstrated benefit in the metastatic setting, these strategies are nowadays being evaluated in the perioperative setting. This chapter review the current landscape of locally advanced GC treatment, focusing on the role of targeted therapies and immunotherapy, with a special consideration to selected populations of GC (MSI and HER2-positive), and to the immune biomarkers of response.

Keywords

Gastric cancer · Gastro-oesophageal junction cancer · Immune checkpoints · perioperative treatment · MSI

1 Introduction

Gastric cancer (GC) remains a worldwide problem. More than 1 million people were diagnosed with gastric cancer worldwide in 2020, ranking the fifth in incidence considering all tumors [1]. It remains also an important leading cause of cancer death, being responsible for almost 770,000 deaths (768,793) in 2020 [1].

Incidence rates show great geographic variations, which correlates at least in part with inherent risk factors distribution. Helicobacter pylori infection, alcohol consumption, tobacco smoking, food preserved by salting, low fruit intake and high consumption of processed meat are the main risk factors of non-cardia gastric cancer. Other risk factors have been related to gastro-oesophageal and cardia gastric cancer, i.e., excess body weight and gastroesophageal reflux disease injury.

Surgery represents the cornerstone of curative treatment although recurrences occur in more than 50% of cases [2]. Indeed, advanced GC (AGC) should be considered a systemic disease from the start of care, as treatment with systemic perioperative chemotherapy significantly potentiates the downstaging and eradication of microscopic metastases. For stages Ib–III, perioperative treatment is mandatory and it requires a multidisciplinary approach [3, 4] (Table 1).

Perioperative chemotherapy became the standard of care since its efficacy had been clearly demonstrated in pivotal phase III trials more than 10 years ago. The MAGIC trial compared face to face surgery versus perioperative chemotherapy plus surgery with a three-drug combination of chemotherapy (epirubicine, cisplatin and 5-fluorouracil) [5]. The main goal was achieved with an increase in 5-years overall survival (OS) of 36% in chemotherapy arm versus 23% in the surgery arm. Similar results were reproduced in the French phase III trial [6] that proposed the same design but with chemotherapy consisting of cisplatin and fluorouracil (5-years overall survival of 38% vs 24%). Recently, the phase II/III FLOT4 trial [2] has shown benefit when adding a taxane to the platin/5-fluorouracil

Table 1 Phase II/III clinical trials assessing the perioperative treatment in locally AGC

Study name	Arms[a]	Phase	Primary end point	Key answer	Reference
MAGIC	(A) Surgery (B) Epirubicine, cisplatin, 5FU	III	Overall survival	Perioperative ECF became the standard of care	[5]
FNCLCC-FFCD	(A) Surgery (B) Cisplatin, 5FU	III	Overall survival	Questions the role of anthracyclines	[6]
FLOT4	(A) Epirubicine, cisplatin, 5FU (B) Docetaxel, oxaliplatin, 5FU	II/III	Overall survival	Benefit adding a taxane	[2]
RESOLVE	(A) Adjuvant oxaliplatin, capecitabine (B) Adjuvant TS-1, oxaliplatin (C) TS-1, oxaliplatin	III	3 years disease-free survival	Evidence of perioperative approach in Asia	[11]
PRODIGY	(A) Adjuvant S1 (B) Docetaxel, oxaliplatin, S1	III	3 years disease-free survival	Evidence of perioperative approach in Asia	[12]
CRITICS	(A) Epirubicin, platin, capecitabine (B) Adding adjuvant radiotherapy with cisplatin, capecitabine	III	Overall survival	No benefit adding adjuvant radiotherapy	[15]
MAGIC-B	(A) Epirubicin, cisplatin, 5FU (B) Adding bevacizumab	II/III	Overall survival	No benefit adding bevacizumab	[21]
NEOPECX	(A) Epirubicin, cisplatin, capecitabine (B) Adding panitumumab	II	Histological response rate	No benefit adding panitumumab	[27]
RAMSES/FLOT	(A) Docetaxel, oxaliplatin, 5FU (B) Adding ramucirumab	II	Histological response rate	Some possible benefit as R0 rate increases	[21]
PETRARCA	(A) Docetaxel, oxaliplatin, 5FU (B) Adding trastuzumab, pertuzumab	II	Pathological complete remission	Significantly improved pCR	[22]
NCT03288350	Docetaxel, cisplatin, 5FU, avelumab	II	Pathological complete remission	Encouraging activity	[69]

[a]All the described treatment with a perioperative approach unless otherwise stated
5FU 5-fluorouracil, *ECF* epirubicine, cisplatin, fluorouracil, *TS-1* titanium silicate 1, *S-1* Tegafur/gimeracil/oteracil, *pCR* pathological complete response, *AGC* advanced gastric cancer

combination. This trial compared perioperative FLOT (fluorouracil, oxaliplatin and docetaxel) vs the "MAGIC regimen" (epirubicine, cisplatin and 5-fluorouracil) demonstrating a better 5-year-OS: 45% vs 36% (median OS of ~50 vs 35 months). With these results, the FLOT regimen has become the Western standard of treatment whenever possible.

Adjuvant chemotherapy has been extensively developed in Asia. The phase III ACTS-GC trial [7] with adjuvant S-1 demonstrated a OS benefit compared with surgery alone (5-year OS 72% vs 61%). With the same trend, the CLASSIC trial [8] tested the combination of capecitabine and oxaliplatin after surgery with improvement in 3-year disease-free survival (DFS) 74% vs 59% in the surgery alone arm. Moreover, the addition of taxanes seems also to be advantageous in this adjuvant strategy. In the JACCRO-GC-07 trial [9], an interim analysis showed increased 3-years DFS with the addition of docetaxel to S1 which resulted in the Japanese approval for high-risk patients [10] (Table 1).

The Chinese RESOLVE trial [11] was proposed to establish the optimal approach in locally AGC, again demonstrating the benefit of the perioperative approach [11]. A total of 1094 patients were randomized in this three-arm multicentre, open-label phase III trial. Patients received adjuvant XELOX (capecitabine and oxaliplatin), arm A; adjuvant SOX (TS-1 and oxaliplatin), arm B; or perioperative SOX, arm C. Perioperative chemotherapy improved 3-years DFS: 62% in arm C versus 54.8% in arm A (HR 0.79, 95% CI [0.62–0.99]; $p = 0.045$). Comparably, the Korean PRODIGY trial [12] endorsed the role of neoadjuvant chemotherapy (docetaxel, oxaliplatin and S-1) over to the standard treatment of surgery followed by S-1 adjuvant treatment. Three-years DFS rate was 66.3% in experimental arm versus 60.2% in standard arm; hazard ratio 0.70 (95% CI 0.52–0.95; $p = 0.023$). With these results, the standard of care in Asia could shift towards perioperative chemotherapy [10, 13] (Table 1).

Despite the adjuvant chemoradiotherapy (RCTX) was initially established by the Intergroup 0116 trial [14], this strategy has been dismissed in Europe. Firstly, most of the RCTX benefit in this trial could be due to a suboptimal US surgery, as D2 resections have been clear surgical standards in Europe and Asia. Secondly, two confirmatory phase III trials had also negative results. The CRITICS trial [15] did not show survival difference adding RCTX to a perioperative chemotherapy approach. In fact, the chemotherapy arm showed better OS in the per protocol analysis from those patients who started the allocated post-operative treatment [16]. In the adjuvant setting, both ARTIST and ARTIST-2 trials failed to demonstrate any benefit adding radiotherapy to adjuvant chemotherapy [17, 18] (Table 1). Thus, this approach is only recommended in European guidelines for patients with insufficient surgical resection. In contrast, the role of the preoperative radiotherapy is still being analysed, the randomized phase III EORTC TOPGEAR (Trial Of Preoperative therapy for Gastric and Esophagogastric junction AdenocaRcinoma) trial has showed the safety and feasibility of adding preoperative chemoradiation to perioperative chemotherapy [19]. The efficacy results will elucidate the true benefit of this strategy.

2 Role of Targeted Therapies

The efficacy of combinations with targeted therapies is still under evaluation, and definitive conclusions are yet to be expected. So far, the addition of the anti-angiogenic bevacizumab to the standard MAGIC protocol could not show any benefit [20]. Still, the combination of ramucirumab with FLOT (RAMSES/FLOT7 trial) [21] may add additional efficacy, especially in the diffuse type and signet cell histology.

Interestingly, the addition of the anti-HER2 targeted therapy with trastuzumab and pertuzumab has demonstrated an improvement in the perioperative outcome in the AIO Phase II/III PETRARCA Trial [22] although with increased toxicity. The results of the still recruiting INNOVATION Phase III trial [23], which randomize patients in three arms to receive standard perioperative chemotherapy ± trastuzumab ± pertuzumab would elucidate the reliable value of targeting HER2.

Epidermal growth factor receptor (EGFR) is overexpressed in more than 30% of GC, and it is associated with a poor prognosis [24]. Nevertheless, neither the use of anti-EGFR agents in the metastatic setting [25, 26] nor in the perioperative [27] has shown efficacy, in an unselected GC population.

Fibroblast growth factor receptor-2 (*FGFR2*) gene is amplified in up to 15% of patients GC, and its amplification has been correlated with an adverse prognostic factor in GC [28]. The role of targeting FGFR2 in metastatic GC is still under evaluation, and if positive it should be explored in the neoadjuvancy.

3 Rational for Immunotherapy

Finally, and supported by the recent data demonstrating the efficacy of the immunotherapy in the metastatic setting, enough rational has led to test these immune approaches in localized GC patients, inquiring for survival improvement.

The rationale for treating GC patients with immunotherapy comes from the recognized link with precursor chronic inflammatory lesions and the high mutational rates [29].

Although the type of risk factor varies, tumours of the oesophagus and stomach generally arise over an inflammatory niche. The recent publication of "The Cancer Genome Atlas Research Network" (TCGA) [30] clearly shows how distal oesophageal adenocarcinomas have almost the same molecular profile as junction carcinomas with a progressive shifting of these molecular subtypes within the different stomach localizations. Actually, not only the TCGA [31] but also other molecular classifications [32] demonstrated a strong rationale to presume an immune deregulation in some subtypes, mainly in those associated with EBV infection and those with a high mutational rate (the MSI subtype).

In addition, Secrier et al. [33] demonstrated the existence of a higher mutational profile within oesophageal adenocarcinomas when performing whole-genome sequencing analysis. This mutational profile is characterized by a domination of a T > G mutational pattern, and it is associated with a high mutational load, neoantigen burden and an increased CD8+ T-cell density. Finally, Maron et al. [34] considered a re-categorization of the TCGA subtypes based on T-cell inflamed phenotype signatures. By analysing almost 500 oesophageal adenocarcinomas and gastric adenocarcinomas, they demonstrated inflamed phenotypes differently represented within the 4 molecular subtypes, mainly over-represented in the EBV and MSI subtypes, and also in the genomically stable subtype.

4 Biomarkers of Immunotherapy

The efficacy of immune checkpoints (ICIs) in metastatic GC has been well recognized, but only with reliable durable responses in selected subgroups of patients. Identification of valid biomarkers able to predict good responders is crucial, and the comprehensive analysis of the data from the reported clinical trials identifies different biomarkers, primary linked to the tumour cell and stroma (Table 2).

MSI or mismatch repair deficiency (MMRD) is identified in 22% of localized GC [31]. It is nowadays the most robust biomarker, with consistent positive correlation demonstrated in all metastatic treatment lines [35]. In localized GC, the MSI status has a prognostic and predictive role, which will be further developed within the next subchapter [36, 37].

EVB-positive status is identified in 4–9% of localized GC [31]. EBV-positive tumours are often accompanied by more extensive lymphocyte infiltration [38] and associate higher PD-L1 and PD-L2 expression [31]. EVB-positivity represents a potential biomarker of immune response. This efficacy has been reported in the metastatic setting in different series of cases and in early clinical trials [39–41], and with pembrolizumab in the phase 2 Korean trial [42].

The role of PD-L1 as a predictive biomarker has been widely assessed. Whereas the PD-L1 expression in the tumour do not correlate with the response to nivolumab nor to avelumab [43, 44], it does when assessed with the combined positive score (CPS) in metastatic GC patients treated with pembrolizumab, nivolumab and

Table 2 Biomarkers of immune response in gastric cancer

Biomarker	Type	Confidence	Evidence	Reference
MSI or MMRD	Prognostic and predictive	Strong	Meta-analysis of the main phase III clinical trials in locally AGC	[36, 37]
EBV	Predictive	Mild	Series of cases and one phase II clinical trial in stage IV AGC	[39–42]
PD-L1 CPS	Predictive	Mild	Phase III clinical trials in stage IV AGC	[45–48]
TMB	Predictive	Mild	Retrospective analysis of clinical trials	[39, 55, 56]
TILs	Predictive	Mild	Pre-clinical data	[58]
Microbiota	Predictive	Mild	Observational analyses	[60]

MSI microsatellite instability, *MMRD* mismatch repair deficiency, *AGC* advanced gastric cancer, *EBV* Epstein Barr virus, *PD-L1* programmed-cell ligand-1, *CPS* combined positive score, *TMB* tumour mutational load, *TILs* tumour infiltrating lymphocytes avelumab [45, 46–48]. Moreover, higher cut-off levels of PD-L1 CPS correlate with better responses to pembrolizumab and nivolumab [46, 49–52].

The tumour mutational burden (TMB) reflects the load of neoantigens expressed on the tumour cells, which can stimulate the patient's immune response against cancer. Although still controversial [53], TMB has been accepted as a biomarker by the FDA [54]. The reported TMB in GC is moderate, and the majority of these cases are from patients with MSI tumours [29]. Retrospective analyses on metastatic GC showed a positive correlation of TMB with immunotherapy [39, 55, 56].

Tumour infiltrating lymphocytes (TILs) are considered a manifestation of the host immune response against tumour cells [57]. A recent publication has demonstrated the value of determining T-cell subsets (CD3+ and CD8+) and macrophages (CD68+ and CD163+) in paired GC samples from patients treated with neoadjuvant chemotherapy, which correlated with response. Actually, this study demonstrated how chemotherapy may play a role in tumour immune microenvironment remodeling [58].

In contrast, a systemic immune-inflammation stroma consistent on peripheral neutrophil, lymphocytes, and platelet counts has being identified as an independent adverse prognostic factor to neoadjuvant chemotherapy in esophagogastric adenocarcinoma patients [59].

Finally, microbiota represents the newest area of research. Gut microbiota plays a fundamental role in the maintenance of host physiology and immune homeostasis. The use of antibiotics that could disrupt the microbiota, the *H. pylori* chronic infection, and different bacteria are in the spotlight of these analyses. Actually, a more diverse microbiome has been observed in metastatic GC patients that better respond to nivolumab, in the recently reported DELIVER trial [60].

5 Immunotherapy for MSI Locally AGC

The analysis of the MSI status of the patients included in the two historical, practice defining, MAGIC (European) and CLASSIC (Asian) trials showed two main findings [61, 62]. Firstly, as expected with an immunogenic, high neoantigen expressing tumour, the 8–10% of patients who were diagnosed with operable MSI tumours had excellent survival with surgery alone. Secondly, neither perioperative (MAGIC) nor adjuvant (CLASSIC) chemotherapy improved survival when added to surgery for patients with MSI GC. These results were consistent with in-vitro studies showing chemoresistance in mismatch repair deficient tumours and poor outcomes in patients with advanced MSI gastric cancer treated with chemotherapy. Moreover, a combined meta-analysis of these trials with two others (ITACA-S and ARTIST trials) showed no benefit for adjuvant chemotherapy in patients with operable MSI GC [36].

Considering these finding, together with large retrospective GC datasets with same conclusions [63], one might wonder how much evidence is required to change practice. If MSI is a tumour agnostic driver, as suggested by prognosis and the predictive value of MSI status for immunotherapy response across tumour types [64] and specifically in GC [35], then an evidence-based reason to continue treating patients with operable MSI GC is at least doubtable.

Oncologists individualize treatment for patients, and common sense suggests that never treating any operable MSI GC with chemotherapy would be neither feasible nor correct. Although requiring a frameshift in thinking, this biologically defined patient group could benefit from a different, non-chemotherapy approach.

6 Immunotherapy for HER2+ GC

The addition of pembrolizumab to trastuzumab with cisplatin plus capecitabine has demonstrated to effectively increase survival in metastatic HER2-positive GC patients in two phase 2 trials [65, 66], being this benefit maintained regardless of the PD-L1 status in the PANTERA trial [65]. Actually, a randomized phase 3 clinical trial is assessing this efficacy in the first-line HER2-positive metastatic GC [67]. Other antibodies are currently testing the efficacy in the same setting, as the phase II/III MAHOGANY trial that evaluates margetuximab, an Fc-optimized monoclonal antibody that binds HER2, plus the anti-PD1 retifanlimab with/without chemotherapy and margetuximab plus tebotelimab, a bispecific DART molecule, with chemotherapy in first-line AGC [68].

Whether this synergic activity is due to an intrinsic higher expression of PD-L1 within the HER2-positive tumours, or in all the CIN subtype tumours, or because the co-stimulation of the antibody-dependent cellular cytotoxicity (ADCC) is still unanswered. Nevertheless, the combination of checkpoint inhibitors with trastuzumab and chemotherapy in the perioperative treatment of HER2-positive GC remains challenging and probably will be assessed in the next future.

7 Immune Strategies for Resectable Non-MSI Non-HER2+ GC

Immunotherapy is also being tested in locoregional non-MSI non-HER2+ GC. Alcindor and colleagues [69] reported the interim analysis of their phase II study with avelumab, an anti-PD-L1 antibody, added to perioperative chemotherapy (modified DCF; docetaxel, cisplatin a 5-fluorouracil). They included locally advanced gastric or oesophageal adenocarcinoma patients. Until March 2019 18 patients had been enrolled, of which 13 had undergone surgery. Two patients showed near pathologic complete response (pCR). The combination regimen was safe, and the study met the requirement of enough pCR to go keep on recruiting patients.

In a phase II trial of Zhengzhou University [70], China, camrelizumab (anti-PD-L1 antibody) combined with FOLFOX as neoadjuvant therapy was tested. Sixteen patients with resectable locally advanced gastric and gastroesophageal junction adenocarcinoma were enrolled, and 13 received radical surgery after neoadjuvant treatment. Four patients experienced pCR or nearby. In all operated patients R0 resection was confirmed. Toxicity and surgical complications were as expected [71]. Interestingly, in this study PDL1 was tested as CPS (combined positive score). CPS was positive (>1) in 56% of patients and CPS was >5 in 31% of the patients [70].

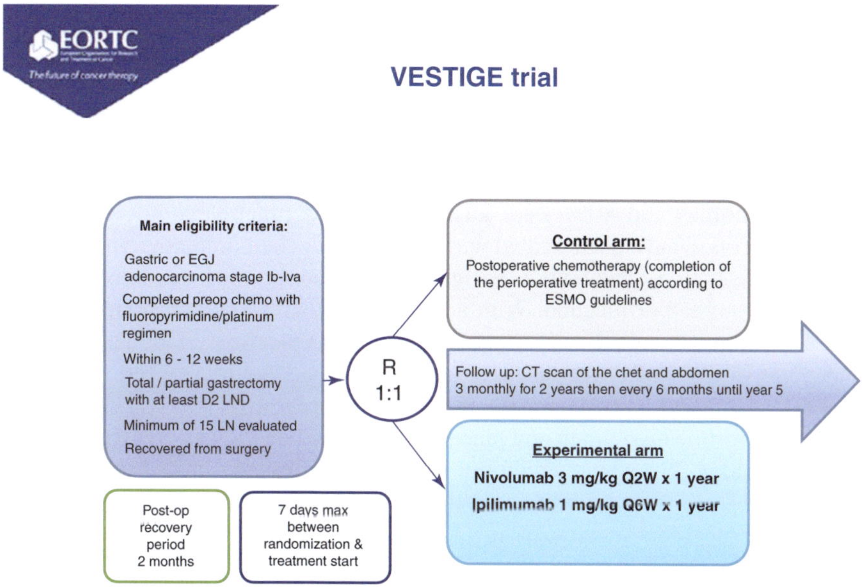

Fig. 1 Design of the EORTC phase III VESTIGE trial; Smyth Frontiers in Oncology 2020; 9 (with permission)

The NeoChance Study [72] was proposed in Korea as a phase II study of IMC-001 (PD-L1 targeting fully human monoclonal antibody) in the neoadjuvant setting for resectable gastric cancer, oesophageal cancer and hepatocellular carcinoma. The primary endpoint was major pathologic response rate defined as <10% of viable tumour. Fourteen patients were enrolled (5 patients with GC, 3 with oesophageal cancer and 6 with hepatocellular carcinoma). Preliminary results have been reported, with acceptable adverse events. All patients were operated with R0 resection. Lymphocyte infiltration in intratumoral or peritumoral areas ranges from 10% to 90%, being increased compared to pre-treatment biopsies.

These three studies demonstrate a good tolerability with encouraging results. These results together with the ones from the other phase 2 trials that are nowadays being conducted in other Germany, Spain and United Kingdom would elucidate the value of the combination of immune checkpoints with chemotherapy in the perioperative setting of GC [73–75]. Finally, the two randomized placebo-control phase III trials with pembrolizumab [76] and durvalumab [77] will set the real role of the combination.

Apart from the described strategies that evaluate the immunotherapy in the perioperative setting, without being guided by any biomarker, the currently recruiting randomized phase III VESTIGE trial [78] explores the novelty of offering adjuvant immunotherapy in GC patients with a poor response to the neoadjuvant chemotherapy (Fig. 1). After receiving neoadjuvant chemotherapy and surgery, GC patients that have an incomplete (R1) resection or have metastatic lymph nodes in the resection specimen (N+) are randomized to receive adjuvant nivolumab plus low dose ipilimumab or standard chemotherapy.

8 Adjuvant Immunotherapy in Oesophageal-Gastric Cancer

In the adjuvant setting immunotherapy has improved disease-free survival in a phase III trial. The CheckMate 577 trial [52]enrolled patients with oesophageal cancer or gastroesophageal junction cancer stage II/III. Most of them (71%) were adenocarcinomas and 40% were gastroesophageal junction tumours. All 794 patients enrolled have been treated with neoadjuvant chemoradiotherapy and surgical R0 resection. They were assigned in a double-blind randomization to receive nivolumab or placebo. With a median follow-up of 24.4 months (range, 6.2–44.9 months), results were reported in ESMO meeting 2020. The primary end point of the study was disease-free survival and the hazard ratio achieved was 0.69 (*p* value 0.0003) with a median of disease-free survival of 22.4 vs 11 months for the nivolumab and placebo arms. The benefit was greater for squamous histology, but adenocarcinoma remains a difference in disease-free survival of 19.4 vs 11.11 months in favour of the nivolumab arm in the subgroup analysis.

Compliance with Ethical Standards

Disclosures Virginia Arrazubi reports financial interest in form of scientific consultancy role for BMS, MSD and Lilly.

Maria Alsina reports financial interest in form of scientific consultancy role for BMS, Merck Serono, MSD, Lilly and Servier.

References

1. Sung H, Ferlay J, Siegel RL et al (2021) Global cancer statistics 2020: GLOBOCAN estimates of incidence and mortality worldwide for 36 cancers in 185 countries. CA Cancer J Clin. https://doi.org/10.3322/caac.21660
2. Al-Batran SE, Homann N, Pauligk C et al (2019) Perioperative chemotherapy with fluorouracil plus leucovorin, oxaliplatin, and docetaxel versus fluorouracil or capecitabine plus cisplatin and epirubicin for locally advanced, resectable gastric or gastro-oesophageal junction adenocarcinoma (FLOT4): a randomised, phase 2/3 trial. Lancet 393(10184):1948–1957. https://doi.org/10.1016/S0140-6736(18)32557-1
3. Smyth EC, Verheij M, Allum W et al (2016) Gastric cancer: ESMO clinical practice guidelines for diagnosis, treatment and follow-up. Ann Oncol 27(Suppl_5):v38–v49. https://doi.org/10.1093/annonc/mdw350
4. Moehler M, Baltin CTH, Ebert M et al (2015) International comparison of the German evidence-based S3-guidelines on the diagnosis and multimodal treatment of early and locally advanced gastric cancer, including adenocarcinoma of the lower esophagus. Gastric Cancer 18(3):550–563. https://doi.org/10.1007/s10120-014-0403-x
5. Cunningham D, Allum WH, Stenning SP et al (2006) Perioperative chemotherapy versus surgery alone for resectable gastroesophageal cancer. N Engl J Med 355(1):11–20. https://doi.org/10.1056/NEJMoa055531
6. Ychou M, Boige V, Pignon J-P et al (2011) Perioperative chemotherapy compared with surgery alone for resectable gastroesophageal adenocarcinoma: an FNCLCC and FFCD multicenter phase III trial. J Clin Oncol 29(13):1715–1721. https://doi.org/10.1200/JCO.2010.33.0597

7. Sasako M, Sakuramoto S, Katai H et al (2011) Five-year outcomes of a randomized phase III trial comparing adjuvant chemotherapy with S-1 versus surgery alone in stage II or III gastric cancer. J Clin Oncol 29(33):4387–4393. https://doi.org/10.1200/JCO.2011.36.5908
8. Bang Y-J, Kim Y-W, Yang H-K et al (2012) Adjuvant capecitabine and oxaliplatin for gastric cancer after D2 gastrectomy (CLASSIC): a phase 3 open-label, randomised controlled trial. Lancet (Lond, Engl) 379(9813):315–321. https://doi.org/10.1016/S0140-6736(11)61873-4
9. Yoshida K, Kodera Y, Kochi M et al (2019) Addition of docetaxel to oral fluoropyrimidine improves efficacy in patients with stage III gastric cancer: interim analysis of JACCRO GC-07, a randomized controlled trial. J Clin Oncol 37(15):1296–1304. https://doi.org/10.1200/JCO.18.01138
10. Japanese Gastric Cancer Association (2021) Japanese gastric cancer treatment guidelines 2018 (5th edition). Gastric Cancer 24(1):1–21. https://doi.org/10.1007/s10120-020-01042-y
11. Ji J, Shen L, Li Z et al (2019) Perioperative chemotherapy of oxaliplatin combined with S-1 (SOX) versus postoperative chemotherapy of SOX or oxaliplatin with capecitabine (XELOX) in locally advanced gastric adenocarcinoma with D2 gastrectomy: a randomized phase III trial (RESOLVE trial). Ann Oncol 30:v877. https://doi.org/10.1093/annonc/mdz394.033
12. Kang Y-K, Yook JH, Park Y-K et al (2019) Phase III randomized study of neoadjuvant chemotherapy (CT) with docetaxel(D), oxaliplatin(O) and S-1(S) (DOS) followed by surgery and adjuvant S-1, vs surgery and adjuvant S-1, for resectable advanced gastric cancer (GC) (PRODIGY). Ann Oncol 30:v876–v877. https://doi.org/10.1093/annonc/mdz394.032
13. Ryu KW, Park YS, Kwon OK et al (2019) Korean practice guideline for gastric cancer 2018: an evidence-based, multi-disciplinary approach. J Gastric Cancer 19(1):1–48. https://doi.org/10.5230/jgc.2019.19.e8
14. Macdonald JS, Smalley SR, Benedetti J et al (2001) Chemoradiotherapy after surgery compared with surgery alone for adenocarcinoma of the stomach or gastroesophageal junction. N Engl J Med 345(10):725–730. https://doi.org/10.1056/NEJMoa010187
15. Cats A, Jansen EPM, van Grieken NCT et al (2018) Chemotherapy versus chemoradiotherapy after surgery and preoperative chemotherapy for resectable gastric cancer (CRITICS): an international, open-label, randomised phase 3 trial. Lancet Oncol 19(5):616–628. https://doi.org/10.1016/S1470-2045(18)30132-3
16. de Steur WO, van Amelsfoort RM, Hartgrink HH et al (2020) Adjuvant chemotherapy is superior to chemoradiation after D2 surgery for gastric cancer in the per-protocol analysis of the randomized CRITICS trial. Ann Oncol 32(3). https://doi.org/10.1016/j.annonc.2020.11.004
17. Lee J, Lim DH, Kim S et al (2012) Phase III trial comparing capecitabine plus cisplatin versus capecitabine plus cisplatin with concurrent capecitabine radiotherapy in completely resected gastric cancer with D2 lymph node dissection: the ARTIST trial. J Clin Oncol 30(3):268–273. https://doi.org/10.1200/JCO.2011.39.1953
18. Park SH, Lim DH, Sohn TS et al (2021) A randomized phase III trial comparing adjuvant single-agent S1, S-1 with oxaliplatin, and postoperative chemoradiation with S-1 and oxaliplatin in patients with node-positive gastric cancer after D2 resection: the ARTIST 2 trial. Ann Oncol 32(3). https://doi.org/10.1016/j.annonc.2020.11.017
19. Leong T, Smithers BM, Haustermans K et al (2017) TOPGEAR: a randomized, phase III trial of perioperative ECF chemotherapy with or without preoperative chemoradiation for resectable gastric cancer: interim results from an international, intergroup trial of the AGITG, TROG, EORTC and CCTG. Ann Surg Oncol 24(8):2252–2258. https://doi.org/10.1245/s10434-017-5830-6
20. Cunningham D, Stenning SP, Smyth EC et al (2017) Peri-operative chemotherapy with or without bevacizumab in operable oesophagogastric adenocarcinoma (UK Medical Research Council ST03): primary analysis results of a multicentre, open-label, randomised phase 2–3 trial. Lancet Oncol 18(3):357–370. https://doi.org/10.1016/S1470-2045(17)30043-8
21. Al-Batran S-E, Hofheinz RD, Schmalenberg H et al (2020) 1424MO perioperative FLOT plus ramucirumab versus FLOT alone for resectable esophagogastric adenocarcinoma—updated results and subgroup analyses of the randomized phase II/III trial RAMSES/FLOT7

of the German AIO and Italian GOIM. Ann Oncol 31:S901. https://doi.org/10.1016/j.annonc.2020.08.1930
22. Al-Batran S-E, Haag GM, Ettrich TJ et al (2020) 1421MO final results and subgroup analysis of the PETRARCA randomized phase II AIO trial: perioperative trastuzumab and pertuzumab in combination with FLOT versus FLOT alone for HER2 positive resectable esophagogastric adenocarcinoma. Ann Oncol 31:S899. https://doi.org/10.1016/j.annonc.2020.08.1927
23. Wagner AD, Grabsch HI, Mauer M et al (2019) EORTC-1203-GITCG-the "INNOVATION"-trial: effect of chemotherapy alone versus chemotherapy plus trastuzumab, versus chemotherapy plus trastuzumab plus pertuzumab, in the perioperative treatment of HER2 positive, gastric and gastroesophageal junction adenocarcinoma on pathologic response rate: a randomized phase II-intergroup trial of the EORTC-Gastrointestinal Tract Cancer Group, Korean Cancer Study Group and Dutch Upper GI-Cancer Group. BMC Cancer 19(1). https://doi.org/10.1186/s12885-019-5675-4
24. Kim BJ, Kim JH, Jang HJ, Kim HS (2017) The role of anti-EGFR agents in the first-line treatment of advanced esophago-gastric adenocarcinoma: a meta-analysis. Oncotarget 8(58):99033–99040. https://doi.org/10.18632/oncotarget.20958
25. Lordick F, Kang YK, Chung HC et al (2013) Capecitabine and cisplatin with or without cetuximab for patients with previously untreated advanced gastric cancer (EXPAND): a randomised, open-label phase 3 trial. Lancet Oncol 14(6):490–499. https://doi.org/10.1016/S1470-2045(13)70102-5
26. Waddell T, Chau I, Cunningham D et al (2013) Epirubicin, oxaliplatin, and capecitabine with or without panitumumab for patients with previously untreated advanced oesophagogastric cancer (REAL3): a randomised, open-label phase 3 trial. Lancet Oncol 14(6):481–489. https://doi.org/10.1016/S1470-2045(13)70096-2
27. Stahl M, Maderer A, Lordick F et al (2018) Perioperative chemotherapy with or without epidermal growth factor receptor blockade in unselected patients with locally advanced oesophagogastric adenocarcinoma: randomized phase II study with advanced biomarker program of the German Cancer Society (AIO/CAO STO-0801). Eur J Cancer 93:119–126. https://doi.org/10.1016/j.ejca.2018.01.079
28. Kim HS, Kim JH, Jang HJ (2019) Pathologic and prognostic impacts of FGFR2 amplification in gastric cancer: a meta-analysis and systemic review. J Cancer 10(11):2560–2567. https://doi.org/10.7150/jca.29184
29. Lawrence MS, Stojanov P, Polak P et al (2013) Mutational heterogeneity in cancer and the search for new cancer-associated genes. Nature 499(7457):214–218. https://doi.org/10.1038/nature12213
30. Cancer Genome Atlas Research Network, Analysis Working Group: Asan University, BC Cancer Agency et al (2017) Integrated genomic characterization of oesophageal carcinoma. Nature 541(7636):169–175. https://doi.org/10.1038/nature20805
31. Bass AJ, Thorsson V, Shmulevich I et al (2014) Comprehensive molecular characterization of gastric adenocarcinoma. Nature 513(7517):202–209. https://doi.org/10.1038/nature13480
32. Cristescu R, Lee J, Nebozhyn M et al (2015) Molecular analysis of gastric cancer identifies subtypes associated with distinct clinical outcomes. Nat Med 21(5):449–456. https://doi.org/10.1038/nm.3850
33. Secrier M, Li X, De Silva N et al (2016) Mutational signatures in esophageal adenocarcinoma define etiologically distinct subgroups with therapeutic relevance. Nat Genet 48(10):1131–1141. https://doi.org/10.1038/ng.3659
34. Maron SB, Luke JJ, Hovey R et al (2017) Identification of T-cell-inflamed gastric adenocarcinoma in The Cancer Genome Atlas (TCGA). J Clin Oncol 35(7_Suppl):16. https://doi.org/10.1200/jco.2017.35.7_suppl.16
35. Chao J, Fuchs CS, Shitara K et al (2021) Assessment of pembrolizumab therapy for the treatment of microsatellite instability–high gastric or gastroesophageal junction cancer among patients in the KEYNOTE-059, KEYNOTE-061, and KEYNOTE-062 clinical trials. JAMA Oncol. https://doi.org/10.1001/jamaoncol.2021.0275

36. Pietrantonio F, Miceli R, Raimondi A et al (2019) Individual patient data meta-analysis of the value of microsatellite instability as a biomarker in gastric cancer. J Clin Oncol 37(35):3392–3400. https://doi.org/10.1200/JCO.19.01124
37. Smyth EC (2020) Chemotherapy for resectable microsatellite instability-high gastric cancer? Lancet Oncol 21(2):204. https://doi.org/10.1016/S1470-2045(20)30025-5
38. Kawazoe A, Kuwata T, Kuboki Y et al (2017) Clinicopathological features of programmed death ligand 1 expression with tumor-infiltrating lymphocyte, mismatch repair, and Epstein–Barr virus status in a large cohort of gastric cancer patients. Gastric Cancer 20(3):407–415. https://doi.org/10.1007/s10120-016-0631-3
39. Janjigian YY, Sanchez-Vega F, Jonsson P et al (2018) Genetic predictors of response to systemic therapy in esophagogastric cancer. Cancer Discov 8(1):49–58. https://doi.org/10.1158/2159-8290.CD-17-0787
40. Xie T, Liu Y, Zhang Z et al (2020) Positive status of Epstein-Barr virus as a biomarker for gastric cancer immunotherapy: a prospective observational study. J Immunother 43(4):139–144. https://doi.org/10.1097/CJI.0000000000000316
41. Wang F, Wei XL, Wang FH et al (2019) Safety, efficacy and tumor mutational burden as a biomarker of overall survival benefit in chemo-refractory gastric cancer treated with toripalimab, a PD-1 antibody in phase Ib/II clinical trial NCT02915432. Ann Oncol 30(9):1479–1486. https://doi.org/10.1093/annonc/mdz197
42. Kim ST, Cristescu R, Bass AJ et al (2018) Comprehensive molecular characterization of clinical responses to PD-1 inhibition in metastatic gastric cancer. Nat Med 24(9):1449–1458. https://doi.org/10.1038/s41591-018-0101-z
43. Kang Y-K, Boku N, Satoh T et al (2017) Nivolumab in patients with advanced gastric or gastro-oesophageal junction cancer refractory to, or intolerant of, at least two previous chemotherapy regimens (ONO-4538-12, ATTRACTION-2): a randomised, double-blind, placebo-controlled, phase 3 trial. Lancet 390(10111):2461–2471. https://doi.org/10.1016/S0140-6736(17)31827-5
44. Bang YJ, Yañez Ruiz E, Van Cutsem E et al (2018) Phase III, randomised trial of avelumab versus physician's choice of chemotherapy as third-line treatment of patients with advanced gastric or gastro-oesophageal junction cancer: primary analysis of JAVELIN gastric 300. Ann Oncol 29(10):2052–2060. https://doi.org/10.1093/annonc/mdy264
45. Shitara K, Van Cutsem E, Bang YJ et al (2020) Efficacy and safety of pembrolizumab or pembrolizumab plus chemotherapy vs chemotherapy alone for patients with first-line, advanced gastric cancer: the KEYNOTE-062 phase 3 randomized clinical trial. JAMA Oncol 6(10):1571–1580. https://doi.org/10.1001/jamaoncol.2020.3370
46. Shitara K, Özgüroğlu M, Bang YJ et al (2018) Pembrolizumab versus paclitaxel for previously treated, advanced gastric or gastro-oesophageal junction cancer (KEYNOTE-061): a randomised, open-label, controlled, phase 3 trial. Lancet 392(10142):123–133. https://doi.org/10.1016/S0140-6736(18)31257-1
47. Fuchs CS, Doi T, Jang RW et al (2018) Safety and efficacy of pembrolizumab monotherapy in patients with previously treated advanced gastric and gastroesophageal junction cancer: phase 2 clinical KEYNOTE-059 trial. JAMA Oncol 4(5). https://doi.org/10.1001/jamaoncol.2018.0013
48. Moehler MH, Dvorkin M, Ozguroglu M et al (2020) Results of the JAVELIN Gastric 100 phase 3 trial: avelumab maintenance following first-line (1L) chemotherapy (CTx) vs continuation of CTx for HER2−advanced gastric or gastroesophageal junction cancer (GC/GEJC). J Clin Oncol 38(4_Suppl):278. https://doi.org/10.1200/jco.2020.38.4_suppl.278
49. Lei M, Siemers N, Pandya D et al (2019) Abstract 2673: association of PD-L1 combined positive score and immune gene signatures with efficacy of nivolumab (NIVO) ± ipilimumab (IPI) in patients with metastatic gastroesophageal cancer (mGEC). In: American Association for Cancer Research (AACR), p 2673. https://doi.org/10.1158/1538-7445.am2019-2673
50. Moehler M, Shitara K, Garrido M et al (2020) LBA6_PR Nivolumab (nivo) plus chemotherapy (chemo) versus chemo as first-line (1L) treatment for advanced gastric

cancer/gastroesophageal junction cancer (GC/GEJC)/esophageal adenocarcinoma (EAC): first results of the CheckMate 649 study. Ann Oncol 31:S1191. https://doi.org/10.1016/j.annonc.2020.08.2296
51. Boku N, Ryu MH, Oh D-Y et al (2020) LBA7_PR nivolumab plus chemotherapy versus chemotherapy alone in patients with previously untreated advanced or recurrent gastric/gastroesophageal junction (G/GEJ) cancer: ATTRACTION-4 (ONO-4538-37) study. Ann Oncol 31:S1192. https://doi.org/10.1016/j.annonc.2020.08.2297
52. Kelly RJ, Ajani JA, Kuzdzal J et al (2021) Adjuvant nivolumab in resected esophageal or gastroesophageal junction cancer. N Engl J Med 384(13):1191–1203. https://doi.org/10.1056/nejmoa2032125
53. Rousseau B, Foote MB, Maron SB et al (2021) The spectrum of benefit from checkpoint blockade in hypermutated tumors. N Engl J Med 384(12):1168–1170. https://doi.org/10.1056/NEJMc2031965
54. Smolle E, Leithner K, Olschewski H (2020) Oncogene addiction and tumor mutational burden in non-small-cell lung cancer: clinical significance and limitations. Thorac Cancer 11(2):205–215. https://doi.org/10.1111/1759-7714.13246
55. Kim J, Kim B, Kang SY et al (2020) Tumor mutational burden determined by panel sequencing predicts survival after immunotherapy in patients with advanced gastric cancer. Front Oncol 10. https://doi.org/10.3389/fonc.2020.00314
56. Shitara K, Özgüroğlu M, Bang Y-J et al (2020) The association of tissue tumor mutational burden (tTMB) using the foundation medicine genomic platform with efficacy of pembrolizumab versus paclitaxel in patients (pts) with gastric cancer (GC) from KEYNOTE-061. J Clin Oncol 38(15_Suppl):4537. https://doi.org/10.1200/jco.2020.38.15_suppl.4537
57. Kang BW, Kim JG, Lee IH, Bae HI, Seo AN (2017) Clinical significance of tumor-infiltrating lymphocytes for gastric cancer in the era of immunology. World J Gastrointest Oncol 9(7):293–299. https://doi.org/10.4251/wjgo.v9.i7.293
58. Wei Q, Xu Q, Yuan X et al (2021) Immunological impact of chemotherapy on the tumor microenvironment in gastric cancer. J Surg Oncol. https://doi.org/10.1002/jso.26449
59. Jomrich G, Paireder M, Kristo I et al (2021) High systemic immune-inflammation index is an adverse prognostic factor for patients with gastroesophageal adenocarcinoma. Ann Surg 273(3):532–541. https://doi.org/10.1097/SLA.0000000000003370
60. Sunakawa Y, Matoba R, Inoue E et al (2021) Genomic pathway of gut microbiome to predict efficacy of nivolumab in advanced gastric cancer: DELIVER trial (JACCRO GC-08). J Clin Oncol 39(3_Suppl):161. https://doi.org/10.1200/jco.2021.39.3_suppl.161
61. Smyth EC, Wotherspoon A, Peckitt C et al (2017) Mismatch repair deficiency, microsatellite instability, and survival: An exploratory analysis of the Medical Research Council Adjuvant Gastric Infusional Chemotherapy (MAGIC) trial. JAMA Oncol 3(9):1197–1203. https://doi.org/10.1001/jamaoncol.2016.6762
62. Choi YY, Kim H, Shin SJ et al (2019) Microsatellite instability and programmed cell death-ligand 1 expression in stage II/III gastric cancer: post hoc analysis of the CLASSIC randomized controlled study. Ann Surg 270(2):309–316. https://doi.org/10.1097/SLA.0000000000002803
63. Kim SY, Choi YY, An JY et al (2015) The benefit of microsatellite instability is attenuated by chemotherapy in stage II and stage III gastric cancer: results from a large cohort with subgroup analyses. Int J Cancer 137(4):819–825. https://doi.org/10.1002/ijc.29449
64. Le DT, Kim TW, van Cutsem E et al (2020) Phase II open-label study of pembrolizumab in treatment-refractory, microsatellite instability-high/mismatch repair-deficient metastatic colorectal cancer: KEYNOTE-164. J Clin Oncol 38:11–19. https://doi.org/10.1200/JCO.19.02107
65. Rha SY, Lee C, Kim HS et al (2021) A multi-institutional phase Ib/II trial of first-line triplet regimen (Pembrolizumab, Trastuzumab, Chemotherapy) for HER2-positive advanced gastric and gastroesophageal junction cancer (PANTHERA Trial): molecular profiling and clinical update. J Clin Oncol 39(3_Suppl):218. https://doi.org/10.1200/jco.2021.39.3_suppl.218
66. Janjigian YY, Maron SB, Chatila WK et al (2020) First-line pembrolizumab and trastuzumab in HER2-positive oesophageal, gastric, or gastro-oesophageal junction cancer: an

open-label, single-arm, phase 2 trial. Lancet Oncol 21(6):821–831. https://doi.org/10.1016/S1470-2045(20)30169-8
67. Chung HC, Bang YJ, S Fuchs C, et al. (2021) First-line pembrolizumab/placebo plus trastuzumab and chemotherapy in HER2-positive advanced gastric cancer: KEYNOTE-811. Future Oncol 17(5):491–501. https://doi.org/10.2217/fon-2020-0737
68. Catenacci DVT, Rosales M, Chung HC et al (2021) MAHOGANY: margetuximab combination in HER2+ unresectable/metastatic gastric/gastroesophageal junction adenocarcinoma. Future Oncol 17(10):1155–1164. https://doi.org/10.2217/fon-2020-1007
69. Alcindor T, Opu T, Mueller C et al (2019) Interim analysis of a phase II trial of perioperative chemotherapy plus avelumab in esophagogastric and gastric adenocarcinoma. Ann Oncol 30:v299–v300. https://doi.org/10.1093/annonc/mdz247.102
70. Liu Y, Han G, Li H et al (2020) Camrelizumab combined with FOLFOX as neoadjuvant therapy for resectable locally advanced gastric and gastroesophageal junction adenocarcinoma. J Clin Oncol 38(15_Suppl):4536. https://doi.org/10.1200/jco.2020.38.15_suppl.4536
71. Zhao Y, Han G, Zhuang J et al (2020) Efficacy and safety of camrelizumab combined with FOLFOX as neoadjuvant therapy for patients with resectable locally advanced gastric and gastroesophageal junction adenocarcinoma who received D2 radical gastrectomy. J Clin Oncol 38(15_Suppl):e16549. https://doi.org/10.1200/jco.2020.38.15_suppl.e16549
72. Im H-S, Song JS, Jo WR et al (2020) Preliminary results of a phase II study of neoadjuvant immune checkpoint inhibitor IMC-001 (anti-PD-L1 monoclonal antibody) in patients with resectable gastrointestinal cancers (NeoChance Study). J Clin Oncol 38(15_Suppl):e16542. https://doi.org/10.1200/jco.2020.38.15_suppl.e16542
73. Peri-operative immuno-chemotherapy in operable oesophageal and gastric cancer. Full text view: ClinicalTrials.gov. https://clinicaltrials.gov/ct2/show/NCT03399071. Accessed 5 Apr 2021
74. Phase II study of avelumab plus chemotherapy in the peri-operative treatment for patients with resectable gastric cancer (GC) or gastroesophageal junction cancer (GEJC). Full text view: ClinicalTrials.gov. https://clinicaltrials.gov/ct2/show/NCT03979131. Accessed 5 Apr 2021
75. Perioperative chemotherapy vs immunotherapy vs. chemo-immunotherapy in patients with advanced GC and AEG. Full text view: ClinicalTrials.gov. https://clinicaltrials.gov/ct2/show/NCT04062656. Accessed 5 Apr 2021
76. Bang YJ, Van Cutsem E, Fuchs CS et al (2019) KEYNOTE-585: phase III study of perioperative chemotherapy with or without pembrolizumab for gastric cancer. Future Oncol 15(9):943–952. https://doi.org/10.2217/fon-2018-0581
77. Assessing durvalumab and FLOT chemotherapy in resectable gastric and gastroesophageal junction cancer. Full text view: ClinicalTrials.gov. https://clinicaltrials.gov/ct2/show/NCT04592913. Accessed 5 Apr 2021
78. Smyth E, Knödler M, Giraut A et al (2020) VESTIGE: adjuvant immunotherapy in patients with resected esophageal, gastroesophageal junction and gastric cancer following preoperative chemotherapy with high risk for recurrence (N+ and/or R1): an open label randomized controlled phase-2-study. Front Oncol 9. https://doi.org/10.3389/fonc.2019.01320

Stomach: The Standard of Care ± HER2

Ryan H. Moy and Yelena Y. Janjigian

Contents

Abstract

Gastric cancer represents the fifth most common cancer and third leading cause of cancer mortality worldwide. The mainstay of treatment for metastatic gastric cancer is systemic therapy, and recent advances have led to the validation of key molecular biomarkers including microsatellite instability (MSI) status, PD-L1 expression and HER2 positivity that impact treatment selection and sequencing. While immune checkpoint inhibitors have modest activity in gastric cancer as monotherapy, recent studies reveal enhanced activity of immunotherapy when combined with chemotherapy or targeted therapy. Here, we review current standard approaches for the treatment of metastatic gastric cancer including chemotherapy, angiogenesis blockade, HER2-directed therapy, and immunotherapy.

R. H. Moy
Department of Medicine, Memorial Sloan Kettering Cancer Center, New York, NY, USA

Y. Y. Janjigian (✉)
Department of Medicine, Gastrointestinal Oncology Service, Memorial Sloan Kettering Cancer Center and Weill Cornell Medical College, New York, NY, USA
e-mail: janjigiy@mskcc.org

Cancer Immunotherapy (2021)

https://doi.org/10.1007/13905_2021_4,
Published Online: 25 August 2021

Keywords

Gastric cancer · Stomach cancer · Immunotherapy · HER2 · Targeted therapy · Angiogenesis

1 Introduction

Representing the third leading cause of cancer mortality worldwide, gastric cancer is a major contributor to global disease burden [1]. While the overall incidence of gastric cancer has declined steadily over the past century, incidence rates among young adults under the age of 50 have been rising, particularly in developed countries [2]. For patients who present with localized disease, surgical resection is the mainstay of curative treatment; however, even with aggressive standard of care perioperative therapy, the majority of patients experience disease recurrence. In the metastatic setting, biomarker assessment including HER2 expression, PD-L1 positivity, and microsatellite instability (MSI)/mismatch repair (MMR) deficiency status is critical for optimizing treatment decisions (Fig. 1). While overall prognosis for metastatic gastric cancer remains poor with median overall survival (OS) of approximately 1 year, significant advances over the past decade have led to

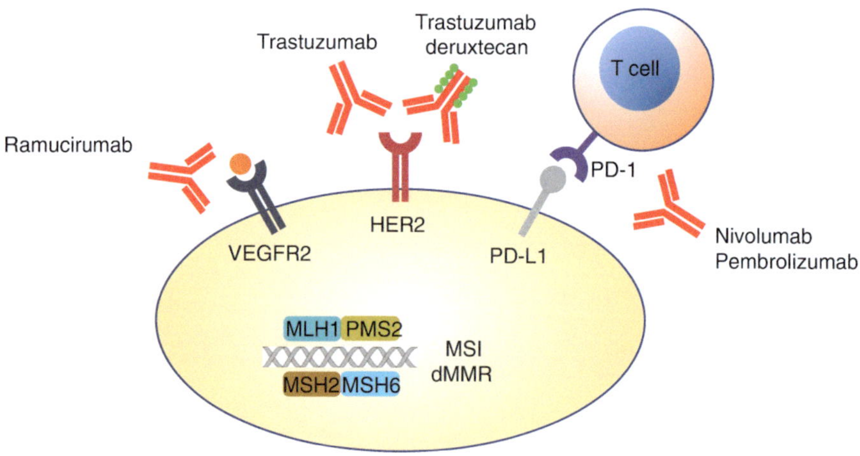

Fig. 1 Standard biomarkers and approved targeted or immune-based therapies in metastatic gastric cancer. Routine biomarker testing in advanced gastric cancer includes HER2, PD-L1, and mismatch repair deficiency (dMMR)/microsatellite instability (MSI). For patients with HER2-positive gastric cancer, trastuzumab is added to first-line fluoropyrimidine- and platinum-based chemotherapy. The antibody-drug conjugate trastuzumab deruxtecan has recently been approved for later lines of therapy in patients who have trastuzumab-refractory HER2-positive disease. Anti-PD-1 agents like pembrolizumab and nivolumab have shown activity, particularly in patients with PD-L1-positive tumors by combined positive score (CPS), as well as in patients with dMMR/MSI tumors. In addition, the VEGFR2 antibody ramucirumab is active in the second-line setting either as monotherapy or in combination with paclitaxel

paradigm changes in gastric cancer treatment, including emerging roles for immunotherapy as both monotherapy and in novel combinations.

2 Molecular Subtypes in Gastric Cancer

Comprehensive molecular analysis has led to the classification of gastric cancers into distinct genomic subtypes. The Asian Cancer Research Group (ACRG) performed deep molecular analysis in conjunction with clinical outcome data, yielding four gastric cancer genotypes: tumors that are microsatellite stable (MSS) with intact *TP53* (MSS/*TP53*$^{+}$), MSS with *TP53* alterations (MSS/*TP53*$^{-}$), MSS with epithelial-mesenchymal transition signature (MSS/EMT), and MSI-high [3]. In addition, through DNA copy number analysis, whole exome sequencing, DNA methylation profiling, messenger RNA sequencing, microRNA profiling, and proteomic analysis, The Cancer Genome Atlas (TCGA) research network defined four molecular subtypes: genomically stable (GS), chromosomal unstable (CIN), MSI, and Epstein–Barr virus-positive [4]. While these studies have enhanced our understanding of the biological pathways driving tumorigenesis and progression of gastric cancers, the actionable biomarkers utilized in routine clinical practice are limited. CIN tumors are enriched for *TP53* mutations and amplifications in receptor tyrosine kinases (RTKs) such as HER2, which can be selectively targeted by anti-HER2 drugs to varying effect [5]. Several other RTKs are overexpressed or activated in gastric cancers, such as EGFR, MET, and FGFR2. While late-phase trials assessing drugs targeting EGFR and MET have been negative [6–9], recent data suggest promising activity for the anti-FGFR2b antibody bemarituzumab in FGFR2-positive gastric cancer [10]. GS tumors, which are frequently of diffuse histology, are enriched for *RHOA* alterations, *CDH1* mutations, and *CLDN18-ARHGAP* fusions. These tumors lack aneuploidy and have low mutational load, making them difficult to target although studies are underway with novel agents such as the Claudin 18.2 (CLDN 18.2) antibody zolbetuximab [11]. Finally, the MSI and EBV-positive gastric cancer subtypes have been shown to be more responsiveness to immunotherapy with checkpoint inhibitors [12].

3 Chemotherapy for Advanced Gastric Cancer

Palliative chemotherapy has long been the foundation of first-line treatment for metastatic gastric adenocarcinoma and is associated with improved survival and quality of life compared to supportive care alone [13, 14]. For most patients, first-line treatment consists of a combination of two drugs, typically a fluoropyrimidine plus a platinum agent (cisplatin or oxaliplatin). 5-fluorouracil (5-FU) is associated with single-agent activity of 10–30% [15–17], and the addition of other cytotoxic agents yields improved efficacy with response rates of approximately 40–50% for doublet regimens. Compared with 5-FU and cisplatin, 5-FU and oxaliplatin (FOLFOX) was found to be non-inferior in terms of OS, with reduced rates of grade 3–4 neutropenia and nephrotoxicity [18]. Regimens combining capecitabine with platinum agents are also active and well-tolerated in patients with advanced gastric cancer [19]. In Asian patients, the oral fluoropyrimidine S-1 is frequently used, but this drug is poorly metabolized in non-Asian populations due to pharmacogenomic differences [20]. Thus, a fluoropyrimidine combined with oxaliplatin or cisplatin is the preferred first-line regimen for patients with non-MSI-H metastatic gastric cancer, with additional agents added depending on biomarker status as will be discussed.

Triplet chemotherapy regimens have also been widely studied in metastatic gastric cancer. While FLOT (5-FU, leucovorin, oxaliplatin, docetaxel) is now standard in the perioperative setting [21], the addition of a third cytotoxic agent is generally avoided for most patients with metastatic disease due to excessive toxicity and questionable survival benefit. In a randomized phase 3 trial comparing docetaxel, cisplatin and 5-FU (DCF) versus cisplatin and 5-FU, the triplet regimen was associated with improved time-to-progression, survival and overall response rate but demonstrated a higher rate of grade 3–4 toxicities, particularly neutropenia (82% vs. 57%) and febrile neutropenia (29% vs. 12%) [22]. In contrast, a phase 3 trial of docetaxel plus cisplatin and S-1 compared with cisplatin and S-1 in 741 Japanese patients with chemotherapy-naïve advanced gastric cancer found no improvement in OS with the addition of docetaxel [23]. While epirubicin has historically been used to treat esophagogastric cancer in combination with fluoropyrimidine and platinum, studies have demonstrated no added efficacy of epirubicin in combination with contemporary chemotherapy [24, 25]. Thus, platinum doublet chemotherapy has remained the standard of care first-line reference regimen, with triplet chemotherapy regimens usually reserved for younger patients with excellent functional status or patients with high disease burden requiring a rapid treatment response.

Besides fluoropyrimidines and platinum agents, several other cytotoxic drugs have demonstrated activity in esophagogastric cancers including taxanes (paclitaxel, docetaxel) and irinotecan, which can be considered as chemotherapeutic options after progression on first-line treatment. Second-line chemotherapy is associated with improved survival compared to best supportive care although the benefit is limited with median survival of approximately 6 months [13, 26–28]. Recent data suggest benefit for trifluridine-tipiracil (an oral cytotoxic chemotherapy consisting of a thymidine-based nucleoside analog and a thymidine phosphorylase inhibitor) in patients with acceptable performance status after progression on two prior lines of therapy. The randomized, placebo-controlled phase 3 TAGS trial demonstrated a modest OS advantage (5.7 versus 3.6 months) of trifluridine-tipiracil compared to best supportive care [29].

4 Role of Angiogenesis Blockade in Metastatic Gastric Cancer

Both preclinical and clinical studies have established that pathologic angiogenesis and extracellular matrix remodeling through the vascular endothelial growth factor (VEGF)-VEGF receptor 2 (VEGFR2) pathway facilitates gastric cancer growth and metastasis (Table 1) [30–32]. Ramucirumab, an anti-VEGFR2 antibody that blocks

Table 1 Select trials of anti-angiogenic agents in advanced gastric cancer

Study	Line	Treatment	OS (months)
AVAGAST	1st	Bevacizumab + fluoropyrimidine + cisplatin vs. fluoropyrimidine + cisplatin	12.1 vs. 10.1 ($p = 0.1002$)
REGARD	2nd	Ramucirumab vs. placebo	5.2 vs. 3.8 ($p = 0.047$)
RAINBOW	2nd	Ramucirumab + paclitaxel vs. paclitaxel	9.6 vs. 7.4 ($p = 0.017$)
RAINFALL	1st	Ramucirumab + capecitabine + cisplatin vs. capecitabine + cisplatin	11.2 vs. 10.7 ($p = 0.6757$)

tumor angiogenesis is active in the second-line setting, either as monotherapy or in combination with paclitaxel. The phase 3 REGARD trial randomized 472 patients with progression on first-line chemotherapy in a 2:1 ratio to either single-agent ramucirumab or best supportive care [33]. Ramucirumab was associated with an improvement in OS (5.2 vs. 3.8 months) and was well-tolerated, with mildly increased rates of hypertension compared to placebo. In the phase 3 RAINBOW trial, 665 patients who had progressed on first-line therapy were randomized to either paclitaxel plus ramucirumab or paclitaxel plus placebo [34]. OS was significantly prolonged in the paclitaxel plus ramucirumab arm (9.6 vs. 7.4 months), and the objective response rate was higher (28% vs. 16%). Thus, paclitaxel plus ramucirumab is a standard second-line option for advanced gastric cancer.

Notably, increased numbers of patients are exposed to taxanes prior to second-line therapy for metastatic disease, particularly with the acceptance of FLOT as a global standard perioperative regimen. The use of oxaliplatin in initial therapy for esophagogastric cancer is also associated with a risk of peripheral neuropathy, with rates of neurotoxicity with FOLFOX ranging from 30% to 70%. Therefore, second-line paclitaxel plus ramucirumab may not be ideal for patients with early disease recurrence after perioperative FLOT or significant neuropathy. Irinotecan as a single agent or in combination with 5-FU (FOLFIRI) has established activity in esophagogastric cancer [25, 27]. Given potential limitations with second-line paclitaxel, recent studies have shown safety of combined FOLFIRI plus ramucirumab, with better efficacy seen among patients previously exposed to taxanes in the phase 2 RAMIRIS trial [35, 36]. Hence, FOLFIRI/ramucirumab is a reasonable option, and a randomized phase 3 study is underway (NCT03081143) comparing paclitaxel/ramucirumab to FOLFIRI/ramucirumab.

While angiogenesis inhibitors have demonstrated activity in the second-line setting, several studies have failed to show a benefit of the addition of angiogenesis inhibitors to first-line chemotherapy. Ramucirumab did not add to the efficacy of first-line 5-FU/cisplatin or S1/oxaliplatin in the phase 3 RAINFALL [37] and phase 2 RAINSTORM study [38]. Similarly, the phase 3 AVAGAST study in which the anti-VEGF antibody bevacizumab was added to standard first-line chemotherapy failed to show a survival benefit with bevacizumab [39]. Given these findings, there is no proven role for anti-angiogenic agents when combined with chemotherapy in the first-line setting for advanced gastric cancer.

5 Targeting HER2

Receptor tyrosine kinase (RTK) HER2 (also known as ERBB2) is a member of the EGFR family of RTKs and is overexpressed in approximately 15–20% of gastric and GEJ adenocarcinomas, typically through *ERBB2* gene amplifications [4, 40]. In the metastatic setting, the anti-HER2 antibody trastuzumab was the first targeted therapy approved for gastric cancers based on results from the Trastuzumab for Gastric Cancer (ToGA) trial [5]. In this double-blind phase 3 trial, 594 patients were randomized to receive chemotherapy with or without trastuzumab. The primary endpoint was achieved with a superior median OS of 13.8 vs. 11.1 months when trastuzumab was added. Importantly, the survival benefit with trastuzumab was increased in patients meeting HER2 positivity by current standard clinical criteria (i.e., IHC 3+ or 2+ in combination with FISH positivity). As a result of this study, the addition of trastuzumab to first-line chemotherapy is established as a global standard.

Given this critical role of HER2, several subsequent studies investigated additional HER2 targeting agents in metastatic gastric cancer (Table 2). The LOGiC trial evaluated first-line capecitabine and oxaliplatin in combination with the oral HER2 and EGFR inhibitor lapatinib versus placebo in patients with advanced HER2-positive esophagogastric cancer [41]. However, there was no significant improvement in median OS with the addition of lapatinib (12.2 versus 10.5 months). Another HER2-targeting antibody pertuzumab (in combination with first-line trastuzumab and chemotherapy) also did not significantly improve outcome (JACOB trial) [42]. In addition, several studies assessing the role of HER2 targeting in the second-line setting were negative. For example, lapatinib failed to show a survival benefit in combination with second-line paclitaxel in the TyTAN study [43]. The GATSBY trial evaluated the antibody-drug conjugate trastuzumab emtansine (T-DM1) also did not observe a survival benefit compared to investigator's choice taxane (paclitaxel or docetaxel) [44]. Compared to HER2-positive breast cancer, in which trastuzumab has been shown to be effective when continued beyond progression, there is no established role for continuing trastuzumab after progression in HER2-positive gastric cancer. This may be due to multiple reasons including tumor heterogeneity,

Table 2 Select trials of HER2-targeting agents in metastatic gastric cancer

Study	Line	Treatment	OS (months)
ToGA	1st	Trastuzumab + fluoropyrimidine + cisplatin vs. fluoropyrimidine + cisplatin	13.8 vs. 11.1 ($p = 0.0046$)
LOGiC	1st	Lapatinib + CAPOX vs. CAPOX	12.2 vs. 10.5 ($p = 0.349$)
TyTAN	2nd	Lapatinib + paclitaxel vs. paclitaxel	11.0 vs. 8.9 ($p = 0.104$)
JACOB	1st	Pertuzumab + trastuzumab + fluoropyrimidine + cisplatin vs. trastuzumab + fluoropyrimidine + cisplatin	17.5 vs. 14.2 ($p = 0.057$)
GATSBY	2nd	Trastuzumab emtansine vs. taxane	7.9 vs. 8.6 ($p = 0.86$)
DESTINY-Gastric01	3rd	Trastuzumab deruxtecan vs. chemotherapy	12.5 vs. 8.4 ($p = 0.01$)

loss of HER2 expression due to selection of non-*ERBB2*-amplified clones, alterations in downstream signaling (including the RTK-RAS-PI3K pathway) and acquisition of alterations in bypass pathways (such as EGFR and MET) [45, 46]. The phase 2 T-ACT study investigated the continuation of trastuzumab with paclitaxel versus paclitaxel alone after progression on first-line trastuzumab-containing therapy, finding no improvement in PFS with trastuzumab beyond progression [47]. Notably, among 16 patients with evaluable tissue for exploratory analysis, 11 patients (69%) had lost HER2 positivity, highlighting the importance of confirming HER2 retention after progression.

Despite these subsequent negative studies, recent trials have shown promising activity with newer HER2-targeted agents. Trastuzumab deruxtecan (T-DXd) is a novel antibody-drug conjugate consisting of a humanized, monoclonal, anti-HER2 antibody conjugated to a DNA topoisomerase I inhibitor payload by a cleavage, tetrapeptide-based linker, with a high drug-to-antibody ratio of 8 [48]. The phase 2 DESTINY-Gastric01 randomized 187 patients in Japan and Korea with advanced HER2-positive gastric cancer and prior progression on at least two therapies including trastuzumab to either T-DXd 6.4 mg/kg or physician's choice chemotherapy in a 2:1 ratio. Impressively, patients receiving trastuzumab deruxtecan demonstrated significant improvement in objective response rate (51% vs. 14%) and OS (12.5 vs. 8.4 months) [49]. One notable toxicity of T-DXd is interstitial lung disease, which was observed in 10% of patients with 2.4% grade 3–4 toxicity and no grade 5 toxicities. Additional studies are underway in Asian and non-Asian populations evaluating T-DXd in the second-line setting as well as in combination with chemotherapy and/or immunotherapy. Based on these unprecedented results from DESTINY-Gastric01, T-DXd was approved in Japan for patients with advanced HER2-positive gastric cancer after progression on chemotherapy, and more recently by the FDA for patients who have received a prior trastuzumab-containing regimen. Other promising HER2-targeted agents include the Fc-optimized monoclonal HER2 antibody margetuximab, the bispecific HER2-targeting antibody ZW25, and novel HER2-specific tyrosine kinase inhibitors such as tucatinib [50–52]. Thus, while trastuzumab had previously been the alone approved HER2-targeted agent in advanced HER2-positive gastric cancer, newer targeted agents such as T-DXd are now being implemented into standard therapy.

6 Immunotherapy for Gastric Cancer

Checkpoint inhibitors have established activity in advanced gastric cancer and have been incorporated into standard treatment paradigms, with recent data revealing emerging roles for immunotherapy in combination regimens (Table 3). In the single-arm phase 2 KEYNOTE-059 study, 259 patients with advanced gastric or gastroesophageal junction (GEJ) cancer refractory to standard chemotherapy received pembrolizumab monotherapy [53]. Patients with PD-L1-positive and PD-L1-negative tumors were included, with PD-L1 positivity evaluated by the combined positive score (CPS), which assesses PD-L1 on both tumor cells and

Table 3 Immunotherapy trials in advanced gastric cancer

Study	Line	Treatment	OS (months)
ATTRACTION-2	3rd	Nivolumab vs. placebo	5.26 vs. 4.14 ($p < 0.0001$)
KEYNOTE-059	3rd	Pembrolizumab	5.6
KEYNOTE-061	2nd	Pembrolizumab vs. paclitaxel (CPS ≥1)	9.1 vs. 8.3 (one-sided $p = 0.0421$)
KEYNOTE-062	1st	Pembrolizumab vs. fluoropyrimidine + cisplatin (CPS ≥1)	10.6 vs. 11.1
		Pembrolizumab + fluoropyrimidine + cisplatin vs. fluoropyrimidine + cisplatin (CPS ≥1)	12.5 vs. 11.1 ($p = 0.05$)
CheckMate 649	1st	Nivolumab + fluoropyrimidine + oxaliplatin vs. fluoropyrimidine + oxaliplatin (CPS ≥5)	14.4 vs. 11.1 ($p < 0.0001$)
ATTRACTION-4	1st	Nivolumab + fluoropyrimidine + oxaliplatin vs. fluoropyrimidine + oxaliplatin	17.5 vs. 17.2 ($p = 0.257$)

tumor-infiltrating lymphocytes. Tumors were considered to be PD-L1-positive if the CPS was ≥1. This study demonstrated an objective response rate of 12% regardless of PD-L1 status, which improved to 16% in the PD-L1-positive population, leading to the FDA approval of pembrolizumab for patients with PD-L1-positive tumors refractory to chemotherapy.

Assessing the role of pembrolizumab in the second-line setting, KEYNOTE-061 randomized 395 patients with PD-L1-positive (CPS ≥1) gastric or GEJ cancers to either pembrolizumab or paclitaxel monotherapy [54]. While pembrolizumab demonstrated a favorable safety profile relative to chemotherapy, there was no improvement in median OS (9.1 months vs. 8.3 months) or median PFS (1.5 vs. 4.1 months). Pembrolizumab was also studied in the first-line setting in the phase 3 KEYNOTE-062 trial, in which patients with PD-L1 CPS ≥1 gastric cancer were randomized 1:1:1 to either pembrolizumab alone, pembrolizumab plus chemotherapy (cisplatin with 5-FU or capecitabine), or chemotherapy plus placebo [55]. In the CPS ≥1 population, there was no improvement in median OS comparing pembrolizumab to chemotherapy (10.6 vs. 11.1 months). In patients with high PD-L1 expressing tumors (CPS ≥10), there was a numerical but not statistical improvement in median OS with pembrolizumab vs. chemotherapy (17.4 vs. 10.8 months).

In addition to pembrolizumab, the anti-PD-1 agent nivolumab has also shown single-agent activity in advanced gastric cancer. ATTRACTION-2 was a multicenter, double-blind phase 3 study of Asian patients with advanced gastric or GEJ cancer with prior progression on at least two prior chemotherapy regimens randomized to either placebo or nivolumab [56]. This study demonstrated an improvement in median OS with nivolumab (5.3 vs. 4.1 months), with an objective response rate (ORR) of 11.2%. Following these results, nivolumab was approved in Japan for the treatment of advanced gastric cancer after progression on chemotherapy.

While immune checkpoint blockade is active as monotherapy with some long-term response, the percentage of patients who benefit is modest. Until recently, anti-PD-1 agents have been limited to later lines of therapy in metastatic gastric cancer. More recently, several studies have assessed the role of immunotherapy in combination with first-line chemotherapy. The first phase 3 trial to report combination chemotherapy and immunotherapy in gastric cancer was KEYNOTE-062 [55]; however, the addition of pembrolizumab to chemotherapy did not improve outcomes. In contrast, the recently reported CheckMate 649 and ATTRACTION-4 studies indicate a clinical benefit for the addition of nivolumab to first-line chemotherapy. The phase 2/3 ATTRACTION-4 study evaluated first-line chemotherapy with or without nivolumab in Asian patients with untreated advanced gastric or GEJ cancer, demonstrating an improvement in median PFS but not OS with the combination [57]. The exact reason for the lack of OS benefit is not known although it has been speculated that the high rate of patients receiving later lines of therapy including immunotherapy may have contributed. In the global phase 3 CheckMate-649 study, patients with previously untreated advanced esophagogastric adenocarcinoma were randomized to standard chemotherapy or chemotherapy plus nivolumab [58]. While the trial enrolled patients regardless of PD-L1 status, the dual primary endpoints were OS and PFS in patients with CPS ≥5 tumors, which made up approximately 60% of the study population. The combination of chemotherapy and nivolumab led to improved median OS (14.4 vs. 11.1 months) and PFS (7.7 vs. 6.1 months) in patients with PD-L1 CPS ≥5 tumors. Based on these results, as of January 2021 the combination of FOLFOX and nivolumab is included in NCCN guidelines for patients with PD-L1 CPS ≥5 disease.

In addition to combinations with chemotherapy, immunotherapy has been evaluated in combination with targeted therapies such as trastuzumab. In a phase 2 trial of patients with previously untreated advanced HER2-positive esophagogastric cancer, the combination of first-line fluoropyrimidine- and platinum-based chemotherapy with trastuzumab and pembrolizumab demonstrated an objective response rate of 91%, with 17% of patients achieving a complete response and 26/37 patients (70%) progression-free at 6 months [59]. Notably, patients on this trial could receive an induction phase of trastuzumab and pembrolizumab alone, resulting in tumor shrinkage for several patients. Another phase 1b/2 study of first-line chemotherapy, pembrolizumab and trastuzumab (PANTHERA trial) also showed similar activity with an objective response rate of 76.7% [60]. These data showing potential synergistic activity of immunotherapy and trastuzumab have led to the randomized, double-blind international phase 3 KEYNOTE 811 trial evaluating pembrolizumab versus placebo in combination with chemotherapy [61].

While biomarkers to identify patients with gastric cancer who are most likely to respond to immunotherapy are under intense study, it is quite clear that patients with MSI-H/dMMR disease derive significant benefit [62]. Pembrolizumab has been approved in a tissue- and site-agnostic manner for patients with metastatic MSI-H or dMMR tumors after progression on standard therapies. In exploratory analysis of patients with MSI-H tumors in KEYNOTE-062, median OS was markedly improved with pembrolizumab compared to chemotherapy (not reached vs. 8.5 months, hazard ratio = 0.29) [55]. These data are consistent with improved outcomes for first-line pembrolizumab compared to chemotherapy in metastatic advanced colorectal cancer [63]. Thus, current data suggest that for MSI-H gastric cancer, immunotherapy should be incorporated into first-line therapy.

7 Conclusion

Immunotherapy is transforming the landscape for advanced gastric cancer. Nevertheless, major questions must be addressed as only a modest percentage of patients benefit with current strategies. In particular, it is critical to elucidate better predictive biomarkers to identify patients that will most likely respond to immunotherapy, as the utility of current biomarkers like PD-L1 is limited. Ongoing and future research will reveal enhanced combinations of immunotherapy and targeted agents that augment anti-tumor immunity, leading to deeper and more durable treatment responses for patients.

Compliance with Ethical Standards

Disclosures Y.Y.J. has received research funding provided to the institution from Rgenix, Boehringer Ingelheim, Bayer, Genentech/Roche, Bristol-Myers Squibb, Eli Lilly, and Merck, served on advisory boards for Rgenix, Merck Serono, Bristol-Myers Squibb, Eli Lilly, Pfizer, Bayer, Imugene, Merck, Daiichi-Sankyo, Zymeworks, Basilea Pharmaceutica and AstraZeneca, and holds stock options for Rgenix.

References

1. Bray F, Ferlay J, Soerjomataram I, Siegel RL, Torre LA, Jemal A (2018) Global cancer statistics 2018: GLOBOCAN estimates of incidence and mortality worldwide for 36 cancers in 185 countries. CA Cancer J Clin 68:394–424
2. Bergquist JR, Leiting JL, Habermann EB, Cleary SP, Kendrick ML, Smoot RL et al (2019) Early-onset gastric cancer is a distinct disease with worrisome trends and oncogenic features. Surgery 166:547–555
3. Cristescu R, Lee J, Nebozhyn M, Kim K-M, Ting JC, Wong SS et al (2015) Molecular analysis of gastric cancer identifies subtypes associated with distinct clinical outcomes. Nat Med 21:449–456
4. Cancer Genome Atlas Research Network (2014) Comprehensive molecular characterization of gastric adenocarcinoma. Nature 513:202–209
5. Bang Y-J, Van Cutsem E, Feyereislova A, Chung HC, Shen L, Sawaki A et al (2010) Trastuzumab in combination with chemotherapy versus chemotherapy alone for treatment of HER2-positive advanced gastric or gastro-oesophageal junction cancer (ToGA): a phase 3, open-label, randomised controlled trial. Lancet 376:687–697
6. Waddell T, Chau I, Cunningham D, Gonzalez D, Okines AFC, Frances A et al (2013) Epirubicin, oxaliplatin, and capecitabine with or without panitumumab for patients with previously untreated advanced oesophagogastric cancer (REAL3): a randomised, open-label phase 3 trial. Lancet Oncol 14:481–489
7. Lordick F, Kang Y-K, Chung H-C, Salman P, Oh SC, Bodoky G et al (2013) Capecitabine and cisplatin with or without cetuximab for patients with previously untreated advanced gastric cancer (EXPAND): a randomised, open-label phase 3 trial. Lancet Oncol 14:490–499

8. Catenacci DVT, Tebbutt NC, Davidenko I, Murad AM, Al-Batran S-E, Ilson DH et al (2017) Rilotumumab plus epirubicin, cisplatin, and capecitabine as first-line therapy in advanced MET-positive gastric or gastro-oesophageal junction cancer (RILOMET-1): a randomised, double-blind, placebo-controlled, phase 3 trial. Lancet Oncol 18:1467–1482
9. Shah MA, Bang Y-J, Lordick F, Alsina M, Chen M, Hack SP et al (2017) Effect of fluorouracil, leucovorin, and oxaliplatin with or without onartuzumab in HER2-negative, MET-positive gastroesophageal adenocarcinoma: the METGastric randomized clinical trial. JAMA Oncol 3:620–627
10. Wainberg ZA, Enzinger PC, Kang Y-K, Yamaguchi K, Qin S, Lee K-W et al (2021) Randomized double-blind placebo-controlled phase 2 study of bemarituzumab combined with modified FOLFOX6 (mFOLFOX6) in first-line (1L) treatment of advanced gastric/gastroesophageal junction adenocarcinoma (FIGHT). JCO 39:160
11. Türeci O, Sahin U, Schulze-Bergkamen H, Zvirbule Z, Lordick F, Koeberle D et al (2019) A multicentre, phase IIa study of zolbetuximab as a single agent in patients with recurrent or refractory advanced adenocarcinoma of the stomach or lower oesophagus: the MONO study. Ann Oncol 30:1487–1495
12. Kim ST, Cristescu R, Bass AJ, Kim K-M, Odegaard JI, Kim K et al (2018) Comprehensive molecular characterization of clinical responses to PD-1 inhibition in metastatic gastric cancer. Nat Med 24:1449–1458
13. Kang JH, Lee SI, Lim DH, Park K-W, Oh SY, Kwon H-C et al (2012) Salvage chemotherapy for pretreated gastric cancer: a randomized phase III trial comparing chemotherapy plus best supportive care with best supportive care alone. J Clin Oncol 30:1513–1518
14. Glimelius B, Ekström K, Hoffman K, Graf W, Sjödén PO, Haglund U et al (1997) Randomized comparison between chemotherapy plus best supportive care with best supportive care in advanced gastric cancer. Ann Oncol 8:163–168
15. Cocconi G, DeLisi V, Di Blasio B (1982) Randomized comparison of 5-FU alone or combined with mitomycin and cytarabine (MFC) in the treatment of advanced gastric cancer. Cancer Treat Rep 66:1263–1266
16. De Lisi V, Cocconi G, Tonato M, Di Costanzo F, Leonardi F, Soldani M (1986) Randomized comparison of 5-FU alone or combined with carmustine, doxorubicin, and mitomycin (BAFMi) in the treatment of advanced gastric cancer: a phase III trial of the Italian Clinical Research Oncology Group (GOIRC). Cancer Treat Rep 70:481–485
17. Ohtsu A, Shimada Y, Shirao K, Boku N, Hyodo I, Saito H et al (2003) Randomized phase III trial of fluorouracil alone versus fluorouracil plus cisplatin versus uracil and tegafur plus mitomycin in patients with unresectable, advanced gastric cancer: the Japan Clinical Oncology Group Study (JCOG9205). J Clin Oncol 21:54–59
18. Al-Batran S-E, Hartmann JT, Probst S, Schmalenberg H, Hollerbach S, Hofheinz R et al (2008) Phase III trial in metastatic gastroesophageal adenocarcinoma with fluorouracil, leucovorin plus either oxaliplatin or cisplatin: a study of the Arbeitsgemeinschaft Internistische Onkologie. J Clin Oncol 26:1435–1442
19. Kang Y-K, Kang W-K, Shin D-B, Chen J, Xiong J, Wang J et al (2009) Capecitabine/cisplatin versus 5-fluorouracil/cisplatin as first-line therapy in patients with advanced gastric cancer: a randomised phase III noninferiority trial. Ann Oncol 20:666–673
20. Yamada Y, Higuchi K, Nishikawa K, Gotoh M, Fuse N, Sugimoto N et al (2015) Phase III study comparing oxaliplatin plus S-1 with cisplatin plus S-1 in chemotherapy-naïve patients with advanced gastric cancer. Ann Oncol 26:141–148
21. Al-Batran S-E, Homann N, Pauligk C, Goetze TO, Meiler J, Kasper S et al (2019) Perioperative chemotherapy with fluorouracil plus leucovorin, oxaliplatin, and docetaxel versus fluorouracil or capecitabine plus cisplatin and epirubicin for locally advanced, resectable gastric or gastro-oesophageal junction adenocarcinoma (FLOT4): a randomised, phase 2/3 trial. Lancet 393:1948–1957
22. Van Cutsem E, Moiseyenko VM, Tjulandin S, Majlis A, Constenla M, Boni C et al (2006) Phase III study of docetaxel and cisplatin plus fluorouracil compared with cisplatin and fluo-

rouracil as first-line therapy for advanced gastric cancer: a report of the V325 Study Group. J Clin Oncol 24:4991–4997

23. Yamada Y, Boku N, Mizusawa J, Iwasa S, Kadowaki S, Nakayama N et al (2019) Docetaxel plus cisplatin and S-1 versus cisplatin and S-1 in patients with advanced gastric cancer (JCOG1013): an open-label, phase 3, randomised controlled trial. Lancet Gastroenterol Hepatol 4:501–510
24. Enzinger PC, Burtness BA, Niedzwiecki D, Ye X, Douglas K, Ilson DH et al (2016) CALGB 80403 (Alliance)/E1206: a randomized phase II study of three chemotherapy regimens plus cetuximab in metastatic esophageal and gastroesophageal junction cancers. J Clin Oncol 34:2736–2742
25. Guimbaud R, Louvet C, Ries P, Ychou M, Maillard E, André T et al (2014) Prospective, randomized, multicenter, phase III study of fluorouracil, leucovorin, and irinotecan versus epirubicin, cisplatin, and capecitabine in advanced gastric adenocarcinoma: a French intergroup (Fédération Francophone de Cancérologie Digestive, Fédération Nationale des Centres de Lutte Contre le Cancer, and Groupe Coopérateur Multidisciplinaire en Oncologie) study. J Clin Oncol 32:3520–3526
26. Ford HER, Marshall A, Bridgewater JA, Janowitz T, Coxon FY, Wadsley J et al (2014) Docetaxel versus active symptom control for refractory oesophagogastric adenocarcinoma (COUGAR-02): an open-label, phase 3 randomised controlled trial. Lancet Oncol 15:78–86
27. Thuss-Patience PC, Kretzschmar A, Bichev D, Deist T, Hinke A, Breithaupt K et al (2011) Survival advantage for irinotecan versus best supportive care as second-line chemotherapy in gastric cancer—a randomised phase III study of the Arbeitsgemeinschaft Internistische Onkologie (AIO). Eur J Cancer 47:2306–2314
28. Hironaka S, Ueda S, Yasui H, Nishina T, Tsuda M, Tsumura T et al (2013) Randomized, open-label, phase III study comparing irinotecan with paclitaxel in patients with advanced gastric cancer without severe peritoneal metastasis after failure of prior combination chemotherapy using fluoropyrimidine plus platinum: WJOG 4007 trial. J Clin Oncol 31:4438–4444
29. Shitara K, Doi T, Dvorkin M, Mansoor W, Arkenau H-T, Prokharau A et al (2018) Trifluridine/tipiracil versus placebo in patients with heavily pretreated metastatic gastric cancer (TAGS): a randomised, double-blind, placebo-controlled, phase 3 trial. Lancet Oncol 19:1437–1448
30. Lieto E, Ferraraccio F, Orditura M, Castellano P, Mura AL, Pinto M et al (2008) Expression of vascular endothelial growth factor (VEGF) and epidermal growth factor receptor (EGFR) is an independent prognostic indicator of worse outcome in gastric cancer patients. Ann Surg Oncol 15:69–79
31. Ebos JML, Kerbel RS (2011) Antiangiogenic therapy: impact on invasion, disease progression, and metastasis. Nat Rev Clin Oncol 8:210–221
32. Maeda K, Chung YS, Ogawa Y, Takatsuka S, Kang SM, Ogawa M et al (1996) Prognostic value of vascular endothelial growth factor expression in gastric carcinoma. Cancer 77:858–863
33. Fuchs CS, Tomasek J, Yong CJ, Dumitru F, Passalacqua R, Goswami C et al (2014) Ramucirumab monotherapy for previously treated advanced gastric or gastro-oesophageal junction adenocarcinoma (REGARD): an international, randomised, multicentre, placebo-controlled, phase 3 trial. Lancet 383:31–39
34. Wilke H, Muro K, Van Cutsem E, Oh S-C, Bodoky G, Shimada Y et al (2014) Ramucirumab plus paclitaxel versus placebo plus paclitaxel in patients with previously treated advanced gastric or gastro-oesophageal junction adenocarcinoma (RAINBOW): a double-blind, randomised phase 3 trial. Lancet Oncol 15:1224–1235
35. Lorenzen S, Thuss-Patience PC, Pauligk C, Goekkurt E, Ettrich TJ, Lordick F et al (2020) FOLFIRI plus ramucirumab versus paclitaxel plus ramucirumab as second-line therapy for patients with advanced or metastatic gastroesophageal adenocarcinoma with or without prior docetaxel: results from the phase II RAMIRIS study of the AIO. JCO 38:4514
36. Klempner SJ, Maron SB, Chase L, Lomnicki S, Wainberg ZA, Catenacci DVT (2019) Initial report of second-line FOLFIRI in combination with ramucirumab in advanced gastroesophageal adenocarcinomas: a multi-institutional retrospective analysis. Oncologist 24:475–482

37. Fuchs CS, Shitara K, Di Bartolomeo M, Lonardi S, Al-Batran S-E, Van Cutsem E et al (2019) Ramucirumab with cisplatin and fluoropyrimidine as first-line therapy in patients with metastatic gastric or junctional adenocarcinoma (RAINFALL): a double-blind, randomised, placebo-controlled, phase 3 trial. Lancet Oncol 20:420–435
38. Yoshikawa T, Muro K, Shitara K, Oh D-Y, Kang Y-K, Chung HC et al (2019) Effect of first-line S-1 plus oxaliplatin with or without ramucirumab followed by paclitaxel plus ramucirumab on advanced gastric cancer in East Asia: the phase 2 RAINSTORM randomized clinical trial. JAMA Netw Open 2:e198243
39. Ohtsu A, Shah MA, Van Cutsem E, Rha SY, Sawaki A, Park SR et al (2011) Bevacizumab in combination with chemotherapy as first-line therapy in advanced gastric cancer: a randomized, double-blind, placebo-controlled phase III study. J Clin Oncol 29:3968–3976
40. Gravalos C, Jimeno A (2008) HER2 in gastric cancer: a new prognostic factor and a novel therapeutic target. Ann Oncol 19:1523–1529
41. Hecht JR, Bang Y-J, Qin SK, Chung HC, Xu JM, Park JO et al (2016) Lapatinib in combination with Capecitabine plus oxaliplatin in human epidermal growth factor receptor 2-positive advanced or metastatic gastric, esophageal, or gastroesophageal adenocarcinoma: TRIO-013/LOGiC—a randomized phase III trial. J Clin Oncol 34:443–451
42. Tabernero J, Hoff PM, Shen L, Ohtsu A, Shah MA, Cheng K et al (2018) Pertuzumab plus trastuzumab and chemotherapy for HER2-positive metastatic gastric or gastro-oesophageal junction cancer (JACOB): final analysis of a double-blind, randomised, placebo-controlled phase 3 study. Lancet Oncol 19:1372–1384
43. Satoh T, Xu R-H, Chung HC, Sun G-P, Doi T, Xu J-M et al (2014) Lapatinib plus paclitaxel versus paclitaxel alone in the second-line treatment of HER2-amplified advanced gastric cancer in Asian populations: TyTAN—a randomized, phase III study. J Clin Oncol 32:2039–2049
44. Thuss-Patience PC, Shah MA, Ohtsu A, Van Cutsem E, Ajani JA, Castro H et al (2017) Trastuzumab emtansine versus taxane use for previously treated HER2-positive locally advanced or metastatic gastric or gastro-oesophageal junction adenocarcinoma (GATSBY): an international randomised, open-label, adaptive, phase 2/3 study. Lancet Oncol 18:640–653
45. Janjigian YY, Sanchez-Vega F, Jonsson P, Chatila WK, Hechtman JF, Ku GY et al (2018) Genetic predictors of response to systemic therapy in esophagogastric cancer. Cancer Discov 8:49–58
46. Sanchez-Vega F, Hechtman JF, Castel P, Ku GY, Tuvy Y, Won H et al (2019) EGFR and MET amplifications determine response to HER2 inhibition in ERBB2-amplified esophagogastric cancer. Cancer Discov 9:199–209
47. Makiyama A, Sukawa Y, Kashiwada T, Kawada J, Hosokawa A, Horie Y et al (2020) Randomized, phase II study of trastuzumab beyond progression in patients with HER2-positive advanced gastric or gastroesophageal junction cancer: WJOG7112G (T-ACT study). J Clin Oncol 38:1919–1927
48. Ogitani Y, Aida T, Hagihara K, Yamaguchi J, Ishii C, Harada N et al (2016) DS-8201a, a novel HER2-targeting ADC with a novel DNA topoisomerase I inhibitor, demonstrates a promising antitumor efficacy with differentiation from T-DM1. Clin Cancer Res 22:5097–5108
49. Shitara K, Bang Y-J, Iwasa S, Sugimoto N, Ryu M-H, Sakai D et al (2020) Trastuzumab deruxtecan in previously treated HER2-positive gastric cancer. N Engl J Med 382:2419–2430
50. Meric-Bernstam F, Beeram M, Mayordomo JI, Hanna DL, Ajani JA, Blum Murphy MA et al (2018) Single agent activity of ZW25, a HER2-targeted bispecific antibody, in heavily pre-treated HER2-expressing cancers. JCO 36:2500
51. Catenacci DVT, Kang Y-K, Park H, Uronis HE, Lee K-W, Ng MCH et al (2020) Margetuximab plus pembrolizumab in patients with previously treated, HER2-positive gastro-oesophageal adenocarcinoma (CP-MGAH22-05): a single-arm, phase 1b-2 trial. Lancet Oncol 21:1066–1076
52. Gambardella V, Fleitas T, Tarazona N, Cejalvo JM, Gimeno-Valiente F, Martinez-Ciarpaglini C et al (2019) Towards precision oncology for HER2 blockade in gastroesophageal adenocarcinoma. Ann Oncol 30:1254–1264

53. Fuchs CS, Doi T, Jang RW, Muro K, Satoh T, Machado M et al (2018) Safety and efficacy of pembrolizumab monotherapy in patients with previously treated advanced gastric and gastroesophageal junction cancer: phase 2 clinical KEYNOTE-059 trial. JAMA Oncol 4:e180013
54. Shitara K, Özgüroğlu M, Bang Y-J, Di Bartolomeo M, Mandalà M, Ryu M-H et al (2018) Pembrolizumab versus paclitaxel for previously treated, advanced gastric or gastro-oesophageal junction cancer (KEYNOTE-061): a randomised, open-label, controlled, phase 3 trial. Lancet 392:123–133
55. Shitara K, Van Cutsem E, Bang Y-J, Fuchs C, Wyrwicz L, Lee K-W et al (2020) Efficacy and safety of pembrolizumab or pembrolizumab plus chemotherapy vs chemotherapy alone for patients with first-line, advanced gastric cancer: the KEYNOTE-062 phase 3 randomized clinical trial. JAMA Oncol 6:1571–1580
56. Kang Y-K, Boku N, Satoh T, Ryu M-H, Chao Y, Kato K et al (2017) Nivolumab in patients with advanced gastric or gastro-oesophageal junction cancer refractory to, or intolerant of, at least two previous chemotherapy regimens (ONO-4538-12, ATTRACTION-2): a randomised, double-blind, placebo-controlled, phase 3 trial. Lancet 390:2461–2471
57. Boku N, Ryu MH, Oh D-Y, Oh SC, Chung HC, Lee K-W et al (2020) LBA7_PR nivolumab plus chemotherapy versus chemotherapy alone in patients with previously untreated advanced or recurrent gastric/gastroesophageal junction (G/GEJ) cancer: ATTRACTION-4 (ONO-4538-37) study. Ann Oncol 31:S1192
58. Moehler M, Shitara K, Garrido M, Salman P, Shen L, Wyrwicz L et al (2020) LBA6_PR nivolumab (nivo) plus chemotherapy (chemo) versus chemo as first-line (1L) treatment for advanced gastric cancer/gastroesophageal junction cancer (GC/GEJC)/esophageal adenocarcinoma (EAC): first results of the CheckMate 649 study. Ann Oncol 31:S1191
59. Janjigian YY, Maron SB, Chatila WK, Millang B, Chavan SS, Alterman C et al (2020) First-line pembrolizumab and trastuzumab in HER2-positive oesophageal, gastric, or gastro-oesophageal junction cancer: an open-label, single-arm, phase 2 trial. Lancet Oncol 21:821–831
60. Rha SY, Lee C, Kim HS, Kang B, Jung M, Kwon WS et al (2021) A multi-institutional phase Ib/II trial of first-line triplet regimen (pembrolizumab, trastuzumab, chemotherapy) for HER2-positive advanced gastric and gastroesophageal junction cancer (PANTHERA trial): molecular profiling and clinical update. JCO 39:218
61. Chung HC, Bang Y-J, Fuchs CS, Qin S-K, Satoh T, Shitara K, et al (2021) First-line pembrolizumab/placebo plus trastuzumab and chemotherapy in HER2-positive advanced gastric cancer: KEYNOTE-811. Future Oncol (Future Med 2020). Available from: https://doi.org/10.2217/fon-2020-0737
62. Le DT, Durham JN, Smith KN, Wang H, Bartlett BR, Aulakh LK et al (2017) Mismatch repair deficiency predicts response of solid tumors to PD-1 blockade. Science 357:409–413
63. André T, Shiu K-K, Kim TW, Jensen BV, Jensen LH, Punt C et al (2020) Pembrolizumab in microsatellite-instability-high advanced colorectal cancer. N Engl J Med 383:2207–2218

Perspective on the Immunotherapy of Gastric Cancer

Yohei Kubota, Akihito Kawazoe, and Kohei Shitara

Contents

Y. Kubota · A. Kawazoe
Department of Gastrointestinal Medical Oncology, National Cancer Center Hospital East, Kashiwa, Chiba, Japan

K. Shitara (✉)
Department of Gastrointestinal Medical Oncology, National Cancer Center Hospital East, Kashiwa, Chiba, Japan

Department of Gastroenterology and Gastrointestinal Oncology, National Cancer Center Hospital East, Kashiwa, Chiba, Japan
e-mail: kshitara@east.ncc.go.jp

Cancer Immunotherapy (2021)
https://doi.org/10.1007/13905_2021_5,
Published Online: 25 August 2021

Abstract

Recently, immune checkpoint inhibitors (ICIs) have emerged as new standard treatment in various cancer types including advanced gastric cancer (AGC), showing favor clinical benefit in some population. More recently, ICIs combined with cytotoxic agents or molecular targeted agents also have emerged as promising strategies in some cancer types, and results of some pivotal trials of combined therapies with ICIs plus standard chemotherapy for AGC patients were also shown. Furthermore, various therapies related to immunotherapy are under verification in AGC, including new treatments such as oncolytic therapy, photoimmunotherapy, chimeric antigen receptor T (CAR-T) cell therapies, and bispecific T-cell engagers (BiTEs). This chapter will mainly introduce future perspective on the immunotherapy of AGC, including biomarkers and novel combination therapies.

Keywords

Biomarkers of immunotherapy · Combined immunotherapy · Gastric cancer · Immune checkpoint inhibitors · Immunotherapy

1 Biomarkers of ICIs in Gastric Cancer

1.1 PD-L1 CPS

No predictive value of PD-L1 expression on tumor cells was observed in the phase III ATTRACTION-2 of nivolumab and the phase III JAVELIN 300 of avelumab [1, 2], which is consistent with the subgroup analyses in CheckMate 649 and ATTRACTION-4 [3, 4].

Based on the results of several phase II and phase III trials, one of possible biomarkers for ICIs is PD-L1 combined positive score (CPS), which was defined as number of PD-L1-positive cells including tumor cells, macrophages, and lymphocytes divided by the total number of tumor cells, multiplied by 100. In the phase II KEYNOTE-059 of pembrolizumab as a third or later-line treatment in patients with AGC, the objective response rate (ORR) was 11.6% in the entire population [5]. In the third-line setting, ORR was 15.5% for patients with PD-L1-positive tumors (CPS ≥1) as determined by the pharmDx immunohistochemistry assay (PD-L1 IHC 22 C3; Agilent Technologies), while ORR was 6.4% for those with PD-L1-negative tumor (CPS <1), resulting in the FDA approval of pembrolizumab for PD-L1-positive AGC and PD-L1 22C3 IHC as a companion diagnostic assay. Although KEYNOTE-061 and 062 did not show significant improvement of OS with pembrolizumab compared with first- or second-line chemotherapy, a correlation between higher PD-L1 CPS and higher treatment effect was suggested [6, 7]. Moreover, patients with PD-L1 CPS <1 tumor showed worse survival with pembrolizumab than that of chemotherapy in the KEYNOTE-061, which suggest CPS is a negative marker to exclude patients without benefit of pembrolizumab. An update results of KEYNOTE-061 demonstrated that ORRs of pembrolizumab in patients with CPS ≥10, CPS ≥5, CPS ≥1 and CPS <1 tumor were 25%, 20%, 16%, and 2%, respectively [8]. In addition, a higher CPS determined by PD-L1 IHC 28-8 pharmDx assay (Dako) was associated with favorable efficacy of nivolumab with chemotherapy for AGC patients in the CheckMate 649 [3] (see detail in Sect. 3.1). Regarding the difference in frequency, the prevalence of CPS ≥5 was about 30% using PD-L1 IHC 22C3 pharmDx assay in KEYNOTE-061, whereas it was about 50–60% using PD-L1 IHC 28-8 pharmDx assay in the CheckMate 649 and CheckMate 032 [3, 6, 9]. Further investigations are needed to clarify the difference between IHC antibodies for CPS evaluation.

1.2 Microsatellite Instability-High

The prevalence of microsatellite instability-high/mismatch repair deficiency (MSI-H/MMR-D) is approximately 3–6% of stage IV AGC [3, 7, 10, 11]. As shown in TCGA 2014 and ACRG 2015 reports, the MSI-H subtype shows elevated mutation rates (including frameshifts or missense mutations) and hypermethylation (including hypermethylation at the MLH1 promoter), which result in the enhanced expression of neoantigens [12, 13]. MSI-H/MMR-D tumors showed hypermutation loads and displayed high infiltration with CD8+ T cells presumably due to the recognition enhanced tumor neoantigens and its corresponding expression of immune checkpoints in the tumor microenvironment [14].

According to the higher ORR and durable response in several trials [15–17], FDA approved pembrolizumab for patients with previously treated MSI-H/MMR-D solid tumors including AGC. In the phase II KEYNOTE-158 trial of pembrolizumab for MSI-H/MMR-D tumors, the ORR was 46.2% (6 of 13 patients) in AGC patients [15]. Consistent efficacies of pembrolizumab for AGC patients with MSI-H/MMR-D were also demonstrated in the subgroup analyses of KEYNOTE-059, KEYNOTE-061, and KEYNOTE-062 trials: the ORR was 57%, 47%, and 57%, respectively [5–7]. MSI-H/MMR-D is one of the most consistent predictive biomarkers for ICIs. However, considering that approximately half of MSI-H/MMR-D patients did not respond to ICIs, further biomarker analysis is needed in the future.

1.3 Tumor Mutation Burden

It has been reported that tumor mutation burden (TMB)-high is a predictive biomarker for ICIs across several cancer types [18]. In the phase II KEYNOTE-158 trial of pembrolizumab, patients with TMB-H solid tumors (≥10 mut/Mb determined by FoundationOne CDx™ assay) showed higher ORR of 29% (28% after excluding MSI-H vs. non-TMB-high 6%) and higher 6-, 12-, and 24-months PFS rates compared with non-TMB-high tumors, which led to approval of pembrolizumab by FDA for patients with TMB-H solid tumors [19]. In an exploratory analysis of KEYNOTE-061, a stronger association between TMB-high and favorable clinical efficacy with pembrolizumab compared to PD-L1 CPS was observed, which was maintained after exclusion of MSI-H patients [20, 21]. An exploratory analysis of KEYNOTE-062 also suggested the association between TMB-high and better clinical outcome with pembrolizumab or pembrolizumab plus chemotherapy although impact of TMB after exclusion of MSI-H was not reported [22]. Impact of TMB on the efficacies of ICIs for AGC patients' needs further evaluations in pivotal clinical trials.

1.4 Epstein–Barr Virus (EBV)

The prevalence of EBV is approximately 5% of stage IV AGC [10, 11]. EBV-positive AGC shows higher infiltration with CD8+ T cells and mature dendritic cells compared with EBV-negative AGC [10]. As shown in the TCGA report, amplification of the CD274 gene (which encodes PD-L1) and the PDCD1LG2 gene (which encodes PD-L2) was frequently observed in EBV-positive AGC [12]. Based on these clinicopathological features, EBV-positive AGC was considered to be potentially sensitive to ICIs. Actually, high ORR (25–100%) of ICIs has been reported in several small studies [11, 23, 24], which warrants further investigations in larger cohorts.

1.5 Others

1.5.1 Hyperprogressive Disease

Several studies in various cancer types have reported that anti-PD-1/PD-L1 antibodies cause hyperprogressive disease (HPD), which is characterized as an unexpected and rapid tumor progression [25, 26]. It was reported that clinical features such as ECOG PS of 1 or more, liver metastasis and a large tumor size at baseline were predictive factors of HPD in AGC after nivolumab treatment [25], meanwhile another report showed no clinical features which predicted HPD [26]. It has been also reported in preclinical study that PD-1 blockade amplifies not only PD-1 positive effector T cells but also PD-1 positive regulatory T cells which result in HPD [27]. In connection with this, the PD-1 expression balance between effector and regulatory T cells has been reported to be useful to predict efficacy of PD-1 blockade [28]. Because HPD has been suggested to cause poor prognoses, further investigations are important to identify predictive factors of HPD.

1.5.2 Gene Expression Signatures

Several studies have indicated that gene expression profiling may predict the efficacy of ICIs in some cancer types [29]. An exploratory analysis of KETNOTE-012 of pembrolizumab suggested interferon γ gene expression score might be associated with the response although it was not statistically significant [30]. CheckMate 032 also demonstrated that an immune gene signature score was associated with response to ICIs [31]. Recently, it has been reported that the burden of copy-number alterations (CNAs) was a superior predictor of ICI in gastrointestinal (GI) cancer compared with other signatures such as PD-L1, MSI, and TMB [32]. It might be result from association between somatic CNA levels and cytotoxic immune cell infiltration. It has been also demonstrated that high alternate promoter utilization was associated with lower T-cell cytolytic activity and lower response rates in AGC patients treated with ICIs [33]. These biomarkers are better to be further investigated in larger studies.

2 Combined Immunotherapy

2.1 ICIs Plus Chemotherapy

Recently, results of three pivotal phase III studies (KEYNOTE-062, ATTRACTION-4, and CheckMate 649) have been reported, which investigated the efficacy of anti-PD-1 antibodies in combination with fluoropyrimidine and platinum-based chemotherapy for AGC in first-line setting. In KEYNOTE-062 trial, chemotherapy in combination with pembrolizumab was not superior to chemotherapy alone for OS in both CPS ≥1 and CPS ≥10 populations [7]. In ATTRACTION-4, nivolumab plus chemotherapy showed statistically superiority for progression free survival (PFS) (HR 0.68; $p < 0.001$) but not OS (HR 0.90; $p = 0.26$) compared with chemotherapy alone in Asian countries without patient selection based on PD-L1 expression [4]. Meanwhile, in CheckMate 649, nivolumab plus chemotherapy improved both OS (median 14.4 vs. 11.1 months; HR 0.71; $p < 0.0001$) and PFS (median 7.7 vs. 6.0 months; HR 0.68; $p < 0.0001$) compared with chemotherapy alone in patients with PD-L1 CPS ≥5. Statistically significant OS benefit was also observed in patients with PD-L1 CPS ≥1 (median 14.0 vs. 11.3 months; HR 0.77; $p < 0.0001$) and the all-randomized population (median 13.8 vs. 11.6 months; HR 0.80; $p = 0.0002$) [3]. A higher proportion of patients in control arm receiving subsequent therapy in ATTRACTION-4 (68% including 27% with anti-PD-1 therapy) than in CheckMate 649 (41% including 8% with anti-PD-1 therapy) might blur positive effects on OS in ATTRACTION-4. These results are expected to change the standard of care in first-line setting for AGC.

2.2 ICI Doublet: Anti-PD-1/PD-L1 Antibody Plus Anti-CTLA4 Antibody

Cytotoxic T lymphocyte antigen 4 (CTLA-4), a key immune checkpoint other than the PD-1/PD-L1 axis, restricts the antitumor immune response. Anti-CTLA-4 antibody exerts anti-tumor activity during initial stage of cancer-immunity cycles; it binds to CTLA-4 on activated T cells or regulatory T cells (Tregs; one of the immune suppressive cells) and prevents T cell inactivation in lymph nodes [34–36]. Meanwhile, anti-PD-1/PD-L1 antibodies inhibit T cell inactivation in tumor tissue during effector stage [34–36]. Although ipilimumab (anti-CTLA4 antibody) monotherapy as maintenance after first-line chemotherapy did not improve immune-related PFS of AGC patients [37], the combination therapy with anti-PD-1/PD-L1 antibody plus anti-CTLA-4 antibody was considered to have synergistic effect because of the differences in action mechanism between two antibodies. Actually, the combination therapy with ipilimumab (anti-CTLA-4 antibody) and nivolumab (anti-PD-1 antibody) demonstrated anti-tumor activities in other cancer types, leading to FDA approval of this combination for metastatic melanoma, renal cell carcinoma, non-small cell lung carcinoma, malignant pleural mesothelioma, and metastatic colorectal cancer with MMR-D/MSI-H [38–42].

In the AGC cohort of the phase I/II CheckMate 032 trial, ORR was higher in nivolumab (1 mg/kg) plus ipilimumab (3 mg/kg) group compared with nivolumab (3 mg/kg) plus ipilimumab (1 mg/kg) group and nivolumab (3 mg/kg) group (24%, 8% and 12%, respectively) [43] although grade 3 or worse treatment related adverse events (TRAEs) were higher in nivolumab (1 mg/kg) plus ipilimumab (3 mg/kg) group (47%, 27%, and 17%, respectively). According to this result, the phase III CheckMate 649 trial included nivolumab (1 mg/kg) plus ipilimumab (3 mg/kg) cohort, but the enrollment of this arm was closed earlier. Detailed results of this combination in this trial are awaited in the future. Another combination therapy with durvalumab (anti-PD-L1 antibody) and tremelimumab (anti-CTLA-4 antibody) did not show higher ORR compared with monotherapy [44].

2.3 Anti-HER2 Antibody Plus Immune Checkpoint Inhibitors

Preclinical studies indicated that anti-HER2 antibody upregulated PD-1 or PD-L1 and enhanced HER2-specific T-cell responses [45–47], which could augment the efficacy of ICIs. Phase II trials, evaluating the efficacy of first-line chemotherapy plus trastuzumab combined with pembrolizumab, showed promising results with ORR of 76.7–91% and median PFS of 8.6–13.0 months [48, 49], which warrants further evaluation in an ongoing phase III KEYNOTE-811 trial (NCT03615326). Furthermore, a phase II trial of margetuximab (an Fc-optimized, anti-HER2 monoclonal antibody) plus pembrolizumab in second-line setting demonstrated favorable results with ORR of 24% and DCR of 62% in AGC patients with HER2 IHC3+ tumor [50]. A phase II/III MAHOGANY trial (NCT04082364), evaluating the efficacy of combination therapy including margetuximab plus anti-PD1 antibody arm, is undergoing.

Recently, trastuzumab deruxtecan (T-DXd), a next-generation antibody-drug conjugate composed of an anti-HER2 antibody and a topoisomerase I inhibitor, demonstrated survival benefit in HER2 positive trastuzumab treated AGC patients compared with standard chemotherapy (irinotecan or paclitaxel) [51]. In mouse model, T-DXd enhanced anti-tumor immunity: T-DXd increased expression markers of dendritic cells, enhanced expression of MHC class I on tumor cells, and contributed to enhancement of tumor recognition by T cells [52]. A phase Ib/II DESTINY-Gastric03 trial (NCT04379596) of several T-DXd combination therapies including T-DXd and durvalumab is underway.

2.4 ICIs and VEGF Inhibitors

In addition to activation of tumor angiogenesis, the vascular endothelial growth factor (VEGF) pathway contributes to suppression of anti-tumor immunity: (1) suppression of maturation of dendritic cells and effector T cells, (2) prevention of migration of effector T cells, (3) promotion of immune suppressive cells such as Tregs, tumor-associated macrophages (TAMs), and myeloid-derived suppressor cells (MDSCs) [53–55]. These suppressions of anti-tumor immunity might reduce anti-tumor activity of ICIs. Also, Treg or TAMs have been reported to be associated with hyperprogressive disease (HPD) during anti-PD-1 antibody [56, 57]. Therefore, ICIs combined with VEGF inhibitors might not only enhanced anti-tumor activity but also reduced HPD.

Ramucirumab is a fully human monoclonal antibody which selectively inhibits the vascular endothelial growth factor receptor 2 (VEGFR-2) and blocks the VEGFR signaling pathways. A phase I/II study of nivolumab plus ramucirumab as a second line treatment for AGC patients demonstrated favorable results with ORR of 26.7% and median PFS (mPFS) of 2.9 months [58]. Similarly, pembrolizumab plus ramucirumab showed anti-tumor activity with ORR of 25% and mPFS with 5.3 months in a first line setting in the AGC cohort of a phase Ia/b trial for solid tumors [59, 60]. A phase Ia/b study of durvalumab plus ramucirumab as second or later line treatment also demonstrated clinical activity with ORR of 21% and mPFS of 2.6 months in the AGC cohort [61]. Moreover, a phase I/II study of nivolumab combined with ramucirumab plus paclitaxel as second line treatment also showed that ORR was 37.2% and 6-month PFS rate was 46.5% for AGC patients in a second-line setting [62].

Most recently, anti-PD-1 antibodies in combination with multi-kinase inhibitors of VEGF receptors and other receptor tyrosine kinases such as regorafenib or lenvatinib also demonstrated promising results for AGC patients [63, 64]. A phase Ib trial of regorafenib plus nivolumab showed that ORR was 44% and median PFS was 5.6 months for AGC patients [63]. Furthermore, 3 of 7 AGC patients refractory to previous PD-1 targeting therapy achieved response with regorafenib plus nivolumab, which support the concept of overcoming resistance of anti-PD-1 targeting therapy using regorafenib. A phase II trial of lenvatinib plus pembrolizumab demonstrated promising anti-tumor activity with ORR of 69% and median PFS of 7.1 months for AGC patients in first- or second-line setting [64], meanwhile another phase II trial (LEAP-005) of lenvatinib plus pembrolizumab showed ORR of only 10% in AGC cohort [65]. These trials were non-randomized phase I/II trials with small sample size, thus the efficacy results are preliminary in nature. Therefore, a further phase III (NCT04662710) is needed to investigate the efficacy of these combinations.

2.5 ICIs and Local Therapies

One of the mechanisms of poor response to ICIs is considered to be lack of CD8+ T cells inside the tumor [66, 67]. Therefore, combined therapy to alter tumor-immune microenvironment to increase CD8+ T cell infiltration within the tumor may improve the anti-tumor effect of ICIs.

Recently, local therapies such as oncolytic therapy and photoimmunotherapy have been developing. The therapies are expected to not only show anti-tumor activity to local lesions by themselves but also increase tumor antigen-specific CD8+ T cells in both the primary tumor and metastatic lesions, which might contribute to synergic effects with ICIs [68]. Actually, a phase Ib clinical trial of oncolytic virotherapy with talimogene laherparepvec combined with pembrolizumab for metastatic melanoma showed higher anti-tumor activity with ORR of 62% [69]. In this study, responders to the combination therapy showed increased CD8+ T cells, elevated PD-L1 expression, and IFN-g gene expression on several cell subsets in tumors after oncolytic virotherapy. Similar strategy has been developing in AGC. Several oncolytic viruses including telomelysin (OB-301) have been identified in previous studies for possible anti-cancer treatments for AGC [70, 71]. Telomelysin is an attenuated adenovirus 5 vector, in which selectively replicate in cancer cells by introducing human telomerase reverse transcriptase (hTERT) promoter. In a preclinical study, telomelysin showed selective replication and antitumor effect in human cancer cells in vitro and in vivo [71]. A phase I study of telomelysin for various tumors showed acceptable safety profile [72], and a phase II study of telomelysin plus pembrolizumab for esophagogastric adenocarcinoma is undergoing (NCT03921021).

Near infrared photoimmunotherapy (NIR-PIT) is a newly developed, molecular targeted cancer therapy based on conjugating a near infrared silica-phthalocyanine dye to a monoclonal antibody, which result in necrotic cell death of targeted cancer cell immediately after exposure to near infrared light. Meanwhile, PD-1 blockade reverses adaptive immune resistance, resulting in activation of tumor infiltrating lymphocyte after NIR-PIT in syngeneic mouse models [73]. A phase IIa trial of NIR-PIT with ASP-1929 (anti-EGFR antibody cetuximab conjugated to IRDye 700DX) demonstrated a favor results with ORR of 50% for recurrent head and neck squamous cell carcinoma [74], which lead to the accelerated approval and a further evaluation in a phase III trial for head and neck squamous cell carcinoma (NCT03769506). A phase Ib study investigating the safety and efficacy of the NIR-PIT using ASP-1929 in combination with nivolumab for AGC or esophageal cancer (GE-PIT study) is undergoing [75] (JapicCTI-194969).

2.6 ICIs and Other Targeted Agents

2.6.1 ICI and PARP Inhibitor

Olaparib, an oral poly (adenosine diphosphate-ribose) polymerase (PARP) inhibitor, demonstrated anti-tumor activity for patients with advanced BRCA-mutated ovarian cancer and breast cancer. In a phase III trial (GOLD), olaparib plus paclitaxel did not demonstrate OS benefit compared with paclitaxel plus placebo in patients with ATM protein negative GC [76]. Meanwhile, preclinical studies indicated that PARP inhibitors could induce an anti-tumor immune response [77, 78], which suggests synergic effect in combination with ICIs. However, in a phase II trial of olaparib and durvalumab (anti-PD-L1 antibody), obvious synergistic effect was not shown (ORR 10% and DCR at 12 weeks 25%), which might result from a high rate of early disease progression following olaparib monotherapy for initial 4 weeks [79]. Several trials of combination therapy with olaparib and ICIs for AGC patients are undergoing (NCT03579784, NCT04209686).

2.6.2 ICI and DKN-01

DKN-01 is a novel humanized monoclonal antibody targeting the DKK1 protein, which regulates Wnt/beta-catenin signaling and contributes to an immune suppressive tumor microenvironment. A phase I/II study (KEYNOTE-731) showed promising anti-tumor activity with ORR of 50% and DCR of 80% in ten patients with DKK1-high and PD-1/PD-L1 naïve AGC patients [80, 81]. A phase II study of DKN-01 in combination with tislelizumab ± chemotherapy in AGC patients is ongoing (NCT04363801).

2.7 Others (CAR-T and BiTEs)

Recently, chimeric antigen receptor T (CAR-T) cell therapies have been urgently developed in solid tumors as well as hematological malignancy. CAR-T cells have been genetically engineered to recognize a specific antigen on cancer cells and selectively kill tumor cells [82, 83]. In CAR-T cell therapy, it is important to select appropriate antigens that exist on tumor cells but not on healthy cells. Possible antigens for CAR-T cell therapy in GC include HER2, mucin1, CEA, claudin18.2, and EPCAM [84]. Recently, a preclinical study indicated that partial or complete tumor elimination was observed in claudin18.2-positive GC patient-derived tumor xenograft models treated with Claudin18.2-specific CAR T cells [85], which warrants further investigation of another phase I studies (NCT04467853, NCT04404595). Meanwhile, CAR-T cells are thought to be reversibly inactivated by multiple mechanisms including the expression of immune checkpoint receptors such as PD1, LAG3, TIM3, and 2B4 [86]. Therefore, ICIs may show to enhance the effect of CAR-T cell therapies.

Bispecific T-cell engagers (BiTEs) are recombinant bispecific monoclonal antibodies without genetic alteration of the T cells which can bind to two antigens simultaneously. BiTEs connect patients' own T cells to malignant cells, which lead T cells' activation and anti-tumor effect [87]. In AGC, phase I studies of BiTEs targeting MUC17 and Claudin18.2 are undergoing (NCT20180290, NCT 04260191).

3 Conclusion

The efficacy of ICI monotherapy for AGC is limited with ORR of approximately 10% without patient's enrichment by biomarkers. Therefore, biomarker research or development of combined therapies expected to have synergistic effect is important to maximize the efficacy of immunotherapy. At this moment, possible biomarkers for ICIs in AGC include CPS, TMB, MSI, and EBV. The combination therapy with ICI plus standard chemotherapy in a first-line setting showed clinical benefit in AGC, which will be a new standard treatment in the near future. Other combination therapies such as ICI doublet, ICI plus anti-HER2 antibody, or anti-VEGF might be promising treatments, which warrants further investigations. It is also important to investigate appropriate treatment sequence, or to clarify the exact changes of tumor microenvironment on immunotherapy or combinations to consider optimal treatments for AGC patients in future.

Compliance with Ethical Standards

Conflicts of Interest Y.K. has no competing interests.

A.K. reports grants and personal fees from Taiho, grants and personal fees from Ono, grants from Sumitomo Dainippon, grants from MSD, outside the submitted work.

K.S. reports paid consulting or advisory roles for Astellas, Eli Lilly, Bristol-Myers Squibb, Takeda, Pfizer, Ono Pharmaceutical, MSD, Taiho, Novartis, AbbVie, and GSK; honoraria from Novartis, AbbVie, and Yakult; and research funding from Astellas, Eli Lilly, Ono Pharmaceutical, Sumitomo Dainippon Pharma, Daiichi Sankyo, Taiho, Chugai, MSD, and Medi Science, outside the submitted work.

Informed Consent Not applicable.

References

1. Kang YK et al (2017) Nivolumab in patients with advanced gastric or gastro-oesophageal junction cancer refractory to, or intolerant of, at least two previous chemotherapy regimens (ONO-4538-12, ATTRACTION-2): a randomised, doubleblind, placebo-controlled, phase 3 trial. Lancet 390:2461–2471
2. Bang YJ et al (2018) Phase III, randomised trial of avelumab versus physician's choice of chemotherapy as third-line treatment of patients with advanced gastric or gastro-oesophageal junction cancer: primary analysis of JAVELIN Gastric 300. Ann Oncol 29:2052–2060
3. Moehler M et al (2020) Nivolumab (NIVO) plus chemotherapy (chemo) versus chemo as first-line (1L) treatment for advanced gastric cancer/gastroesophageal junction cancer (GC/GEJC)/esophageal adenocarcinoma (EAC): first results of the CheckMate 649 study. In: ESMO virtual congress 2020. #LBA6_PR
4. Boku N et al (2020) Nivolumab plus chemotherapy versus chemotherapy alone in patients with previously untreated advanced or recurrent gastric/gastroesophageal junction (G/GEJ) cancer: ATTRACTION-4 (ONO-4538-37) study. In: ESMO virtual congress 2020. #LBA7_PR
5. Fuchs CS et al (2018) Safety and efficacy of pembrolizumab monotherapy in patients with previously treated advanced gastric and gastroesophageal junction cancer: phase 2 clinical KEYNOTE-059 trial. JAMA Oncol 4:e180013
6. Shitara K et al (2018) Pembrolizumab versus paclitaxel for previously treated, advanced gastric or gastro-oesophageal junction cancer (KEYNOTE-061): a randomised, open-label, controlled, phase 3 trial. Lancet 392:123–133
7. Shitara K et al (2020) Efficacy and safety of pembrolizumab or pembrolizumab plus chemotherapy vs chemotherapy alone for patients with first-line, advanced gastric cancer: the KEYNOTE-062 phase 3 randomized clinical trial. JAMA Oncol 6:1571–1580

8. Fuchs S et al (2020) Pembrolizumab versus paclitaxel for previously treated patients with PD-L1–positive advanced gastric or gastroesophageal junction cancer (GC): update from the phase III KEYNOTE-061 trial. J Clin Oncol 38(15):4503
9. Lei M et al (2019) Association of PD-L1 combined positive score and immune gene signatures with efficacy of nivolumab (NIVO) ± ipilimumab (IPI) in patients with metastatic gastroesophageal cancer (mGEC). In: AACR annual meeting 2019. Abstract 2673
10. Kawazoe A et al (2017) Clinicopathological features of programmed death ligand 1 expression with tumour-infiltrating lymphocyte, mismatch repair, and Epstein-Barr virus status in a large cohort of gastric cancer patients. Gastric Cancer 20:407–415
11. Kubota Y et al (2020) The impact of molecular subtype on efficacy of chemotherapy and checkpoint inhibition in advanced gastric cancer. Clin Cancer Res 26:3784–3790
12. The Cancer Genome Atlas Research Network (2014) Comprehensive molecular characterization of gastric adenocarcinoma. Nature 513:202–209
13. Cristescu R et al (2015) Molecular analysis of gastric cancer identifies subtypes associated with distinct clinical outcomes. Nat Med 21:449–456
14. Llosa NJ et al (2015) The vigorous immune microenvironment of microsatellite instable colon cancer is balanced by multiple counter-inhibitory checkpoints. Cancer Discov 5:43–51
15. Marabelle A et al (2020) Efficacy of Pembrolizumab in patients with non-colorectal high microsatellite instability/mismatch repair-deficient cancer: results from the phase II KEYNOTE-158 study. J Clin Oncol 38:1–10
16. Le DT et al (2015) PD-1 blockade in tumors with mismatch repair deficiency. N Engl J Med 372:2509–2520
17. Le DT et al (2017) Mismatch repair deficiency predicts response of solid tumors to PD-1 blockade. Science 357:409–413
18. Samstein RM et al (2019) Tumor mutational load predicts survival after immunotherapy across multiple cancer types. Nat Genet 51:202–206
19. Marabelle A et al (2020) Association of tumour mutational burden with outcomes in patients with advanced solid tumours treated with pembrolizumab: prospective biomarker analysis of the multicohort, open-label, phase 2 KEYNOTE-158 study. Lancet Oncol 21:1353–1365
20. Shitara K et al (2020) The association of tissue tumor mutational burden (tTMB) using the Foundation Medicine genomic platform with efficacy of pembrolizumab versus paclitaxel in patients (pts) with gastric cancer (GC) from KEYNOTE-061. J Clin Oncol 38(15):4537
21. Fuchs CS et al (2020) The association of molecular biomarkers with efficacy of pembrolizumab versus paclitaxel in patients with gastric cancer (GC) from KEYNOTE-061. J Clin Oncol 38(15):4512
22. Wyrwicz LS et al (2020) Association of TMB using the Foundation Medicine Companion Diagnostic (F1CDx) with efficacy of first-line pembrolizumab (pembro) or pembro plus chemotherapy (pembro + chemo) versus chemo in patients with gastric cancer (gc) from KEYNOTE-062. In: ESMO virtual congress 2020. 1442P
23. Kim ST et al (2018) Comprehensive molecular characterization of clinical responses to PD-1 inhibition in metastatic gastric cancer. Nat Med 24:1449–1458
24. Panda A et al (2018) Immune activation and benefit from avelumab in EBV-positive gastric cancer. J Natl Cancer Inst 110:316–320
25. Sasaki A et al (2019) Predictive factors for hyperprogression during nivolumab treatment in patients with advanced gastric cancer. Gastric Cancer 22:793–802
26. Aoki M et al (2019) Hyperprogressive disease during nivolumab or irinotecan treatment in patients with advanced gastric cancer. ESMO Open 4:e000488
27. Kamada T et al (2019) PD-1 + regulatory T cells amplified by PD-1 blockade promote hyperprogression of cancer. Proc Natl Acad Sci U S A 116:9999–10008
28. Kumagai S et al (2020) The PD-1 expression balance between effector and regulatory T cells predicts the clinical efficacy of PD-1 blockade therapies. Nat Immunol 21: 1346–1358

29. Tong M et al (2018) Predictive biomarkers for tumor immune checkpoint blockade. Cancer Manag Res 10:4501–4507
30. Muro K et al (2016) Pembrolizumab for patients with PD-L1 positive advanced gastric cancer (KEYNOTE-012): a multicentre, open-label, phase 1B trial. Lancet Oncol 17:717–726
31. Lei M et al (2019) Abstract 2673: association of PD-L1 combined positive score and immune gene signatures with efficacy of nivolumab (NIVO) ± ipilimumab (IPI) in patients with metastatic gastroesophageal cancer (mGEC). Cancer Res 79:2673
32. Zhihao L et al (2020) Tumor copy-number alterations predict response to immune-checkpoint-blockade in gastrointestinal cancer. J Immunother Cancer 8:e000374
33. Sundar R et al (2019) Epigenomic promoter alterations predict for benefit from immune checkpoint inhibition in metastatic gastric cancer. Ann Oncol 30:424–430
34. Wei SC et al (2018) Fundamental mechanisms of immune checkpoint blockade therapy. Cancer Discov 8:1069–1086
35. Daniel SC et al (2013) Oncology meets immunology: the cancer-immunity cycle. Immunity 39:1–10
36. Rotte A et al (2019) Combination of CTLA-4 and PD-1 blockers for treatment of cancer. J Exp Clin Cancer Res 38:255
37. Bang YJ et al (2017) Efficacy of sequential ipilimumab monotherapy versus best supportive care for unresectable locally advanced/metastatic gastric or gastroesophageal junction cancer. Clin Cancer Res 23:5671–5678
38. Larkin J et al (2019) Five-year survival with combined nivolumab and ipilimumab in advanced melanoma. N Engl J Med 381:1535–1546
39. Cella D et al (2019) Patient-reported outcomes of patients with advanced renal cell carcinoma treated with nivolumab plus ipilimumab versus sunitinib (CheckMate 214): a randomised, phase 3 trial. Lancet Oncol 20:297–310
40. Hellmann MD et al. (2019) Nivolumab plus Ipilimumab in Advanced Non-Small-Cell Lung Cancer. N Engl J Med 381:2020–2031
41. Baas P et al (2021) First-line nivolumab plus ipilimumab in unresectable malignant pleural mesothelioma (CheckMate 743): a multicentre, randomised, open-label, phase 3 trial. Lancet 397:375–386
42. Overman DMJ et al (2018) Durable Clinical Benefit With Nivolumab Plus Ipilimumab in DNA Mismatch Repair-Deficient/Microsatellite Instability-High Metastatic Colorectal Cancer. J Clin Oncol 36:773–779
43. Janjigian YY et al (2018) CheckMate-032 study: efficacy and safety of nivolumab and nivolumab plus ipilimumab in patients with metastatic esophagogastric cancer. J Clin Oncol 36:2836–2844
44. Kelly RJ et al (2020) Safety and efficacy of durvalumab and tremelimumab alone or in combination in patients with advanced gastric and gastroesophageal junction adenocarcinoma. Clin Cancer Res 26:846–854
45. Varadan V et al (2016) Immune signatures following single dose trastuzumab predict pathologic response to preoperative trastuzumab and chemotherapy in HER2-positive early breast cancer. Clin Cancer Res 22:3249–3259
46. Chaganty BKR et al (2018) Trastuzumab upregulates PD-L1 as a potential mechanism of trastuzumab resistance through engagement of immune effector cells and stimulation of IFNγ secretion. Cancer Lett 430:47–56
47. Taylor C et al (2007) Augmented HER-2 specific immunity during treatment with trastuzumab and chemotherapy. Clin Cancer Res 13:5133–5143
48. Janjigian YY et al (2020) First-line pembrolizumab and trastuzumab in HER2-positive oesophageal, gastric, or gastro-oesophageal junction cancer: an open-label, single-arm, phase 2 trial. Lancet Oncol 21:821–831
49. Rha SY et al (2020) Targeting HER2 in combination with anti-PD-1 and chemotherapy confers a significant tumor shrinkage of gastric cancer: a multi-institutional phase Ib/II trial of first-line triplet regimen (pembrolizumab, trastuzumab, chemotherapy) for HER2-positive advanced gastric cancer (AGC). J Clin Oncol 38(15):3081

50. Catenacci DVT et al (2020) Margetuximab plus pembrolizumab in patients with previously treated, HER2-positive gastro-oesophageal adenocarcinoma (CP-MGAH22-05): a single-arm, phase 1b-2 trial. Lancet Oncol 21:1066–1076
51. Shitara K et al (2020) Trastuzumab deruxtecan in previously treated HER2-positive gastric cancer. N Engl J Med 382:2419–2430
52. Iwata T et al (2018) A HER2-targeting antibody-drug conjugate, trastuzumab deruxtecan (DS-8201a), enhances anti-tumour immunity in a mouse model. Mol Cancer Ther 17:1494–1503
53. Ott PA et al (2015) Inhibition of immune checkpoints and vascular endothelial growth factor as combination therapy for metastatic melanoma: an overview of rationale, preclinical evidence, and initial clinical data. Front Oncol 5:202
54. Terme M et al (2013) VEGFA-VEGFR pathway blockade inhibits tumor-induced regulatory T-cell proliferation in colorectal cancer. Cancer Res 73:539–549
55. Roland CL et al (2009) Cytokine levels correlate with immune cell infiltration after anti-VEGF therapy in preclinical mouse models of breast cancer. PLoS One 4:e7669
56. Kamada T et al (2019) PD-1 + regulatory T cells amplified by PD-1 blockade promote hyper progression of cancer. Proc Natl Acad Sci U S A 116:9999–10008
57. Lo Russo G et al (2019) Antibody-fc/FcR interaction on macrophages as a mechanism for hyperprogressive disease in non-small cell lung cancer subsequent to PD-1/PD-L1 blockade. Clin Cancer Res 25:929–999
58. Hara H et al (2019) Phase I/II study of ramucirumab plus nivolumab in patients in second-line treatment for advanced gastric adenocarcinoma (NivoRam study). J Clin Oncol 37(4):129
59. Herbst RS et al (2019) Ramucirumab plus pembrolizumab in patients with previously treated advanced non-small-cell lung cancer, gastro-oesophageal cancer, or urothelial carcinomas (JVDF): a multicohort, non-randomised, open-label, phase 1a/b trial. Lancet Oncol 20:1109–1123
60. Chau I et al (2020) Ramucirumab in combination with pembrolizumab in treatment-naïve advanced gastric or GEJ adenocarcinoma: safety and antitumor activity from the phase 1a/b JVDF trial. Cancers (Basel) 12:2985
61. Bang YJ et al (2020) Ramucirumab and durvalumab for previously treated, advanced nonesmall-cell lung cancer, gastric/gastrooesophageal junction adenocarcinoma, or hepatocellular carcinoma: an open-label, phase Ia/b study. Eur J Cancer 137:272–284
62. Nakajima T et al (2020) Multicenter phase I/II study of nivolumab combined with paclitaxel plus ramucirumab as second-line treatment in patients with advanced gastric cancer. Clin Cancer Res. https://doi.org/10.1158/1078-0432.CCR-20-3559
63. Fukuoka S et al (2020) Regorafenib plus nivolumab in patients with advanced gastric or colorectal cancer: an open-label, dose-escalation, and dose-expansion phase Ib trial (REGONIVO, EPOC1603). J Clin Oncol 38:2053–2061
64. Kawazoe A et al (2020) Lenvatinib plus pembrolizumab in patients with advanced gastric cancer in the first-line or second-line setting (EPOC1706): an open-label, single-arm, phase 2 trial. Lancet Oncol 23:1057–1065
65. Lwin Z (2020) LEAP-005: phase II study of lenvatinib (len) plus pembrolizumab (pembro) in patients (pts) with previously treated advanced solid tumours. In: ESMO virtual congress 2020. Abstract LBA41
66. Pardoll DM et al (2012) The blockade of immune checkpoints in cancer immunotherapy. Nat Rev Cancer 12:252–264
67. Tumeh PC et al (2014) PD-1 blockade induces responses by inhibiting adaptive immune resistance. Nature 515:568–571
68. Ribas A et al (2017) Oncolytic virotherapy promotes intratumoral T cell infiltration and improves anti-PD-1 immunotherapy. Cell 170:1109–1119
69. Gujar S et al (2018) Antitumor benefits of antiviral immunity: an underappreciated aspect of oncolytic virotherapies. Trends Immunol 39:209–221
70. Yokoda R et al (2018) Oncolytic virotherapy in upper gastrointestinal tract cancers. Oncol Virother 7:13–24

71. Kawashima T et al (2004) Telomerase-specific replication-selective virotherapy for human cancer. Clin Cancer Res 10:285–292
72. Nemunaitis J et al (2010) A phase I study of telomerase-specific replication competent oncolytic adenovirus (telomelysin) for various solid tumors. Mol Ther 18:429–434
73. Nagaa T et al (2019) Host immunity following near-infrared photoimmunotherapy is enhanced with PD-1 checkpoint blockade to eradicate established antigenic tumors. Cancer Immunol Res 7:401–413
74. Cognetti DM et al (2019) Results of a phase 2a, multicenter, open-label, study of RM-1929 photoimmunotherapy (PIT) in patients with locoregional, recurrent head and neck squamous cell carcinoma (rHNSCC). J Clin Oncol 37(15):6014
75. Kadota T et al (2020) A phase Ib study of near infrared photoimmunotherapy (NIR-PIT) using ASP-1929 in combination with nivolumab and for patients with advanced gastric or esophageal cancer (GE-PIT study, EPOC1901). J Clin Oncol 38:4
76. Bang YJ et al (2017) Olaparib in combination with paclitaxel in patients with advanced gastric cancer who have progressed following first-line therapy (GOLD): a double-blind, randomised, placebo-controlled, phase 3 trial. Lancet Oncol 18:1637–1651
77. Hodgson DR et al (2018) Candidate biomarkers of PARP inhibitor sensitivity in ovarian cancer beyond the BRCA genes. Br J Cancer 119:1401–1409
78. Gay CM et al (2019) PARP inhibition combined with immune checkpoint blockade in SCLC: oasis in an immune desert or mirage. J Thorac Oncol 14:1323–1326
79. Bang YJ et al (2019) An open-label, phase II basket study of olaparib and durvalumab (MEDIOLA): results in patients with relapsed gastric cancer. J Clin Oncol 37:140
80. Klempner SJ et al (2020) DKN-01 in combination with pembrolizumab in patients with advanced gastroesophageal adenocarcinoma (GEA): tumoral DKK1 expression as a predictor of response and survival. J Clin Oncol 38:357
81. Leap therapeutics presents updated data at the ASCO 2020 gastrointestinal cancers symposium (ASCO GI) global meeting
82. Tian Y et al (2020) Gene modification strategies for next-generation CAR T cells against solid cancers. J Hematol Oncol 13:54
83. Martinez M et al (2019) CAR T cells for solid tumors: new strategies for finding, infiltrating, and surviving in the tumor microenvironment. Front Immunol 10:128. https://doi.org/10.3389/fimmu.2019.00128
84. Bębnowska D et al (2020) CAR-T cell therapy—an overview of targets in gastric cancer. J Clin Med 9:1894. https://doi.org/10.3390/jcm9061894
85. Jiang H et al (2019) Claudin18.2-specific chimeric antigen receptor engineered T cells for the treatment of gastric cancer. J Natl Cancer Inst 111:409–418
86. Edmund KM et al (2014) Multifactorial T-cell hypofunction that is reversible can limit the efficacy of chimeric antigen receptor-transduced human T cells in solid tumors. Clin Cancer Res 20:4262–4273
87. Einsele H et al (2020) The BiTE (bispecific T-cell engager) platform: development and future potential of a targeted immuno-oncology therapy across tumor types. Cancer 126:3192–3201

Part IV

Colon

Immunotherapy in dMMR/MSI-H Colon Cancer

Joseph Tintelnot and Alexander Stein

Contents

Abstract

Checkpoint inhibitors (e.g., PD1, PD-L1, or CTLA 4) have revolutionized the treatment algorithm of mismatch repair-deficient (dMMR) or microsatellite instability-high (MSI-H) metastatic colorectal cancer (MCRC). In 2017, two

J. Tintelnot
Department of Internal Medicine II (Oncology Center), University Medical Center Hamburg-Eppendorf, Hamburg, Germany

A. Stein (✉)
Department of Internal Medicine II (Oncology Center), University Medical Center Hamburg-Eppendorf, Hamburg, Germany

Hubertus Wald Tumorcenter—UCCH, University Medical Center Hamburg-Eppendorf, Hamburg, Germany

Hämatoonkologische Praxis Eppendorf, Hamburg, Germany
e-mail: stein@hope-hamburg.de; a.stein@uke.de

Cancer Immunotherapy (2021)
https://doi.org/10.1007/13905_2021_6,
Published Online: 25 August 2021

phase II studies revealed extraordinarily high overall response rates for single-agent PD1-antibodies in treatment-refractory colorectal cancer. Apart from treatment response, PD1-treatment resulted in a remarkable overall survival of 31.4 months. Recently, the phase III KN-177 study set the new standard for first line MCRC treatment by proving immunotherapy with pembrolizumab superior to investigators choice chemotherapy (doublet chemotherapy of FOLFIRI or FOLFOX with or without Bevacizumab or Cetuximab). The progression-free survival at 12 months was almost doubled compared to the former chemotherapy standard. In addition to this, checkpoint inhibitor combinations like PD1/PD-L1 and CTLA 4 showed promising early results in metastatic or resectabel colorectal cancer. Several studies are currently evaluating the benefit of checkpoint inhibitor combinations, checkpoint inhibitor chemotherapy combinations and/or the combination with other agents like anti-angiogenic antibodies. Only randomized controlled trials will tell us whether these combinations will even increase the efficacy of single agent immunotherapy in first line dMMR or MSI-H mCRC.

Keywords

CM-142 · dMMR/MSI-H · Immunotherapy · KN-16 · KN-177 · MCRC · Nivolumab · Pembrolizumab · POLE · TMB

1 Introduction

In colon cancer, the clinical use of checkpoint inhibitors is currently limited to a small subset of patients whose tumors have a high tumor mutational burden (TMB) and infiltration of T cells expressing checkpoint receptors (e.g., PD1, PD-L1, or CTLA 4) which is mainly found in the subset of mismatch repair-deficient (dMMR) or microsatellite instability-high (MSI-H) tumors [1–3]. The frequency of microsatellite instability (MSI-H) highly varies from 20% in stage I and II to only 4–5% in metastatic colorectal cancer (MCRC). One-third of MSI-H tumors is due to germline mutations in mismatch repair genes leading to hereditary non-polyposis colorectal cancer (HNPCC, Lynch Syndrome), the other two-thirds are due to sporadic and mostly (80–90%) epigenetic modification of the MLH1 promoter and are partly associated with BRAFV600E mutations [4]. By this insufficiency in DNA repair, double-strand breaks cannot be re-synthesized properly owing to the accumulation of somatic mutations. However, some mismatch repair proficient tumors even accumulate greater numbers of mutations due to polymerase proofreading domain mutations (POLE) and might be comparable in treatment response to MSI-H tumors [5, 6]. In 2017, extraordinary overall response rates (ORR) of 30–40% in two phase II studies, namely Keynote (KN)-16 (pembrolizumab) and Check-Mate (CM)-142 (nivolumab), led to the approval of both PD-1 inhibitors for the treatment of dMMR or MSI-H treatment-refractory MCRC in the United States (US).

2 Evidence for Immunotherapy in dMMR/MSI-H CRC

2.1 Monotherapy with PD-1 Inhibitors

Metastatic First data regarding the efficacy of immunotherapy in dMMR/MSI-H MCRC came from the phase II Keynote (KN)-16 trial testing pembrolizumab (anti-PD1) in different treatment refractory tumors. The first interim analysis showed an ORR of 40% in ten dMMR/MSI-H patients compared to 0% in proficient (pMMR/MSS) patients. Overall, this cohort included 40 dMMR/MSI-H MCRC patients and led to the first ever agnostic approval of a cancer drug in 2017 in the US [7]. Two other phase II studies added evidence for the efficacy of checkpoint inhibitor monotherapy in previously treated MSI-H MCRC patients, namely KN-164 (pembrolizumab) and Check-Mate (CM)-142 (nivolumab). An ORR of 31% in the CM-142 study and 28% in the KN-164 study and a progression free survival (PFS) of 50% or 34%, respectively, at 1-year was reached. Despite the slightly increased PFS interval in the KN-164 study, both studies revealed a comparable 1-year overall survival (OS) rate of 73% and 72% which also led to the approval of nivolumab in 2017 in the US [8]. The KN-164 study included two cohorts (A $\geq$ 1 therapy and B $\geq$ 2 therapies) with a comparable overall response rate (ORR) of 32.8% (A) and 34.9% (B). A recent update of this study showed a remarkable high median overall survival of 31.4 months (21.4-NR) with a 3-year OS rate of 49% in cohort A and an unreached median overall survival (19.2-NR) with a 3-year OS rate of 52% in cohort B [9]. Apart from these appealing results, there was a trend towards increased efficacy in early therapy lines comparing cohort B to A. Following up on this, the phase III KN-177 study compared the efficacy of first line pembrolizumab with investigators choice chemotherapy (doublet chemotherapy of FOLFIRI or FOLFOX with or without Bevacizumab or Cetuximab). Strikingly, PFS at 12 months was almost doubled with 55% (median OS 16.5 months) compared to 37% (median OS 8.5 months) and 48% compared to 19% at 24 months favoring pembrolizumab (HR 0.60 95% CI 0.45–0.80, $p = 0.0002$) [10]. As expected, pembrolizumab treatment had lower grade 3/4 adverse events (AEs) with 22% compared to 66% with diarrhea being the most prevalent. In contrast, 30% of patients directly progressed with pembrolizumab in the first staging, thus further evaluation on predictive factors is urgently required [10]. Response to pembrolizumab was irrespective of concurrent BRAFV600E mutations, but the subgroup of RAS mutated and left-sided tumors were not benefitting compared to standard of care. Although these preliminary results on subgroups need to be validated in other cohorts, understanding the tumor microenvironment of colorectal cancer mediated by sidedness or RAS mutation might be important to tailor therapy. Even though, a comparable PFS in RAS mutated or left-sided tumor patients might be also beneficial regarding better tolerability of pembrolizumab. Taken together, the outstanding PFS rates for first line single-agent pembrolizumab in dMMR/MSI-H MCRC patients within the KN-177 study will build the groundwork for a new standard of care.

In analogy to the results observed in dMMR/MSI-H MCRC, a recently published study testing nivolumab in pMMR/MSS, but POLE mutated and thus hypermutated tumors, showed comparable results for this subset of patients. In total 16 patients with colorectal, gastric, endometrial, pancreatic, glial or biliary tract tumors were treated with an ORR of 36% at 84 days. The study included a promising outlook for colorectal cancer patients with 1 CR, 3PR, 1 PD, and 1 non-evaluable patient, despite being preliminary due to the low patient numbers ($n = 6$; [11]) other studies like the POLEM trial (NCT 03827044) will further evaluate the susceptibility of POLE mutated tumors to checkpoint inhibitors (Table 1).

2.2 Combination of PD-1 and CTLA-4 Inhibitors

Neoadjuvant In the non-metastatic setting, 4 weeks of neoadjuvant treatment with nivolumab 3 mg/kg (day 1 and 15) and ipilimumab 1 mg/kg (day 1) was tested in 21 dMMR/MSI-H and 20 pMMR/MSS (stage II and III) colorectal cancer patients [12, 13]. All analyzed tumors from dMMR/MSI-H patients showed a pathological response with 19 major pathological responses (<10% viable tumor cells) and 12 complete responses (out of 21). In patients with pMMR/MSS tumors, 4 pathological responses (27%) with 3 major pathological responses and 1 partial response were observed. Despite these fascinating results, randomized comparison of immunotherapy and chemotherapy is still missing in the perioperative treatment of this subgroup with a very good overall prognosis. Several trials are ongoing.

Metastatic Evidence for the combination of nivolumab and ipilimumab in dMMR/MSI-H MCRC patients came from two cohorts of the CM-142 study. In the treatment refractory cohort, comprising 119 patients with at least two prior therapies (76%), an iORR of 55% and a 12-week disease control-rate of 80% were reported. Moreover, PFS rates of 71% and OS of 85% after 1-year were reached independent of KRAS or BRAF mutational status, PD-L1 expression on tumors or inherited family history of Lynch syndrome. Although no randomized data is currently available, an ORR of 55% and 1-year OS of 85% compares numerically favorable to an ORR of 31% and 1-year OS of 72% in single-agent PD-1 inhibitor treatment. Despite the expected increase in treatment-related grade 3 to 4 AEs that occurred in 32% of all patients, all AEs were manageable in the chosen regimen of nivolumab 3 mg/kg and ipilimumab 1 mg/kg (week 1, 4, 8 and 11), followed by nivolumab every 2 weeks. Recently, a third cohort with 45 previously untreated dMMR/MSI-H MCR patients was presented, confirming the prior results with an ORR of 60% (27/45) and 1-year PFS of 77% and OS of 83% [14]. Notably, a low dose ipilimumab regimen was applied with 1 mg/kg every 6 weeks continuously in combination with nivolumab 3 mg/kg every 2 weeks resulting in a very low rate of treatment-related grade 3/4 AEs (only 16%). Together, a direct comparison to monotherapy with checkpoint inhibitors is missing, however, response rates of combinations are promising independent of the respective therapy line and dosing schedule with a manageable safety profile (Table 1).

Table 1 Clinical trials with checkpoint inhibitors in dMMR/MSI-H CRC

	Drugs	*N*	ORR	PFS at 12 months	Median PFS (months)	OS at 12 months
Neoadjuvant	Nivolumab (3) + Ipilimumab (1)	20	pCR 60% (12/20)	nr	nr	nr
1st line	***Pembrolizumab (randomized)***	**153**	**44%**	**55%**	**16.5**	**78%**
	Nivolumab 3 mg/kg every 2 weeks + Ipilimumab 1 mg/kg every 6 weeks	45	60%	77%		83%
≥2nd line	*Nivolumab*	74	31%	50%	14.3	73%
	Pembrolizumab	61	28%	34%	2.3	72%
	Nivolumab 3 mg/kg + Ipilimumab 1 mg/kg (week 1, 4, 7, 11), followed by Nivolumab 3 mg/kg every 2 weeks	119	55%	71%	*nr*	85%

2.3 Combination of PD-L1 Inhibitor with Anti-angiogenic VEGF-Antibody

The combination of PD-L1 inhibitors and the anti-angiogenic antibody bevacizumab showed favorable results in hepatocellular carcinoma and non-small cell lung cancer and was therefore also evaluated in MCRC. In total, ten dMMR/MSI-H MCRC patients were treated in a phase Ib. study. The combination was proven as well tolerated and disease control was reached in 90% with an ORR of 30% [15]. Since these are only preliminary results, further studies are needed to reveal the relevance of this combination in dMMR/MSI-H MCRC treatment.

2.3.1 Ongoing Clinical Trials

Adjuvant The phase III ATOMIC trial (NCT02912559) is currently comparing standard adjuvant chemotherapy with FOLFOX with the combination of PD-L1 antibody atezolizumab and FOLFOX for stage III lymph node metastasized dMMR/MSI-H colorectal cancer. The phase III POLEM trial is evaluating the addition of PD-L1 antibody avelumab to standard 5-FU based adjuvant chemotherapy in stage III dMMR/MSI-H or POLE mutated colorectal cancer (NCT 03827044). Both studies will evaluate the role of checkpoint inhibitors in the curative setting, further, the POLEM study will substantiate our knowledge about the response of POLE mutated tumors to checkpoint inhibitors.

Metastatic A phase III study is evaluating the addition of checkpoint inhibitor atezolizumab to standard chemotherapy with FOLFOX and bevacizumab compared to FOLFOX and bevacizumab alone in first line treatment of dMMR/MSI-H MCRC (COMMIT-study, NCT02997228). This study will give hypothesis whether the combination of chemotherapy and checkpoint inhibitor treatment may increase the appealing results observed for monotherapy with checkpoint inhibitors. The second open question regarding the potential increase in response and survival observed by the combination of PD-1 and CTLA-4 inhibition in the CM-142 study will be tested in in different disease settings (first, second, and third line of therapy) in dMMR/MSI-H MCRC patients in the CM 8HW study (NCT04008030).

3 Conclusions and Perspective

Monotherapy with checkpoint inhibitors will become the first line standard of care in dMMR/MSI-H MCRC patients due to its impressive PFS rates at 12 months compared to standard chemotherapy. Although much earlier in terms of clinical trials the combination of nivolumab and ipilimumab might be even more effective in terms of response rates at the cost of increased, but manageable AEs. Only randomized controlled trials will show how the combination of nivolumab and ipilimumab, or chemotherapy and checkpoint inhibitor combinations compare to the new standard of checkpoint inhibitor monotherapy in first line MCRC treatment. Finally, long-term follow-up data on checkpoint inhibitor treatment in early stage dMMR/

MSI-H colorectal cancer will show whether the high rates of complete or major pathological response after neoadjuvant treatment will translate into survival and thereby proving the efficacy in other indications than metastatic disease.

Compliance with Ethical Standards

Conflict of Interest AS received institutional research grants from Merck, Bristol-Myers Squibb, Roche, Sanofi and Servier and serves as an advisory board member for Merck, Bristol-Myers Squibb, Merck Sharp and Dohme, Roche, Sanofi and Amgen.

References

1. Giannakis M, Mu XJ, Shukla SA, Qian ZR, Cohen O, Nishihara R et al (2016) Genomic correlates of immune-cell infiltrates in colorectal carcinoma. Cell Rep 15(4):857–865. https://doi.org/10.1016/j.celrep.2016.03.075
2. Llosa NJ, Cruise M, Tam A, Wicks EC, Hechenbleikner EM, Taube JM et al (2015) The vigorous immune microenvironment of microsatellite instable colon cancer is balanced by multiple counter-inhibitory checkpoints. Cancer Discov 5(1):43–51
3. Le DT, Uram JN, Wang H, Bartlett BR, Kemberling H, Eyring AD et al (2016) PD-1 blockade in tumors with mismatch-repair deficiency. N Engl J Med 372(26):2509–2520
4. Haydon AMM, Jass JR (2002) Emerging pathways in colorectal-cancer development. Lancet Oncol 3(2):83–88
5. Gong J, Wang C, Lee PP, Chu P, Fakih M (2017) Response to PD-1 blockade in microsatellite stable metastatic colorectal cancer harboring a POLE mutation. J Natl Compr Cancer Netw 15(2):142–147
6. Bourdais R, Rousseau B, Pujals A, Boussion H, Joly C, Guillemin A et al (2017) Polymerase proofreading domain mutations: new opportunities for immunotherapy in hypermutated colorectal cancer beyond MMR deficiency. Crit Rev Oncol Hematol 113:242–248. https://doi.org/10.1016/j.critrevonc.2017.03.027
7. Le DT, Durham JN, Smith KN, Wang H, Bjarne R, Aulakh LK et al (2017) Mismatch-repair deficiency predicts response of solid tumors to PD-1 blockade. Science 357(6349):409–413
8. Overman MJ, Mcdermott R, Leach JL, Lonardi S, Lenz H, Morse MA et al (2017) Nivolumab in patients with metastatic DNA mismatch repair deficient/microsatellite instability–high colorectal cancer (CheckMate 142): results of an open-label, multicentre, phase 2 study. Lancet Oncol 18(9):1182–1191
9. Diaz LA, Le DT, Kim TW, Van Cutsem E, Geva R, Jaeger D et al (2020) Pembrolizumab monotherapy for patients with advanced MSI-H colorectal cancer: longer-term follow-up of the phase II, KEYNOTE-164 study. J Clin Oncol 38(15_Suppl):4032. https://doi.org/10.1200/JCO.2020.38.15_suppl.4032
10. Andre T, Shiu K-K, Kim TW, Jensen BV, Jensen LH, Punt CJA et al (2020) Pembrolizumab versus chemotherapy for microsatellite instability-high/mismatch repair deficient metastatic colorectal cancer: the phase 3 KEYNOTE-177 Study. J Clin Oncol 38(18_Suppl):LBA4–LBA4. https://doi.org/10.1200/JCO.2020.38.18_suppl.LBA4
11. Rousseau B-C, Bieche I, Pasmant E, Simmet V, Hamzaoui N, Masliah-Planchon J et al (2020) 526O High activity of nivolumab in patients with pathogenic exonucleasic domain POLE (edPOLE) mutated Mismatch Repair proficient (MMRp) advanced tumours. Ann Oncol 31:S463. https://doi.org/10.1016/j.annonc.2020.08.640
12. Grootscholten C, Voest EE, Chalabi M, Kuiper M, Van Leerdam ME, Fanchi LF et al (2018) LBA37_PR_Neoadjuvant ipilimumab plus nivolumab in early stage colon cancer. Ann Oncol. https://doi.org/10.1093/annonc/mdy424.047

13. Chalabi M, Fanchi LF, Dijkstra KK, Van den Berg JG, Aalbers AG, Sikorska K et al (2020) Neoadjuvant immunotherapy leads to pathological responses in MMR-proficient and MMR-deficient early-stage colon cancers. Nat Med 26(4):566–576. https://doi.org/10.1038/s41591-020-0805-8
14. Lenz H-JJ, Cardin D, Dragovich T, Shah U, Atasoy A, Postema R et al (2018) LBA18_PR_ Durable clinical benefit with nivolumab (NIVO) plus low-dose ipilimumab (IPI) as first-line therapy in microsatellite instability-high/mismatch repair deficient (MSI-H/dMMR) metastatic colorectal cancer (mCRC). Ann Oncol. https://doi.org/10.1093/annonc/mdy424.019
15. Hochster HS, Bendell JC, Cleary JM, Foster P, Zhang W, He X et al (2017) Efficacy and safety of atezolizumab (atezo) and bevacizumab (bev) in a phase Ib study of microsatellite instability (MSI)-high metastatic colorectal cancer (mCRC). J Clin Oncol 35(4_Suppl):673. https://doi.org/10.1200/JCO.2017.35.4_suppl.673

Immunotherapy in the Treatment of Advanced Colorectal Cancer

Puneet Raman, Gehan Botrus, and Tanios Bekaii-Saab

Contents

Abstract

Immunotherapy has rapidly evolved in the treatment of select malignancies. In colorectal cancer, response to treatment has varied based on the presence of mismatch repair deficiency (dMMR) and microsatellite instability (MSI-H). Patients with dMMR/MSI-H metastatic colorectal cancer (mCRC) have a favorable tumor microenvironment (TME) resulting in activation of the immune system

Puneet Raman and Gehan Botrus contributed equally with all other contributors.

P. Raman · G. Botrus · T. Bekaii-Saab (✉)
Mayo Clinic College of Medicine and Science, Phoenix, AZ, USA
e-mail: Raman.Puneet@mayo.edu; Botrus.Gehan@mayo.edu; bekaii-saab.tanios@mayo.edu

Cancer Immunotherapy (2022)
https://doi.org/10.1007/13905_2021_12,
Published Online: 19 March 2022

and targeting of the malignancy by T and NK cells leading to a good response to immune checkpoint inhibitors (ICIs). Pembrolizumab and nivolumab are ICIs that target programmed cell death protein 1. Nivolumab is FDA approved for the treatment of dMMR/MSI-H mCRC after initial chemotherapy regimens have failed, while pembrolizumab is now approved for first-line treatment. However, at least 96% of metastatic colorectal cancers are pMMR/MSS and do not exhibit responses to treatment with ICIs. Studies are exploring therapeutic combinations with targets such as BRAF, VEGF, and others that may activate T and NK cells, reduce inhibitory signals, and increase robustness of the immune response.

Keywords
Advanced colorectal cancer · Anti-CTLA-4 · Anti-PD-1 · Colorectal cancer · dMMR/MSI-H · EGFR · Immune checkpoint inhibitor · Immunotherapy · Metastatic colorectal cancer · pMMR/MSS · VEGF

1 Introduction

Colorectal cancer (CRC) is ranked third in cancer diagnoses and second in cancer deaths among men and women in the United States. Approximately 147,950 patients were newly diagnosed with CRC and 53,200 died from the disease in 2020, with the incidence rising at a rate of 2% annually in individuals younger than 50 years old [1]. Significant focus and resources have been allocated for screening to prevent advanced disease, with the National Colorectal Cancer Roundtable (NCCRT) establishing a goal of screening 80% of eligible patients by 2018 [2]. Yet, only 66% of individuals 50 years and older have been currently screened in the USA and less than 50% of those between ages 50 and 54 [1], corresponding with a rise in the incidence of advanced CRC.

Treatment of metastatic CRC (mCRC) with chemotherapy began with 5-fluorouracil and leucovorin in the 1980s with several studies demonstrating a significant increase in RR and PFS [3]. Further development in the early 2000s occurred with the introduction of the topoisomerase I inhibitor irinotecan in combination with fluorouracil and leucovorin, as well as oxaliplatin as a component of cytotoxic combination therapy. In a randomized multicenter trial, patients who received irinotecan, fluorouracil, and leucovorin had longer progression-free survival (PFS), higher overall response rate (ORR), and longer overall survival (OS) compared to those treated with the then-standard fluorouracil and leucovorin [4]. The Intergroup Trial N9741 demonstrated superior OS, RR, and time to progression (TTP) with FOLFOX (5FU/leucovorin and oxaliplatin) compared to bolus treatment with 5FU/leucovorin and irinotecan (IFL) with lower rates of adverse effects [5]. On the other hand, FOLFIRI was shown to be similarly efficacious to FOLFOX in multiple studies [6, 7].

Further evolution included biologics targeting angiogenesis, as a pivotal phase III trial in 2004 demonstrated improved OS, PFS, and RR in patients treated with

IFL and bevacizumab, an anti-vascular endothelial growth factor (VEGF A) monoclonal antibody, compared to IFL alone [8]. Similar findings were noted with bevacizumab and FOLFOX treatment compared to FOLFOX alone [9]. Epidermal growth factor receptor (EGFR) was also explored as a target for therapy with monoclonal antibodies cetuximab and panitumumab, though initial studies including CRYSTAL (cetuximab combined with irinotecan in first-line therapy for mCRC) and PRIME (panitumumab randomized trial in combination with chemotherapy for mCRC to determine efficacy) demonstrated some improvement in progression-free survival (PFS) without significant improvements in OS [3]. Other trials include FIRE-3, in which treatment with FOLFIRI and cetuximab demonstrated no significant difference in ORR or PFS compared with FOLFIRI and bevacizumab as first-line treatment for patients with mCRC and wild-type KRAS [10, 11]. The TRIBE trial showed a significant increase in PFS in patients treated with FOLFOXIRI and bevacizumab compared to FOLFIRI and bevacizumab as first-line therapy in mCRC [12]. Additional evaluation occurred in the TRIBE2 phase III trial, which explored first-line FOLFOXIRI and bevacizumab with reintroduction of the same regimen after disease progression compared to a control group receiving first-line mFOLFOX6 and bevacizumab followed by FOLFIRI and bevacizumab after disease progression. Median PFS was 19.2 months in the experimental group compared to 16.4 months in the control group with a hazard ratio of 0.74 (95% CI: 17.3–21.4; $p = 0.0005$) [13]. This suggests that initial exposure to FOLFOXIRI and bevacizumab with reintroduction after progression improves survival outcomes compared to three cytotoxic agents across two lines of therapy.

Further improvements in the prognosis of advanced CRC have occurred due to identification of genomic markers through next-generation sequencing (NGS) and targeted therapies. Specifically, genes such as KRAS, NRAS, BRAFV600E, HER2, and PI3KCA have been identified in CRC pathogenesis via NGS and targeted in treatment [14]. It is noteworthy that CRC death rates from 2008 to 2017 decreased 3% annually in those over 65 years old and 0.6% in those aged 50–64 years [1]. However, death rates increased 1.3% annually in those younger than 50 years old with 26% of these patients presenting with metastatic disease, indicating the need for continuing evolution of treatment for advanced malignancy.

2 Role of the Immune System in Colorectal Cancer

The survival rate for patients diagnosed with metastatic CRC has increased steadily since the 1990s [1], a change driven by the study and use of various targeted therapies and recent adaptation of immunotherapy in highly select patient groups. The immune system is involved in the pathogenesis of colorectal cancer via immune checkpoints (ICI) and correlates with both the tumor microenvironment (TME) and the mismatch repair (MMR) system. In cells, MMR can recognize damage to DNA as well as insertion, deletion, and/or mis-incorporation of bases that occur during DNA replication and recombination. Proteins involved in MMR include MSH1-6 and PMS1-2 [15], and colon cancer syndromes including hereditary nonpolyposis colorectal cancer (HNPCC) involve germline mutations in MSH1, MSH2, MSH6, and SM2 [16]. One phase II study demonstrated that CRC with deficient MMR (dMMR) was shown to have a rate of 1782 somatic mutations per tumor as compared to 73 in those with proficient MMR (pMMR) in one phase II study [17]. These mutations often occur in microsatellites, small repeating stretches of DNA scattered throughout the genome, resulting in variation in the length of microsatellites termed microsatellite instability high (MSI-H). Identification of dMMR/MSI-H typically occurs by immunohistochemical staining demonstrating loss of MSH1, MSH2, MSH6, PMS2, and PCR showing instability in length variation of the five most common microsatellites (BAT25, BAT26, D2S123, D5S346, D17S250) [18]. The advent of NGS has allowed for more reliably evaluating additional microsatellites throughout the genome with specificity and sensitivity of 100% and 99.3% for 178 patients [19]. The dMMR/MSI-H pathway is responsible for the development of 12–15% of CRC across all stages and less than 4% of mCRC [20], with one-third of these patients inheriting it via HNPCC and the remainder acquiring it via methylation of MLH1 or biallelic somatic mutations [18]. The remainder and large majority of CRC is classified as pMMR with microsatellite stability (MSS), or pMMR/MSS.

In addition to contributing to the development of CRC, there is a known association of dMMR CRC with a unique TME. The microenvironment is typically characterized by infiltrating immune cells that can be responsible for angiogenesis, sustained proliferative signaling, evading growth suppressors, invasion, metastasis, and treatment resistance among other roles [21–23]. dMMR CRC has been associated with a TME characterized as a Crohn's-like lymphoid reaction (CLR). There are a variety of lymphoid aggregates including an initial surplus of CD4+ T cells, antigen-presenting dendritic cells, increasing B cells and follicular dendritic cells with maturation of the CLR, and eventually an environment consistent with functional tertiary lymphoid structures [24]. The robust immune response in the microenvironment is a positive prognostic factor in a variety of solid malignancies [25, 26]. This has led to the development of the Immunoscore, an immunologic assay that quantifies the T-cell presence in the TME and indicates prognosis of CRC [27]. The immune response of the TME is so significant to therapeutic response that the Immunoscore was demonstrated to be superior to the TNM classification in demonstrating the prognosis of patients with CRC [28].

While most dMMR tumors have a robust tumor microenvironment that portends effective response to targeted therapy, including checkpoint inhibitors, most CRC cases have pMMR tumors with lower tumor mutation burden (TMB) and an immune-desert TME with significantly reduced CLR. Effective therapeutic response in these patients relies on exploration of other aspects of the immune response, including the expression of neoantigens. These are completely foreign proteins that are absent from healthy human tissues [29]. Neoantigens are taken up by antigen-presenting cells (APCs), which present peptides to a complex of CD8+ and CD4+ T cells and HLA class I and II molecules to drive a more robust immune system response to tumors [30, 31]. Tumors with a high TMB such as dMMR CRC have high loads of neoantigens [32], priming a significant adaptive immune response correlating with a higher density of tumor-infiltrating lymphocytes (TIL). Though the probability of a neoantigen presenting to T cells is reduced in pMMR cancers [33, 34], they may still play an important role in targeted therapy.

Peptide-MHC class I complexes created by APCs in the presence of neoantigens alone are insufficient to activate T cells. The downstream signaling pathways are mediated by stimulatory or inhibitory signals known as immune checkpoints [35, 36]. In normal physiologic conditions, these checkpoints primarily prevent the immune system from attacking healthy host tissue. However, inhibitory checkpoints include programmed cell death protein 1 (PD-1), programmed death-ligand 1 (PD-L1), programmed death-ligand 2, cytotoxic T-lymphocyte-associated protein 4 (CTLA-4), T-cell immunoglobulin and mucin-domain containing-3 (TIM-3), B- and T-cell lymphocyte attenuator (BTLA), and lymphocyte activation gene-3 (LAG-3) [37, 38]. Upregulation of PD-1 on TILs and PD-L1 on tumor cells has been implicated in tumor evasion due to suppression of tumor-specific CD8+ T cells [39]. Similarly, CTLA-4 single-nucleotide polymorphisms (SNPs) are correlated with an increased risk of developing CRC [40] and occur at higher levels in MSI-H compared to MSS tumors [41]. As immune checkpoints play a key role in the development of malignancy, inhibitors were studied as a potential therapeutic target. ICIs function by disrupting the interaction of the checkpoint receptors on T cells and ligands present on tumor cells. This process results in increased T-cell recognition of tumor cells leading to activation, infiltration, and tumor death [42, 43]. Given the connection between immune checkpoints, MMR, and TME, ICIs have recently come to the forefront in the targeted treatment of CRC. However, ICIs have not been found to be as effective in pMMR/MSS with the immune-desert TME. Thus, alternate targets and strategies have been explored as the majority of CRC is pMMR/MSS.

3 Strategies to Overcome ICI Resistance in pMMR/MSS Colorectal Cancer

While ICIs have demonstrated superiority in the efficacy and tolerability to standard chemotherapy, similar results have been noticeably absent in pMMR tumors which comprise the majority of CRC. As noted earlier, differences identified between dMMR and pMMR tumors may also be the factors driving resistance to immune checkpoint blockade. Reduced tumor mutational burden (TMB) in pMMR CRC reduces the likelihood of the tumor-producing neoantigens and immunogenic peptides via APCs and class I and II MHCs [44]. A clinicopathological study evaluated samples collected from MSI-H patients for TMB and found a predictive cut point for mutation burden, in which 13 cases with high TMB had response to treatment while 6 of 9 cases with low TMB had progressive disease [45]. This was further evaluated in a large MSI-H mCRC population and TMB was validated as an independent biomarker within MSI-H to stratify likely response to ICIs. TME has also been shown to play a role in response to ICI and other immune therapies. The TME is often characterized by either hot or cold, depending on the presence of inflammatory cells, or immune desert (absence of immune cells), immune excluded (immune cells in the stroma but not penetrating the tumor), and immune inflamed (immune cells adjacent to tumor cells) [44]. Preclinical studies have shown that attempts to immunologically enrich the TME by activating interferons, specifically interferon-gamma, can promote T-cell responses and increase tumor sensitivity to cytotoxic T cells [46, 47]. Additionally, genomic defects in genes for the interferon-gamma pathway, including Janus kinase 1 (JAK1) and JAK2, are implicated in primary and acquired resistance to ICI therapy [48]. Ongoing studies are exploring methods of overcoming ICI resistance with current approaches exploring synergy between conventional chemotherapy, immunotherapy, and small-molecule inhibitors.

3.1 BRAF/MAPK

The MAPK signaling cascade is a pathway full of common oncogenes that can promote proliferation of CRC [49]. The pathway includes RAF kinases, three serine/threonine-specific protein kinases, that participate in the RAS-RAF-MEK-ERK signal transduction cascade [50]. BRAF mutations occur in 10–13% of CRC patients [51, 52], resulting in inappropriate activation of MEK and ERK leading to increased proliferation and survival of cancer cells.

BRAF mutations are detectable even in small polyps [53] and as compared with RAS mutations, they are more common in hyperplastic polyps, serrated adenomas, and proximal colon cancers. Tumors with BRAF mutations are characterized by methylation of CpG islands, regions of the genome with tumor-suppressor genes that are silenced by this alteration. Tumors of this type are referred to as CpG island methylator phenotype (CIMP) [54]. The most common mutation is a missense mutation in codon 600 of exon 15 referred to as V600E which accounts for 90% of all BRAF mutations in CRC [55, 56], resulting in MEK activation and bypassing of the EGFR pathway that regulates cellular proliferation. Notably, BRAF and KRAS/NRAS mutations are not present simultaneously in CRC [57, 58], which may indicate that both mutations act as oncogenes via the same pathway. Molecular studies have shown that BRAF mutations are seen in up to 60% of MSI-H tumors while present in only 5–10% of MSS tumors [55, 59, 60]. BRAF mutations result in hypermethylation of the MLH1 gene, among others responsible for DNA mismatch repair [61], increasing microsatellite instability in these tumors.

The presence of BRAF mutations also has prognostic value both alone and in combination with the microsatellite status of the tumor. Data from two large adjuvant trials (PETACC-8, NCT00079274) were pooled to assess disease progression and survival endpoints among 4411 patients treated with standard 5-fluorouracil plus oxaliplatin (FOLFOX)-based adjuvant therapy. Regardless of the microsatellite status, BRAF mutations were associated with shorter time to recurrence (TTR; HR 1.27; 95% CI: 1.04–1.56; $p = 0.02$) and OS (HR 1.49; 95% CI: 1.20–1.86; $p < 0.001$) compared to wild-type tumors [59]. In MSS patients with BRAF mutations, TTR was significantly reduced (HR 1.65; 95% CI: 1.23–1.92; $p < 0.001$) as was OS (HR 2.01; 95% CI: 1.56–2.57; $p < 0.001$) [59]. MSI-H patients harboring BRAF mutations had no significant difference in TTR (HR 0.94; 95% CI: 0.58–1.51; $p = 0.80$)

or OS (HR 1.26; 95% CI: 0.78–2.04, $p = 0.35$) [59]. Other trials have shown similar results, with the trial NCCTG N0147 demonstrating that BRAF mutations were associated with a statistically significant reduction in DFS (HR 1.37; 95% CI: 1.08–1.70; $p = 0.009$) [62]. Mixing a good prognostic factor (MSI-H) and poor prognostic factor (BRAF) does not seem to affect the outcome, while MSS/BRAF phenotype may upregulate genes facilitated by both malignant growth and metastatic spread [63].

Novel agents targeting BRAF have been in use with melanoma, as the FDA approved oral selective BRAF V600E inhibitors such as vemurafenib for surgically unresectable or metastatic disease [64]. Similar success was not found in refractory CRC with V600E mutations, as a pilot phase II study of vemurafenib demonstrated partial response in only 1 patient out of a total 21 (5%) with 7 experiencing stable disease [65]. Theories explaining this poor response to BRAF inhibition include upstream activation of EGFR resulting in activation of MAPK leading to treatment resistance [66, 67].

Attempts to circumvent treatment resistance involve a multitargeted approach with both BRAF and EGFR inhibition, as well as other downstream targets such as MEK and ERK. A nonrandomized phase I/II clinical trial (NCT01750918) evaluated combined inhibition of BRAF and EGFR, respectively, with dabrafenib and panitumumab with or without concomitant MEK inhibition with trametinib in 142 patients with BRAF V600E CRC. Treatment with dabrafenib and panitumumab had a RR of 10% and PFS of 3.5 months (95% CI: 2.8–5.8), while the addition of MEK inhibition with trametinib increased RR to 21% and PFS to 4.2 months (95% CI: 4.0–5.6) [68].

Additional trials include a phase II study (SWOG S1406) of irinotecan and cetuximab with or without vemurafenib in refractory BRAF V600E mCRC. MSI-H tumors were not excluded as this was prior to FDA approval of ICIs in MSI-H tumors. The addition of vemurafenib to cetuximab, an EGFR inhibitor, and irinotecan increased PFS to 4.2 months from 2.0 months with only irinotecan and cetuximab [69].

BEACON is a randomized phase III trial (NCT02928224) investigating cetuximab and encorafenib (BRAF inhibitor) with or without binimetinib vs. standard chemotherapy in patients with BRAF V600E-mutated metastatic colorectal cancer. The median OS was 9 months with triple therapy compared to 5.4 months in those receiving standard chemotherapy (HR 0.52; 95% CI: 0.39–0.70; $p < 0.001$) [70]. Similar changes were noted in RR with 26% (95% CI: 18–35) in the triple-therapy group compared to 2% (95% CI: 0–7) in the control group ($p < 0.001$). All groups had similar rates of adverse events (50–61%) [70]. Updates demonstrated that patients in the cetuximab and encorafenib arm also had improved OS of 9.3 months compared to 5.9 months in the control arm (HR 0.61; 95% CI: 0.48–0.75), nearly identical to the triple-therapy group [71]. As a result, the FDA has approved cetuximab and encorafenib for refractory mCRC with a BRAF V600E mutation. Future trials, including the BREAKWATER trial (NCT04607421), are evaluating cetuximab and encorafenib with or without chemotherapy in treatment-naïve patients as well [72].

Other approaches to BRAF-mutated CRC are derived from the correlation between BRAF and MSI-H status in tumors. Several trials are underway evaluating the efficacy of combining BRAF inhibition with ICIs which have been approved for the treatment of mCRC in dMMR/MSI-H patients. Patients with BRAF V600E CRC were treated with PD-1 inhibitors spartalizumab, dabrafenib, and trametinib, and of 20 patients with restaging scans, the ORR was 35% and DCR was 75%, indicating some response to combination therapy with ICIs [73]. A phase I/II trial of cetuximab, encorafenib, and nivolumab is underway (NCT04017650), while another trial is evaluating various approved novel agents in combination with dabrafenib (NCT04294160).

These trials indicate that the future of treating BRAF-mutated colorectal cancer, particularly those with MSS as well, may lie in combination therapy designed to block multiple oncogenes and more effectively shut down the MAPK signaling cascade. Of note, challenges in studying and treating patients with BRAF-mutated or MSS tumors include that tissue collection is limited by the fact that most patients present with surgically unresectable disease. Circulating tumor DNA (ctDNA) will be of utmost importance for detecting the presence of somatic mutations in these patients. Though most patients with BRAF mutations have MSI-H status as well, conferring neutral to beneficial prognosis, the small subject of patients with BRAF/MSS phenotype may benefit from combination therapy of novel agents designed to block multiple oncogenes and achieve more durable response.

3.2 VEGF Inhibitors

Clinical trials like COMMIT are exploring anti-VEGF mAb like bevacizumab in combination with ICIs and standard chemotherapy. While VEGF has an established role of enhancing tumor vascular growth, it also inhibits T cells, hinders differentiation of dendritic APC cells, and suppresses localized immune response [74]. One of the mechanisms of anti-CTLA-4 antibodies is by reinvigorating tumor-specific CD8+ T cells that are suppressed by Treg cells [75]. Treatment with VEGF inhibitors can suppress the function of Treg cells allowing for a more robust T-cell response to tumors [76]. A previously mentioned phase Ib study evaluated treatment with atezolizumab, bevacizumab, and chemotherapy but unfortunately only MSI-H patients were enrolled. However, updates to the study described elevations in cytotoxic T-cell signatures, increased CD8+ T cells, and increased PD-L1 expression in tumors confirmed by immunohistochemistry stains on pre- and posttreatment biopsies with administration of combination therapy [77]. Further studies could evaluate the efficacy of this treatment regimen in pMMR/MSS mCRC. Bevacizumab is already FDA approved for combination therapy with FOLFOX4 as a second-line treatment of mCRC [78].

ICI as maintenance therapy after cotreatment with standard chemotherapy and VEGF inhibitors has also been explored with the MODUL trial (NCT NCT02291289). This was a phase II randomized trial in which 445 mCRC patients were treated with FOLFOX + bevacizumab for induction with or without maintenance atezolizumab

[79]. Despite a median follow-up of 10.5 months, there was no significant increase in PFS with a hazard ratio of 0.92 (95% CI: 0.72–1.17; $p = 0.48$). In updated analysis with a follow-up of 18.7 months, PFS outcome remained unchanged with a hazard ratio of 0.96 (95% CI: 0.77–1.20; $p = 0.727$). Fifty one percent of patients experienced an event, and with the mature OS endpoint, no differences were observed with maintenance therapy.

Ongoing phase II trials evaluating VEGF inhibition in combination with ICI and chemotherapy include the AtezoTRIBE trial (NCTNCT03721653), a randomized phase II study of FOLFOXIRI and bevacizumab alone or with atezolizumab followed by bevacizumab and 5-fluorouracil/leucovorin maintenance therapy in mCRC irrespective of the microsatellite status [80]. The primary endpoint is PFS with a planned safety run-in phase. A phase III trial, VISNU-1 (NCT01640405), already identified FOLFOXIRI and bevacizumab as a superior first-line treatment compared to FOLFOX and bevacizumab, as the addition of irinotecan to induction therapy improved PFS to 12.4 months (95% CI: 11.2–14.0 months) compared to 9.3 months (95% CI: 8.5–10.7 months) without irinotecan [81]. The stratified hazard ratio was 0.64 (95% CI: 0.49–0.82; $p = 0.0006$). The AtezoTRIBE trial may shed light on the use of VEGF inhibitors in combination with ICI and chemotherapy for pMMR/MSS mCRC.

In addition to atezolizumab, lenvatinib in combination with pembrolizumab has shown antitumor activity and tolerability in patients previously treated for advanced solid tumors including mCRC with pMMR/MSS phenotype. Data was initially presented at the 2020 European Society for Medical Oncology meeting and updated in January 2021 via the Journal of Clinical Oncology from the phase II LEAP-005 trial (NCT03797326). Thirty-two patients were enrolled who had two prior treatment regimens for mCRC, with an ORR of 21.9% (95% CI: 9.3–40%) and grade 3–4 treatment-related AEs occurring in 16 patients [82, 83]. Enrollment and data analysis are ongoing, with this cohort expanded to 100 patients given the promising efficacy and safety preliminarily demonstrated.

Another anti-VEGF agent that was evaluated for therapeutic potential is regorafenib, recently in a phase Ib trial known as REGONIVO (NCT04030260) and given in combination with nivolumab for gastric cancer and CRC [84]. Twenty-five patients were enrolled with all having received at least two prior lines of chemotherapy. Only one patient had MSI-H mCRC with 24 having pMMR/MSS mCRC. The ORR was 33.3% (95% CI: 15.6–55.3%) in patients with MSS mCRC and 36% (95% CI: 18–57.5%) overall in patients with CRC. Median PFS was 7.9 months (95% CI: 2.9 months to NR) and median OS was NR in CRC (95% CI: 9.8 months to NR). Regorafenib monotherapy already has demonstrated an overall survival benefit irrespective of the microsatellite status in the phase III CORRECT trial [85]. Further investigation of regorafenib occurred in a single US center, evaluating the outcome of MSS mCRC patients treated on a compassionate basis with PD-1 inhibitors combined with regorafenib. Out of 18 patients studied, 13 experienced progressive disease while 5 patients experienced stable disease as a best response of which 4 had no liver metastasis [86]. They were unable to replicate the high response rate observed in the REGONIVO trial, possibly related to the presence of liver metastasis, and as such recommended caution implementing this regimen in clinical practice moving forward. However, as the landscape of mCRC continues to evolve, other combinations of ICI, VEGF inhibitors, and chemotherapy show promising results in ongoing trials that may demonstrate efficacy and safety of treatment of pMMR/MSS mCRC.

3.3 EGFR Inhibitors

Another strategy to overcome ICI resistance is with co-treatment with antibodies that inhibit the epidermal growth factor receptor (EGFR). Similar to VEGF inhibitors, EGFR inhibition decreases local immunosuppression by reducing Treg functioning which improves cytotoxicity of CD8+ T cells [87]. ICI combination with cetuximab (anti-EGFR mAb) has been shown to overcome immunosuppression in the TME [88] and promote a more robust host immune response [89, 90]. A phase Ib/II trial evaluated cetuximab in combination with pembrolizumab for 9 RAS RAS wild-type mCRC patients that were initially enrolled (NCT02713373) [91]. Initial phase Ib data demonstrated tolerable safety with common AEs including xerosis, dermatitis acneiform rash, hypomagnesemia, vomiting, and fatigue. Six out of nine patients achieved SD lasting at least 16 weeks. The most recent update included 42 RAS wild-type mCRC patients with peripheral blood and flow cytometry to determine the effects on the TME. Cytotoxic T cells increased by 47% ($p < 0.05$) within the tumor with decreases in PD1+ T cells. Though Treg cells increased, the ratio of Teff to Treg cells increased indicating a shift to a more favorable TME. Endpoint outcomes of PFS, OS, and ORR are pending maturation. Enrolled patients were not differentiated based on the microsatellite status of the tumors, but positive changes in TME with anti-EGFR co-treatment are an encouraging result. An additional phase II study (NCT03442569) has finished recruiting and is investigating treatment with nivolumab, ipilimumab, and panitumumab (anti-EGFR mAB) in patients with refractory RAS wild-type MSS mCRC. While outcome data from both trials are pending, an improvement in survival combined with observed beneficial TME changes could signify EGFR as a potential therapeutic target for immune-desert pMMR CRC. Table 1 summarizes clinical trials evaluating growth factor receptor inhibition in mCRC.

3.4 MEK Inhibitors

The interferon-gamma pathway has already been established as a critical part of T-cell response to malignancy and activity of cytotoxic T cells [46, 47]. Preclinical studies have shown that the mitogen-activated protein kinase (MAPK) pathway is involved in PD-L1 expression via EGFR and interferon-gamma-mediated pathways [92]. When inhibited, MAPK/extracellular signal-regulated kinase (ERK) increases MHC-1 levels, stimulates T-cell expansion, and enhances anti-PD-1 activity [93]. MEK is part of the MAPK/ERK pathway that can be targeted by inhibitors such as

Table 1 Clinical trials evaluating combination therapy with ICI and VEGF/EGFR

ICI	Combination	Disease	Phase	Trial number
Nivolumab	Regorafenib (VEGF) ± CRTX	mCRC	I	NCT04030260
Nivolumab	Bevacizumab (VEGF) ± TFD/TPI + oxaliplatin	mCRC	I	NCT02848443
Nivolumab	Encorafenib (BRAF) + cetuximab (EGFR)	BRAFV600E CRC	I/II	NCT04017650
Nivolumab	Bevacizumab (VEGF) + CTX	rCRC or mCRC	II/III	NCT03414983
Nivolumab + ipilimumab	Panitumumab (EGFR)	RAS wild-type CRC	II	NCT03442569
Pembrolizumab	Nintedanib (VEGF)	mCRC	I/II	NCT02856425
Pembrolizumab	Cetuximab (EGFR)	Pre-treated mCRC	I/II	NCT02713373
Pembrolizumab	Capecitabine + bevacizumab (VEGF)	mCRC	II	NCT03396926
Durvalumab	Cediranib (VEGF)	rCRC	I/II	NCT02484404
Atezolizumab	Capecitabine + bevacizumab (VEGF)	rCRC	II	NCT02873195
Avelumab	Cetuximab (EGFR) + irinotecan	mCRC	II	NCT03608046

CRC colorectal cancer, *CRTX* chemoradiation therapy, *CTX* chemotherapy, *EGFR* epidermal growth factor receptor, *mCRC* metastatic colorectal cancer, *rCRC* refractory colorectal cancer, *VEGF* vascular endothelial growth factor

cobimetinib. A phase Ib clinical study (NCT01988896) was conducted with 84 patients enrolled for mCRC and treated with cobimetinib and atezolizumab [94]. Confirmed responses were present in 8% (7/84) of patients of which 6 were MSS. With some evidence of clinical response, investigators began a phase III randomized international trial known as IMBLAZE370 (NCT02788279) [95]. Three hundred and sixty patients with refractory mCRC were enrolled with more than 90% pMMR/MSS. They were randomized to receive atezolizumab plus cobimetinib, atezolizumab monotherapy, or regorafenib (anti-VEGF mAb). The trial did not meet its primary endpoint of improved OS, with the median OS of the combination treatment cohort and the regorafenib cohort at 8.9 months and 8.5 months, respectively, with a hazard ratio of 1.00 (95% CI: 0.73–1.38; $p = 0.99$). There was also no difference in PFS or ORR observed when comparing cohorts. Though MEK inhibition for pMMR/MSS mCRC in this study was not shown to have efficacy, there are ongoing clinical trials exploring other combinations of ICIs and MEK inhibitors (Table 2).

3.5 POLE Mutations

The POLEM trial as discussed earlier is already exploring the role of POLE mutations in advanced CRC. POLE mutations disrupt proofreading and lead to misincorporation of bases which can drastically increase TMB [96]. As TMB increases, the

Table 2 Clinical trials evaluating combination therapy with ICI and MEK

ICI	Combination	Disease	Phase	Trial number
Nivolumab + ipilimumab	Binimetinib (MEK)	RAS-mutated mCRC	I/II	NCT03271047
Nivolumab + ipilimumab	Trametinib (MEK)	Pre-treated mCRC	I/II	NCT03377361
Nivolumab + ipilimumab	Cobimetinib (MEK) or daratumumab (CD38)	rCRC	II	NCT02060188
Pembrolizumab	MK-8353 (ERK1/2)	mCRC	I	NCT03442569
Atezolizumab	Cobimetinib (MEK) + bevacizumab (VEGF)	mCRC	I	NCT02876224
Atezolizumab	Cobimetinib (MEK)	First-line mCRC	II	NCT02291289
Atezolizumab	Cobimetinib (MEK) + bevacizumab (VEGF)	mCRC	III	NCT02788279
Durvalumab	Trametinib (MEK)	mCRC	II	NCT03428126
PDR001	Dabrafenib (BRAF) + trametinib (MEK)	mCRC	II	NCT03668431

CRC colorectal cancer, *ERK1/2* extracellular signal-regulated kinases, *MEK* Ras-Raf-MEK-ERK pathway, *mCRC* metastatic colorectal cancer, *PDR001* anti-PD-1 mAB; *rCRC* refractory colorectal cancer, *VEGF* vascular endothelial growth factor

likelihood of having a high neoantigen burden and activation of T-cell-mediated response increases. Thus, POLE mutations may modulate the response to ICIs by increasing the likelihood of triggering a strong immune response in CRC. Younger patients are more likely to have POLE mutations, but so far they have only been found in 1–2% of pMMR/MSS CRCs [97]. However, patients who have tumors with POLE mutations have lower rates of recurrence after surgical removal of CRC. Cases have been reported in which patients with POLE mutations have strong response to pembrolizumab with pMMR/MSS phenotype [98]; however, more studies are needed to determine whether POLE mutations can serve as an effective prognostic marker or indicator for ICI-sensitive CRC.

3.6 IDO Inhibitors

Enzymes and markers that can affect the TME have the potential to modulate response to ICI in advanced CRC. Indoleamine 2, 3-dioxygenase (IDO) 1 and IDO 2 catalyze the conversion of tryptophan to kynurenine and are found in immune cells [99]. The accumulation of kynurenine and deficiency in tryptophan arrest T-cell replication and activation, reducing the cytotoxic response to tumors [100]. This is associated with poor prognosis in colorectal cancer as tumor cells are able to avoid immune attack and prevent T-cell invasion by depleting tryptophan [101]. IDO is expressed in high levels in 40% of CRC making it a valuable potential target for therapy [102]. IDO inhibition would prevent accumulation of kynurenine, maintain tryptophan levels, and enhance T-cell activity in the TME, all of which would increase sensitivity to ICIs. A phase I study (NCT01195311) established tolerability of epacadostat (IDO inhibitor) without demonstrating single-agent activity against solid malignancies [103]. However, it is currently being studied in a phase I/II trial, ECHO-206 (NCT02959437), in combination with pembrolizumab and azacitidine (DNA methyltransferase inhibitor) for patients with advanced solid tumors. After establishing tolerability and recommended dosing, subjects with MSS mCRC will be enrolled allowing for the evaluation of whether IDO inhibitors can increase the efficacy of ICIs in patients with pMRR/MSS.

3.7 Carcinoembryonic Antigen T-Cell Bispecific Protein

Carcinoembryonic antigen (CEA) is a marker often associated with gastrointestinal malignancies. It is naturally found on the cell membrane of enterocytes during fetal development, and though it is not useful in detecting early CRC, it is overexpressed in advanced CRC which gives it value as a therapeutic target [104]. CEA CD3 T-cell bispecific protein (CEA-TCB) simultaneously binds the CEA that is abundant on tumor cells and CD3 on T cells which allows for direction of T cells and immune response to cancer [105]. Phase Ia and Ib studies (NCT02324257, NCT02650713) established preliminary efficacy and safety of CEA TCB in patients with advanced CEA+ solid tumors [106]. Sixty-eight patients with mCRC were treated with CEA TCB monotherapy while 28 patients were treated with CEA TCB and atezolizumab. MSS CRC patients on mono- and combination therapy had partial responses to treatment, while the DCR in the monotherapy cohort was 45%. 6% of patients had a PR and 39% had SD. In the most recent update, no treatment-related deaths were reported yet there were several dose-limiting toxicities. While the CEA T-cell engager has good theoretical action demonstrated in preclinical studies, the role it has in conjunction with ICIs in MSS CRC remains to be seen.

3.8 Toll-Like Receptor Agonists

Toll-like receptors (TLR) have had a known role in immunotherapy for several decades. Imiquimod, a TLR7 receptor agonist, has been used for treating HPV since 1997 and was approved for superficial basal cell carcinoma (BCC) in 2004 [107, 108]. Topical TLR7 agonists target dendritic cells resulting in the production of interferon-alpha and increasing antigen-presenting cell capacity to augment the adaptive immune response [109]. TLR9 is expressed in plasmacytoid dendritic cells (pDC) and B cells, with activation resulting in downstream production of proinflammatory cytokines and enhanced response of cytotoxic NK and CD8+ T cells [110, 111]. MGN1703 (Lefitolimod) is a TLR9 agonist that was evaluated in a phase II trial known as the IMPACT trial (NCT01208194) as maintenance treatment in patients with mCRC and disease control after standard chemotherapy regimen. Fifty-nine patients were enrolled and randomized to MGN1703 or placebo with hazard ratio as the primary endpoint. The HR for investigator assessment was 0.55 (95% CI: 0.3–1.0; $p = 0.04$) with a median PFS of 2.8 months (95% CI: 2.8–4.1 months) in those treated with MGN1703 compared to 2.6 months (95% CI: 2.5–2.8 months) with placebo [112]. Of patients in the treatment group, 79% experienced treatment-related AEs with 26% having grade 3 or 4 adverse events. Most common AEs included flu-like symptoms (13.9%), general pain (9.3%), and rash or pruritis (9.3%) while serious events included ileus (9.3%), hypertension (4.7%), and worsening of hypertension (4.7%). Updates to the trial 1 year later did not have mature OS data but indicated that only 35% of MGN1703 patients experienced a disease-related event compared to 50% of placebo patients [113]. A phase III clinical trial, IMPALA, is currently in progress (NCT02077868) [114]. However preliminary data from the trial demonstrates that the overall survival endpoint was not met with a median OS of 22 months with MGN1703 compared to 21.9 months with standard of care (HR 1.12; 95% CI: 0.91–1.38; $p = 0.2765$) [115]. Other TLR agonists have been or are being explored in clinical trials as combination therapy, including poly-ICLC (TLR3) with pembrolizumab in pMMR mCRC (NCT02834052), VTX-2337 (TLR8) with cyclophosphamide and pegfilgrastim in metastatic solid tumors including CRC (NCT02650635; recently closed), and MGN1703 (TLR9) with ipilimumab (NCT02668770) in advanced malignancy including CRC.

3.9 Radiation Therapy

Radiation therapy enhancing chemo- or immunotherapy in local or distant sites is a phenomenon known as the abscopal effect. One of the preliminary studies to establish this effect was in a patient with metastatic melanoma on maintenance therapy with ipilimumab (anti-CTLA-4) who had progressive disease during maintenance phase but a systemic response after a paraspinal mass was treated with palliative radiation [116]. This effect has been demonstrated again preclinically [117] and clinically in melanoma [118, 119] and non-small cell lung cancer [120]. Suggested mechanisms for the abscopal effect include altering the balance between signals activating and suppressing the immune system in the TME, regulation via induction of type I interferon, and activation of DNA damage response promoting further immune system activation [121]. Several studies have evaluated combination radiotherapy with ICIs in mCRC patients. A pilot study (NCT02298946) investigated 17 patients treated with AMP-224 (anti-PD-1) and stereotactic body radiation therapy (SBRT) to the site of liver metastasis. The study failed to record any objective responses to combination therapy, confirmed by biopsy [122]. A following phase II trial (NCT02437071) assessed whether pembrolizumab in combination with RT or ablation enhanced the efficacy in refractory pMMR mCRC patients. While the safety profile was tolerable, the ORR was 9% (1/11) in the radiation therapy cohort [123]. A phase II clinical trial (NCT03122509) is ongoing to evaluate the efficacy of durvalumab (anti-PD-L1) and tremelimumab (anti-CTLA-4) in combination with radiation or ablation in patients with mCRC. There are many clinical trials evaluating the potential of radiation therapy to enhance systemic response to ICI particularly in pMMR CRC but completed studies have demonstrated poor efficacy.

3.10 Costimulatory Receptor Agonists

Novel strategies for immunotherapy in resistant tumors revolve around reversing tumor-related immune system dysfunction and promoting the activity of targeted responses by T cells. Costimulatory receptors are an integral part of T-cell engagement as they lower the activation threshold of T cells secondary to T-cell receptor [124]. CD28 is the primary costimulatory receptor present on T cells, as it initiates IL-2 production and clonal T-cell expansion. Other well-studied costimulatory targets include members of the TNF receptor (TNFR) family, 4-1BB (CD137), glucocorticoid-induced TNFR (GITR), and OX40 (CD134) [124]. OX40 is expressed mainly on Treg and activated effector T cells, and preclinical studies demonstrate that agonism with monoclonal antibodies increases clonal expansion of CD4+ and CD8+ T cells [125, 126]. A completed phase I trial (NCT01644968) evaluated the tolerability and efficacy of treatment with OX40 mAb in patients with metastatic refractory solid malignancies. Investigators noted regression of one or more metastatic lesions in 40% (12/30) of patients, thought to be due to upregulation of OX40 on regulatory T cells in TIL resulting in increased T- and B-cell antitumor activity [127]. Preclinical studies in murine models further assessed OX40 mAb in combination with anti-CTLA-4 mAb. Enhanced effector T-cell expansion and function, induced Th2 cytokine production, and improved survival were all observed in these studies indicating that OX40 is a potential target for co-treatment. An ongoing phase I clinical trial (NCT02559024), MEDI6469, is evaluating an OX40 mAb in mCRC prior to surgical treatment to determine an immune score, clinical survival, and immunologic data [128].

GITR is a costimulatory receptor that is basally expressed at low levels on T cells, and the interaction between GITR and its ligand signals CD4+ and CD8+ cells resulting in enhanced proliferation and effector functioning [129]. A GITR agonist, MEDI1873, is currently being investigated in a phase I clinical trial (NCT02583165) treating patients with refractory advanced solid tumors. The best initial response was stable disease in 42.5% (17/40) patients including 1 unconfirmed PR [130]. Twenty percent (8/40) patients had SD for at least 24 weeks. Treatment was well tolerated with only three dose-limiting toxicities, and the most common treated-related AEs were headache (25%), infusion-related reaction (17.5%), and decreased appetite (17.5%). Further studies are investigating GITR agonists in a variety of metastatic malignancies.

4-1BB (CD137) is a TNF family receptor expressed on primed T and NK cells that provides a strong costimulatory signal when ligand activated [131]. Preclinical models demonstrated that the combination of anti-CTLA-4 and 4-1BB antibodies increased infiltration of CD8+ T cells and CD4+ effector T cells and reduced Treg cell infiltration of tumors, all promoting antitumor activity [132]. A phase Ib study (NCT02179918) evaluated treatment with utomilumab (anti-4-1BB) and pembrolizumab (anti-PD-1) in patients with advanced solid tumors, with 6 out of 23 patients (26.1%) achieving complete or partial responses with a tolerable safety profile. Future evaluation in advanced-phase clinical trials of costimulatory signals, including OX40, GITR, and 4-1BB, in combination with ICIs may lead to better therapeutic options in pMMR/MSS mCRC.

4 Conclusion and Future Direction

Immunotherapy in mCRC is a changing landscape with the evolution of immune checkpoint inhibitors and potential effectiveness of combination therapy. ICIs have been so effective at treating dMMR/MSI-H mCRC that they are currently being evaluated in phase III clinical trials as neoadjuvant chemotherapy with preliminary data indicating increased effectiveness compared to standard chemotherapy. They are also being evaluated in early-stage CRC, as in the ATOMIC trial (NCT02912559), a study evaluating whether patients with resected stage III colon carcinomas and MSI-H tumors will benefit from the addition of atezolizumab (anti-PD-L1 mAb) to adjuvant FOLFOX therapy with a primary endpoint of DFS [133]. However, dMMR/MSI-H mCRC makes up only 12–15% across stages of colorectal cancer, which is why initial unselected studies with ICIs in CRC demonstrated minimal clinical effectiveness. This absence of meaningful outcome is likely due to a suboptimal immunosuppressed tumor microenvironment, absence of identifiable biomarkers, and resistance to ICIs. Several clinical trials are underway with an aim to evaluate how combination therapy with other immune targets or immunomodulatory agents, such as BRAF, VEGF, EGFR, MEK, and TLR, may provide a pathway to overcome resistance in pMMR/MSS mCRC. Further investigation of molecular mechanisms of immunity and innovative targets to activate cellular immunity and suppress inhibitory signaling may lead to advancements in the treatment of mCRC. Advances in ICI therapy have been recent and continued evolution of this promising therapy may create a new era in the treatment of advanced colorectal cancer.

Compliance with Ethical Standards

Conflict of Interest: Puneet Raman, M.D., declares no conflicts of interest that might be relevant to the contents of this manuscript.

Gehan Botrus, M.D., Ph.D., declares no conflicts of interest that might be relevant to the contents of this manuscript.

Tanios S. Bekaii-Saab, M.D., declares: Research Funding (to institution): Boston Biomedical, Bayer, Amgen, Merck, Celgene, Lilly, Ipsen, Clovis, Seattle Genetics, Array Biopharma, Genentech, Abgenomics, Incyte, and eBMS. Consulting (to institution): Ipsen, Array Biopharma, Seattle Genetics, Bayer, Genentech, Incyte, and Merck. Consulting (to self): Boehringer Ingelheim, TreosBio, and Sobi. IDMC/DSMB (to self): AstraZeneca, Exelixis, Lilly, PanCan, and 1Globe. Scientific Advisory Board: Imugene, Immuneering, and Sun Biopharma. Inventions/Patents: WO/2018/183488 and WO/2019/055687.

References

1. Siegel RL, Miller KD, Goding Sauer A, Fedewa SA, Butterly LF, Anderson JC et al (2020) Colorectal cancer statistics, 2020. CA Cancer J Clin 70(3):145–164. https://doi.org/10.3322/caac.21601
2. Montminy EM, Karlitz JJ, Landreneau SW (2019) Progress of colorectal cancer screening in United States: past achievements and future challenges. Prev Med 120:78–84. https://doi.org/10.1016/j.ypmed.2018.12.004
3. Gustavsson B, Carlsson G, Machover D, Petrelli N, Roth A, Schmoll HJ et al (2015) A review of the evolution of systemic chemotherapy in the management of colorectal cancer. Clin Colorectal Cancer 14(1):1–10. https://doi.org/10.1016/j.clcc.2014.11.002
4. Saltz LB, Cox JV, Blanke C, Rosen LS, Fehrenbacher L, Moore MJ et al (2000) Irinotecan plus fluorouracil and leucovorin for metastatic colorectal cancer. Irinotecan Study Group. N Engl J Med 343(13):905–914. https://doi.org/10.1056/nejm200009283431302
5. Goldberg RM, Sargent DJ, Morton RF, Fuchs CS, Ramanathan RK, Williamson SK et al (2004) A randomized controlled trial of fluorouracil plus leucovorin, irinotecan, and oxaliplatin combinations in patients with previously untreated metastatic colorectal cancer. J Clin Oncol 22(1):23–30. https://doi.org/10.1200/jco.2004.09.046
6. Tournigand C, André T, Achille E, Lledo G, Flesh M, Mery-Mignard D et al (2004) FOLFIRI followed by FOLFOX6 or the reverse sequence in advanced colorectal cancer: a randomized GERCOR study. J Clin Oncol 22(2):229–237. https://doi.org/10.1200/jco.2004.05.113
7. Colucci G, Gebbia V, Paoletti G, Giuliani F, Caruso M, Gebbia N et al (2005) Phase III randomized trial of FOLFIRI versus FOLFOX4 in the treatment of advanced colorectal cancer: a multicenter study of the Gruppo Oncologico Dell'Italia Meridionale. J Clin Oncol 23(22):4866–4875. https://doi.org/10.1200/jco.2005.07.113
8. Hurwitz H, Fehrenbacher L, Novotny W, Cartwright T, Hainsworth J, Heim W et al (2004) Bevacizumab plus irinotecan, fluorouracil, and leucovorin for metastatic colorectal cancer. N Engl J Med 350(23):2335–2342. https://doi.org/10.1056/NEJMoa032691
9. Giantonio BJ, Catalano PJ, Meropol NJ, O'Dwyer PJ, Mitchell EP, Alberts SR et al (2007) Bevacizumab in combination with oxaliplatin, fluorouracil, and leucovorin (FOLFOX4) for previously treated metastatic colorectal cancer: results from the Eastern Cooperative Oncology Group Study E3200. J Clin Oncol 25(12):1539–1544. https://doi.org/10.1200/jco.2006.09.6305
10. Heinemann V, von Weikersthal LF, Decker T, Kiani A, Vehling-Kaiser U, Al-Batran SE et al (2014) FOLFIRI plus cetuximab versus FOLFIRI plus bevacizumab as first-line treatment for patients with metastatic colorectal cancer (FIRE-3): a randomised, open-label, phase 3 trial. Lancet Oncol 15(10):1065–1075. https://doi.org/10.1016/s1470-2045(14)70330-4
11. Heinemann V, von Weikersthal LF, Decker T, Kiani A, Kaiser F, Al-Batran S-E et al (2021) FOLFIRI plus cetuximab or bevacizumab for advanced colorectal cancer: final survival and per-protocol analysis of FIRE-3, a randomised clinical trial. Br J Cancer 124(3):587–594. https://doi.org/10.1038/s41416-020-01140-9
12. Falcone A, Cremolini C, Masi G, Lonardi S, Zagonel V, Salvatore L et al (2013) FOLFOXIRI/bevacizumab (bev) versus FOLFIRI/bev as first-line treatment in unresectable metastatic colorectal cancer (mCRC) patients (pts): results of the phase III TRIBE trial by GONO group. J Clin Oncol 31(Suppl. 15):3505. https://doi.org/10.1200/jco.2013.31.15_suppl.3505
13. Cremolini C, Antoniotti C, Rossini D, Lonardi S, Loupakis F, Pietrantonio F et al (2020) Upfront FOLFOXIRI plus bevacizumab and reintroduction after progression versus mFOLFOX6 plus bevacizumab followed by FOLFIRI plus bevacizumab in the treatment of patients with metastatic colorectal cancer (TRIBE2): a multicentre, open-label, phase 3, randomised, controlled trial. Lancet Oncol 21(4):497–507. https://doi.org/10.1016/S1470-2045(19)30862-9
14. Del Vecchio F, Mastroiaco V, Di Marco A, Compagnoni C, Capece D, Zazzeroni F et al (2017) Next-generation sequencing: recent applications to the analysis of colorectal cancer. J Transl Med 15(1):246. https://doi.org/10.1186/s12967-017-1353-y

15. Fukui K (2010) DNA mismatch repair in eukaryotes and bacteria. J Nucl Acids 2010. https://doi.org/10.4061/2010/260512
16. Nojadeh JN, Behrouz Sharif S, Sakhinia E (2018) Microsatellite instability in colorectal cancer. EXCLI J 17:159–168. https://doi.org/10.17179/excli2017-948
17. Le DT, Uram JN, Wang H, Bartlett BR, Kemberling H, Eyring AD et al (2015) PD-1 Blockade in tumors with mismatch-repair deficiency. N Engl J Med 372(26):2509–2520. https://doi.org/10.1056/NEJMoa1500596
18. Overman MJ, Ernstoff MS, Morse MA (2018) Where we stand with immunotherapy in colorectal cancer: deficient mismatch repair, proficient mismatch repair, and toxicity management. Am Soc Clin Oncol Educ Book 38:239–247. https://doi.org/10.1200/edbk_200821
19. Stadler ZK, Battaglin F, Middha S, Hechtman JF, Tran C, Cercek A et al (2016) Reliable detection of mismatch repair deficiency in colorectal cancers using mutational load in next-generation sequencing panels. J Clin Oncol 34(18):2141–2147. https://doi.org/10.1200/jco.2015.65.1067
20. Kawakami H, Zaanan A, Sinicrope FA (2015) Microsatellite instability testing and its role in the management of colorectal cancer. Curr Treat Options in Oncol 16(7):30. https://doi.org/10.1007/s11864-015-0348-2
21. Hanahan D, Coussens LM (2012) Accessories to the crime: functions of cells recruited to the tumor microenvironment. Cancer Cell 21(3):309–322. https://doi.org/10.1016/j.ccr.2012.02.022
22. Korneev KV, Atretkhany KN, Drutskaya MS, Grivennikov SI, Kuprash DV, Nedospasov SA (2017) TLR-signaling and proinflammatory cytokines as drivers of tumorigenesis. Cytokine 89:127–135. https://doi.org/10.1016/j.cyto.2016.01.021
23. Mlecnik B, Tosolini M, Kirilovsky A, Berger A, Bindea G, Meatchi T et al (2011) Histopathologic-based prognostic factors of colorectal cancers are associated with the state of the local immune reaction. J Clin Oncol 29(6):610–618. https://doi.org/10.1200/jco.2010.30.5425
24. Maoz A, Dennis M, Greenson JK (2019) The Crohn's-like lymphoid reaction to colorectal cancer-tertiary lymphoid structures with immunologic and potentially therapeutic relevance in colorectal cancer. Front Immunol 10:1884. https://doi.org/10.3389/fimmu.2019.01884
25. Basile D, Garattini SK, Bonotto M, Ongaro E, Casagrande M, Cattaneo M et al (2017) Immunotherapy for colorectal cancer: where are we heading? Expert Opin Biol Ther 17(6):709–721. https://doi.org/10.1080/14712598.2017.1315405
26. Pagès F, Kirilovsky A, Mlecnik B, Asslaber M, Tosolini M, Bindea G et al (2009) In situ cytotoxic and memory T cells predict outcome in patients with early-stage colorectal cancer. J Clin Oncol 27(35):5944–5951. https://doi.org/10.1200/jco.2008.19.6147
27. Pagès F, Mlecnik B, Marliot F, Bindea G, Ou F-S, Bifulco C et al (2018) International validation of the consensus Immunoscore for the classification of colon cancer: a prognostic and accuracy study. Lancet 391(10135):2128–2139. https://doi.org/10.1016/S0140-6736(18)30789-X
28. Bruni D, Angell HK, Galon J (2020) The immune contexture and Immunoscore in cancer prognosis and therapeutic efficacy. Nat Rev Cancer 20(11):662–680. https://doi.org/10.1038/s41568-020-0285-7
29. Jiang T, Shi T, Zhang H, Hu J, Song Y, Wei J et al (2019) Tumor neoantigens: from basic research to clinical applications. J Hematol Oncol 12(1):93. https://doi.org/10.1186/s13045-019-0787-5
30. Trombetta ES, Mellman I (2005) Cell biology of antigen processing in vitro and in vivo. Annu Rev Immunol 23:975–1028. https://doi.org/10.1146/annurev.immunol.22.012703.104538
31. Chen C, Liu S, Qu R, Li B (2020) Recurrent neoantigens in colorectal cancer as potential immunotherapy targets. Biomed Res Int 2020:2861240. https://doi.org/10.1155/2020/2861240
32. Schumacher TN, Schreiber RD (2015) Neoantigens in cancer immunotherapy. Science (New York, NY) 348(6230):69–74. https://doi.org/10.1126/science.aaa4971
33. Rodriguez-Salas N, Dominguez G, Barderas R, Mendiola M, García-Albéniz X, Maurel J et al (2017) Clinical relevance of colorectal cancer molecular subtypes. Crit Rev Oncol Hematol 109:9–19. https://doi.org/10.1016/j.critrevonc.2016.11.007

34. Peltomäki P (2003) Role of DNA mismatch repair defects in the pathogenesis of human cancer. J Clin Oncol 21(6):1174–1179. https://doi.org/10.1200/jco.2003.04.060
35. Sharma P, Allison JP (2015) The future of immune checkpoint therapy. Science (New York, NY) 348(6230):56–61. https://doi.org/10.1126/science.aaa8172
36. Townsend SE, Allison JP (1993) Tumor rejection after direct costimulation of CD8+ T cells by B7-transfected melanoma cells. Science (New York, NY) 259(5093):368–370. https://doi.org/10.1126/science.7678351
37. Wei SC, Duffy CR, Allison JP (2018) Fundamental mechanisms of immune checkpoint blockade therapy. Cancer Discov 8(9):1069–1086. https://doi.org/10.1158/2159-8290.cd-18-0367
38. Khalil DN, Smith EL, Brentjens RJ, Wolchok JD (2016) The future of cancer treatment: immunomodulation, CARs and combination immunotherapy. Nat Rev Clin Oncol 13(5):273–290. https://doi.org/10.1038/nrclinonc.2016.25
39. Jacobs J, Smits E, Lardon F, Pauwels P, Deschoolmeester V (2015) Immune checkpoint modulation in colorectal cancer: what's new and what to expect. J Immunol Res 2015:158038. https://doi.org/10.1155/2015/158038
40. Ge J, Zhu L, Zhou J, Li G, Li Y, Li S et al (2015) Association between co-inhibitory molecule gene tagging single nucleotide polymorphisms and the risk of colorectal cancer in Chinese. J Cancer Res Clin Oncol 141(9):1533–1544. https://doi.org/10.1007/s00432-015-1915-4
41. Llosa NJ, Cruise M, Tam A, Wicks EC, Hechenbleikner EM, Taube JM et al (2015) The vigorous immune microenvironment of microsatellite instable colon cancer is balanced by multiple counter-inhibitory checkpoints. Cancer Discov 5(1):43–51. https://doi.org/10.1158/2159-8290.cd-14-0863
42. Arora SP, Mahalingam D (2018) Immunotherapy in colorectal cancer: for the select few or all? J Gastrointestinal Oncol 9(1):170–179. https://doi.org/10.21037/jgo.2017.06.10
43. Pardoll DM (2012) The blockade of immune checkpoints in cancer immunotherapy. Nat Rev Cancer 12(4):252–264. https://doi.org/10.1038/nrc3239
44. Tran L, Theodorescu D (2020) Determinants of resistance to checkpoint inhibitors. Int J Mol Sci 21(5). https://doi.org/10.3390/ijms21051594
45. Schrock AB, Ouyang C, Sandhu J, Sokol E, Jin D, Ross JS et al (2019) Tumor mutational burden is predictive of response to immune checkpoint inhibitors in MSI-high metastatic colorectal cancer. Ann Oncol 30(7):1096–1103. https://doi.org/10.1093/annonc/mdz134
46. Zemek RM, Chin WL, Nowak AK, Millward MJ, Lake RA, Lesterhuis WJ (2020) Sensitizing the tumor microenvironment to immune checkpoint therapy. Front Immunol 11:223. https://doi.org/10.3389/fimmu.2020.00223
47. Xu L, Pelosof L, Wang R, McFarland HI, Wu WW, Phue JN et al (2020) NGS evaluation of colorectal cancer reveals interferon gamma dependent expression of immune checkpoint genes and identification of novel IFNγ induced genes. Front Immunol 11:224. https://doi.org/10.3389/fimmu.2020.00224
48. Gao J, Shi LZ, Zhao H, Chen J, Xiong L, He Q et al (2016) Loss of IFN-γ pathway genes in tumor cells as a mechanism of resistance to anti-CTLA-4 therapy. Cell 167(2):397–404.e9. https://doi.org/10.1016/j.cell.2016.08.069
49. Koveitypour Z, Panahi F, Vakilian M, Peymani M, Seyed Forootan F, Nasr Esfahani MH et al (2019) Signaling pathways involved in colorectal cancer progression. Cell Biosci 9(1):97. https://doi.org/10.1186/s13578-019-0361-4
50. Roberts PJ, Der CJ (2007) Targeting the Raf-MEK-ERK mitogen-activated protein kinase cascade for the treatment of cancer. Oncogene 26(22):3291–3310. https://doi.org/10.1038/sj.onc.1210422
51. Caputo F, Santini C, Bardasi C, Cerma K, Casadei-Gardini A, Spallanzani A et al (2019) BRAF-mutated colorectal cancer: clinical and molecular insights. Int J Mol Sci 20(21):5369. https://doi.org/10.3390/ijms20215369
52. Markowitz SD, Bertagnolli MM (2009) Molecular origins of cancer: Molecular basis of colorectal cancer. N Engl J Med 361(25):2449–2460. https://doi.org/10.1056/NEJMra0804588

53. Nosho K, Irahara N, Shima K, Kure S, Kirkner GJ, Schernhammer ES et al (2008) Comprehensive biostatistical analysis of CpG island methylator phenotype in colorectal cancer using a large population-based sample. PLoS One 3(11):e3698. https://doi.org/10.1371/journal.pone.0003698
54. Clarke CN, Kopetz ES (2015) BRAF mutant colorectal cancer as a distinct subset of colorectal cancer: clinical characteristics, clinical behavior, and response to targeted therapies. J Gastrointestinal Oncol 6(6):660–667. https://doi.org/10.3978/j.issn.2078-6891.2015.077
55. Rajagopalan H, Bardelli A, Lengauer C, Kinzler KW, Vogelstein B, Velculescu VE (2002) Tumorigenesis: RAF/RAS oncogenes and mismatch-repair status. Nature 418(6901):934. https://doi.org/10.1038/418934a
56. Beeram M, Patnaik A, Rowinsky EK (2005) Raf: a strategic target for therapeutic development against cancer. J Clin Oncol 23(27):6771–6790. https://doi.org/10.1200/jco.2005.08.036
57. Fransén K, Klintenäs M, Osterström A, Dimberg J, Monstein HJ, Söderkvist P (2004) Mutation analysis of the BRAF, ARAF and RAF-1 genes in human colorectal adenocarcinomas. Carcinogenesis 25(4):527–533. https://doi.org/10.1093/carcin/bgh049
58. Tie J, Gibbs P, Lipton L, Christie M, Jorissen RN, Burgess AW et al (2011) Optimizing targeted therapeutic development: analysis of a colorectal cancer patient population with the BRAF(V600E) mutation. Int J Cancer 128(9):2075–2084. https://doi.org/10.1002/ijc.25555
59. Taieb J, Le Malicot K, Shi Q, Penault-Llorca F, Bouché O, Tabernero J et al (2016) Prognostic value of BRAF and KRAS mutations in MSI and MSS stage III colon cancer. J Natl Cancer Inst 109(5):djw272. https://doi.org/10.1093/jnci/djw272
60. Taieb J, Shi Q, Pederson L, Alberts S, Wolmark N, Van Cutsem E et al (2019) Prognosis of microsatellite instability and/or mismatch repair deficiency stage III colon cancer patients after disease recurrence following adjuvant treatment: results of an ACCENT pooled analysis of seven studies. Ann Oncol 30(9):1466–1471. https://doi.org/10.1093/annonc/mdz208
61. Wang L, Cunningham JM, Winters JL, Guenther JC, French AJ, Boardman LA et al (2003) BRAF mutations in colon cancer are not likely attributable to defective DNA mismatch repair. Cancer Res 63(17):5209–5212
62. Sinicrope FA, Shi Q, Smyrk TC, Thibodeau SN, Dienstmann R, Guinney J et al (2015) Molecular markers identify subtypes of stage III colon cancer associated with patient outcomes. Gastroenterology 148(1):88–99. https://doi.org/10.1053/j.gastro.2014.09.041
63. Kim YH, Kakar S, Cun L, Deng G, Kim YS (2008) Distinct CpG island methylation profiles and BRAF mutation status in serrated and adenomatous colorectal polyps. Int J Cancer 123(11):2587–2593. https://doi.org/10.1002/ijc.23840
64. Kim G, McKee AE, Ning YM, Hazarika M, Theoret M, Johnson JR et al (2014) FDA approval summary: vemurafenib for treatment of unresectable or metastatic melanoma with the BRAFV600E mutation. Clin Cancer Res 20(19):4994–5000. https://doi.org/10.1158/1078-0432.ccr-14-0776
65. Kopetz S, Desai J, Chan E, Hecht JR, O'Dwyer PJ, Maru D et al (2015) Phase II Pilot Study of vemurafenib in patients with metastatic BRAF-mutated colorectal cancer. J Clin Oncol 33(34):4032–4038. https://doi.org/10.1200/JCO.2015.63.2497
66. Prahallad A, Sun C, Huang S, Di Nicolantonio F, Salazar R, Zecchin D et al (2012) Unresponsiveness of colon cancer to BRAF(V600E) inhibition through feedback activation of EGFR. Nature 483(7387):100–103. https://doi.org/10.1038/nature10868
67. Corcoran RB, Ebi H, Turke AB, Coffee EM, Nishino M, Cogdill AP et al (2012) EGFR-mediated re-activation of MAPK signaling contributes to insensitivity of BRAF mutant colorectal cancers to RAF inhibition with vemurafenib. Cancer Discov 2(3):227–235. https://doi.org/10.1158/2159-8290.cd-11-0341
68. Corcoran RB, André T, Atreya CE, Schellens JHM, Yoshino T, Bendell JC et al (2018) Combined BRAF, EGFR, and MEK inhibition in patients with BRAF(V600E)-mutant colorectal cancer. Cancer Discov 8(4):428–443. https://doi.org/10.1158/2159-8290.cd-17-1226
69. Kopetz S, Guthrie KA, Morris VK, Lenz H-J, Magliocco AM, Maru D et al (2020) Randomized trial of irinotecan and cetuximab with or without vemurafenib in BRAF-Mutant Metastatic

Colorectal Cancer (SWOG S1406). J Clin Oncol 39(4):285–294. https://doi.org/10.1200/JCO.20.01994
70. Kopetz S, Grothey A, Yaeger R, Van Cutsem E, Desai J, Yoshino T et al (2019) Encorafenib, binimetinib, and cetuximab in BRAF V600E–mutated colorectal cancer. N Engl J Med 381(17):1632–1643. https://doi.org/10.1056/NEJMoa1908075
71. Tabernero J, Grothey A, Van Cutsem E, Yaeger R, Wasan H, Yoshino T et al (2021) Encorafenib Plus Cetuximab as a new standard of care for previously treated BRAF V600E-mutant metastatic colorectal cancer: updated survival results and subgroup analyses from the BEACON study. J Clin Oncol 39(4):273–284. https://doi.org/10.1200/jco.20.02088
72. Kopetz S, Grothey A, Yaeger R, Ciardiello F, Desai J, Kim TW et al (2021) BREAKWATER: randomized phase 3 study of encorafenib (enco) + cetuximab (cetux) ± chemotherapy for first-line (1L) treatment (tx) of BRAF V600E-mutant (BRAFV600E) metastatic colorectal cancer (mCRC). J Clin Oncol 39(Suppl. 15):TPS3619. https://doi.org/10.1200/JCO.2021.39.15_suppl.TPS3619
73. Corcoran R, Giannakis M, Allen J, Chen J, Pelka K, Chao S et al (2020) SO-26 Clinical efficacy of combined BRAF, MEK, and PD-1 inhibition in BRAFV600E colorectal cancer patients. Ann Oncol 31:S226–S2S7. https://doi.org/10.1016/j.annonc.2020.04.041
74. Yang J, Yan J, Liu B (2018) Targeting VEGF/VEGFR to modulate antitumor immunity. Front Immunol 9:978. https://doi.org/10.3389/fimmu.2018.00978
75. Wolchok JD, Saenger Y (2008) The mechanism of anti-CTLA-4 activity and the negative regulation of T-cell activation. Oncologist 13(Suppl. 4):2–9. https://doi.org/10.1634/theoncologist.13-S4-2
76. Zhu P, Hu C, Hui K, Jiang X (2017) The role and significance of VEGFR2(+) regulatory T cells in tumor immunity. Onco Targets Ther 10:4315–4319. https://doi.org/10.2147/ott.s142085
77. Wallin J, Pishvaian MJ, Hernandez G, Yadav M, Jhunjhunwala S, Delamarre L et al (2016) Abstract 2651: clinical activity and immune correlates from a phase Ib study evaluating atezolizumab (anti-PDL1) in combination with FOLFOX and bevacizumab (anti-VEGF) in metastatic colorectal carcinoma. Cancer Res 76(Suppl. 14):2651. https://doi.org/10.1158/1538-7445.am2016-2651
78. Cohen MH, Gootenberg J, Keegan P, Pazdur R (2007) FDA drug approval summary: bevacizumab plus FOLFOX4 as second-line treatment of colorectal cancer. Oncologist 12(3):356–361. https://doi.org/10.1634/theoncologist.12-3-356
79. Grothey A, Tabernero J, Arnold D, De Gramont A, Ducreux MP, O'Dwyer PJ et al (2018) LBA19 - Fluoropyrimidine (FP) + bevacizumab (BEV) + atezolizumab vs FP/BEV in BRAFwt metastatic colorectal cancer (mCRC): findings from Cohort 2 of MODUL—a multicentre, randomized trial of biomarker-driven maintenance treatment following first-line induction therapy. Ann Oncol 29:viii714–viii715. https://doi.org/10.1093/annonc/mdy424.020
80. Antoniotti C, Borelli B, Rossini D, Pietrantonio F, Morano F, Salvatore L et al (2020) AtezoTRIBE: a randomised phase II study of FOLFOXIRI plus bevacizumab alone or in combination with atezolizumab as initial therapy for patients with unresectable metastatic colorectal cancer. BMC Cancer 20(1):683. https://doi.org/10.1186/s12885-020-07169-6
81. Aranda E, Viéitez JM, Gómez-España A, Gil Calle S, Salud-Salvia A, Graña B et al (2020) FOLFOXIRI plus bevacizumab versus FOLFOX plus bevacizumab for patients with metastatic colorectal cancer and ≥3 circulating tumour cells: the randomised phase III VISNÚ-1 trial. ESMO Open 5(6). https://doi.org/10.1136/esmoopen-2020-000944
82. Lwin Z, Gomez-Roca C, Saada-Bouzid E, Yanez E, Muñoz FL, Im SA et al (2020) LBA41 LEAP-005: Phase II study of lenvatinib (len) plus pembrolizumab (pembro) in patients (pts) with previously treated advanced solid tumours. Ann Oncol 31:S1170. https://doi.org/10.1016/j.annonc.2020.08.2271
83. Gomez-Roca C, Yanez E, Im S-A, Castanon Alvarez E, Senellart H, Doherty M, et al. LEAP-005: a phase II multicohort study of lenvatinib plus pembrolizumab in patients with previously treated selected solid tumors—results from the colorectal cancer cohort. J Clin Oncol 2021;39(3_suppl):94-. https://doi.org/10.1200/JCO.2021.39.3_suppl.94

84. Fukuoka S, Hara H, Takahashi N, Kojima T, Kawazoe A, Asayama M et al (2020) Regorafenib Plus Nivolumab in patients with advanced gastric or colorectal cancer: an open-label, dose-escalation, and dose-expansion phase Ib trial (REGONIVO, EPOC1603). J Clin Oncol 38(18):2053–2061. https://doi.org/10.1200/jco.19.03296
85. Grothey A, Van Cutsem E, Sobrero A, Siena S, Falcone A, Ychou M et al (2013) Regorafenib monotherapy for previously treated metastatic colorectal cancer (CORRECT): an international, multicentre, randomised, placebo-controlled, phase 3 trial. Lancet (London, England) 381(9863):303–312. https://doi.org/10.1016/s0140-6736(12)61900-x
86. Wang C, Chevalier D, Saluja J, Sandhu J, Lau C, Fakih M (2020) Regorafenib and nivolumab or pembrolizumab combination and circulating tumor DNA response assessment in refractory microsatellite stable colorectal cancer. Oncologist 25(8):e1188–e1e94. https://doi.org/10.1634/theoncologist.2020-0161
87. MacDonald F, Zaiss DMW (2017) The immune system's contribution to the clinical efficacy of EGFR antagonist treatment. Front Pharmacol 8:575. https://doi.org/10.3389/fphar.2017.00575
88. Ferris RL, Lenz HJ, Trotta AM, García-Foncillas J, Schulten J, Audhuy F et al (2018) Rationale for combination of therapeutic antibodies targeting tumor cells and immune checkpoint receptors: harnessing innate and adaptive immunity through IgG1 isotype immune effector stimulation. Cancer Treat Rev 63:48–60. https://doi.org/10.1016/j.ctrv.2017.11.008
89. Cremolini C, Antoniotti C, Lonardi S, Aprile G, Bergamo F, Masi G et al (2018) Activity and safety of cetuximab plus modified FOLFOXIRI followed by maintenance with cetuximab or bevacizumab for RAS and BRAF wild-type metastatic colorectal cancer: a randomized phase 2 clinical trial. JAMA Oncol 4(4):529–536. https://doi.org/10.1001/jamaoncol.2017.5314
90. Holubec L, Polivka J Jr, Safanda M, Karas M, Liska V (2016) The role of cetuximab in the induction of anticancer immune response in colorectal cancer treatment. Anticancer Res 36(9):4421–4426. https://doi.org/10.21873/anticanres.10985
91. Boland PM, Hutson A, Maguire O, Minderman H, Fountzilas C, Iyer RV (2018) A phase Ib/II study of cetuximab and pembrolizumab in RAS-wt mCRC. J Clin Oncol 36(Suppl. 4):834. https://doi.org/10.1200/JCO.2018.36.4_suppl.834
92. Stutvoet TS, Kol A, de Vries EG, de Bruyn M, Fehrmann RS, Terwisscha van Scheltinga AG et al (2019) MAPK pathway activity plays a key role in PD-L1 expression of lung adenocarcinoma cells. J Pathol 249(1):52–64. https://doi.org/10.1002/path.5280
93. Hatzivassiliou G, Haling JR, Chen H, Song K, Price S, Heald R et al (2013) Mechanism of MEK inhibition determines efficacy in mutant KRAS- versus BRAF-driven cancers. Nature 501(7466):232–236. https://doi.org/10.1038/nature12441
94. Hellmann MD, Kim TW, Lee CB, Goh BC, Miller WH Jr, Oh DY et al (2019) Phase Ib study of atezolizumab combined with cobimetinib in patients with solid tumors. Ann Oncol 30(7):1134–1142. https://doi.org/10.1093/annonc/mdz113
95. Eng C, Kim TW, Bendell J, Argilés G, Tebbutt NC, Di Bartolomeo M et al (2019) Atezolizumab with or without cobimetinib versus regorafenib in previously treated metastatic colorectal cancer (IMblaze370): a multicentre, open-label, phase 3, randomised, controlled trial. Lancet Oncol 20(6):849–861. https://doi.org/10.1016/s1470-2045(19)30027-0
96. Guerra J, Pinto C, Pinto D, Pinheiro M, Silva R, Peixoto A et al (2017) POLE somatic mutations in advanced colorectal cancer. Cancer Med 6(12):2966–2971. https://doi.org/10.1002/cam4.1245
97. Domingo E, Freeman-Mills L, Rayner E, Glaire M, Briggs S, Vermeulen L et al (2016) Somatic POLE proofreading domain mutation, immune response, and prognosis in colorectal cancer: a retrospective, pooled biomarker study. Lancet Gastroenterol Hepatol 1(3):207–216. https://doi.org/10.1016/s2468-1253(16)30014-0
98. Gong J, Wang C, Lee PP, Chu P, Fakih M (2017) Response to PD-1 Blockade in microsatellite stable metastatic colorectal cancer harboring a POLE mutation. J Natl Comp Cancer Netw 15(2):142–147. https://doi.org/10.6004/jnccn.2017.0016
99. Moffett JR, Namboodiri MA (2003) Tryptophan and the immune response. Immunol Cell Biol 81(4):247–265. https://doi.org/10.1046/j.1440-1711.2003.t01-1-01177.x

100. Munn DH, Shafizadeh E, Attwood JT, Bondarev I, Pashine A, Mellor AL (1999) Inhibition of T cell proliferation by macrophage tryptophan catabolism. J Exp Med 189(9):1363–1372. https://doi.org/10.1084/jem.189.9.1363
101. Brandacher G, Perathoner A, Ladurner R, Schneeberger S, Obrist P, Winkler C et al (2006) Prognostic value of indoleamine 2,3-dioxygenase expression in colorectal cancer: effect on tumor-infiltrating T cells. Clin Cancer Res 12(4):1144–1151. https://doi.org/10.1158/1078-0432.ccr-05-1966
102. Ciardiello D, Vitiello PP, Cardone C, Martini G, Troiani T, Martinelli E et al (2019) Immunotherapy of colorectal cancer: challenges for therapeutic efficacy. Cancer Treatment Rev 76:22–32. https://doi.org/10.1016/j.ctrv.2019.04.003
103. Beatty GL, O'Dwyer PJ, Clark J, Shi JG, Bowman KJ, Scherle PA et al (2017) First-in-human phase I study of the oral inhibitor of indoleamine 2,3-dioxygenase-1 epacadostat (INCB024360) in patients with advanced solid malignancies. Clin Cancer Res 23(13):3269–3276. https://doi.org/10.1158/1078-0432.ccr-16-2272
104. Duffy MJ (2001) Carcinoembryonic antigen as a marker for colorectal cancer: is it clinically useful? Clin Chem 47(4):624–630
105. Bacac M, Fauti T, Sam J, Colombetti S, Weinzierl T, Ouaret D et al (2016) A Novel Carcinoembryonic Antigen T-Cell Bispecific Antibody (CEA TCB) for the treatment of solid tumors. Clin Cancer Res 22(13):3286–3297. https://doi.org/10.1158/1078-0432.ccr-15-1696
106. Tabernero J, Melero I, Ros W, Argiles G, Marabelle A, Rodriguez-Ruiz ME et al (2017) Phase Ia and Ib studies of the novel carcinoembryonic antigen (CEA) T-cell bispecific (CEA CD3 TCB) antibody as a single agent and in combination with atezolizumab: preliminary efficacy and safety in patients with metastatic colorectal cancer (mCRC). J Clin Oncol 35(Suppl. 15):3002. https://doi.org/10.1200/JCO.2017.35.15_suppl.3002
107. Chuang YC, Tseng JC, Huang LR, Huang CM, Huang CF, Chuang TH (2020) Adjuvant effect of toll-like receptor 9 activation on cancer immunotherapy using checkpoint blockade. Front Immunol 11:1075. https://doi.org/10.3389/fimmu.2020.01075
108. Kamath P, Darwin E, Arora H, Nouri K (2018) A review on imiquimod therapy and discussion on optimal management of basal cell carcinomas. Clin Drug Investig 38(10):883–899. https://doi.org/10.1007/s40261-018-0681-x
109. Kobold S, Wiedemann G, Rothenfußer S, Endres S (2014) Modes of action of TLR7 agonists in cancer therapy. Immunotherapy 6(10):1085–1095. https://doi.org/10.2217/imt.14.75
110. Gowda NM, Wu X, Gowda DC (2012) TLR9 and MyD88 are crucial for the development of protective immunity to malaria. J Immunol (Baltimore, MD: 1950) 188(10):5073–5085. https://doi.org/10.4049/jimmunol.1102143
111. Chen M, Hu S, Li Y, Jiang TT, Jin H, Feng L (2020) Targeting nuclear acid-mediated immunity in cancer immune checkpoint inhibitor therapies. Signal Transduct Target Ther 5(1):270. https://doi.org/10.1038/s41392-020-00347-9
112. Schmoll HJ, Wittig B, Arnold D, Riera-Knorrenschild J, Nitsche D, Kroening H et al (2014) Maintenance treatment with the immunomodulator MGN1703, a Toll-like receptor 9 (TLR9) agonist, in patients with metastatic colorectal carcinoma and disease control after chemotherapy: a randomised, double-blind, placebo-controlled trial. J Cancer Res Clin Oncol 140(9):1615–1624. https://doi.org/10.1007/s00432-014-1682-7
113. Schmoll H-J, Riera-Knorrenschild J, Kopp H-G, Mayer F, Kroening H, Nitsche D et al (2015) Maintenance therapy with the TLR-9 agonist MGN1703 in the phase II IMPACT study of metastatic colorectal cancer patients: a subgroup with improved overall survival. J Clin Oncol 33(Suppl. 3):680. https://doi.org/10.1200/jco.2015.33.3_suppl.680
114. Cunningham D, Zurlo A, Salazar R, Ducreux M, Waddell TS, Stein A et al (2015) IMPALA, a randomized phase III study in patients with metastatic colorectal carcinoma: immunomodulatory maintenance therapy with TLR-9 agonist MGN1703. J Clin Oncol 33(Suppl. 3):TPS791. https://doi.org/10.1200/jco.2015.33.3_suppl.tps791
115. Cunningham D, Salazar R, Sobrero A, Ducreux MP, Van Cutsem E, Scheithauer W et al (2019) LBA33—Lefitolimod vs standard of care (SOC) for patients with metastatic colorec-

tal cancer (mCRC) responding to first-line standard treatment: results from the randomized phase III IMPALA trial. Ann Oncol 30:v868–v869. https://doi.org/10.1093/annonc/mdz394.022
116. Postow MA, Callahan MK, Barker CA, Yamada Y, Yuan J, Kitano S et al (2012) Immunologic correlates of the abscopal effect in a patient with melanoma. N Engl J Med 366(10):925–931. https://doi.org/10.1056/NEJMoa1112824
117. Deng L, Liang H, Burnette B, Beckett M, Darga T, Weichselbaum RR et al (2014) Irradiation and anti-PD-L1 treatment synergistically promote antitumor immunity in mice. J Clin Invest 124(2):687–695. https://doi.org/10.1172/jci67313
118. Stamell EF, Wolchok JD, Gnjatic S, Lee NY, Brownell I (2013) The abscopal effect associated with a systemic anti-melanoma immune response. Int J Radiat Oncol Biol Phys 85(2):293–295. https://doi.org/10.1016/j.ijrobp.2012.03.017
119. Hiniker SM, Chen DS, Reddy S, Chang DT, Jones JC, Mollick JA et al (2012) A systemic complete response of metastatic melanoma to local radiation and immunotherapy. Transl Oncol 5(6):404–407. https://doi.org/10.1593/tlo.12280
120. Golden EB, Demaria S, Schiff PB, Chachoua A, Formenti SC (2013) An abscopal response to radiation and ipilimumab in a patient with metastatic non-small cell lung cancer. Cancer Immunol Res 1(6):365–372. https://doi.org/10.1158/2326-6066.cir-13-0115
121. Rodríguez-Ruiz ME, Vanpouille-Box C, Melero I, Formenti SC, Demaria S (2018) Immunological mechanisms responsible for radiation-induced abscopal effect. Trends Immunol 39(8):644–655. https://doi.org/10.1016/j.it.2018.06.001
122. Duffy AG, Makarova-Rusher OV, Pratt D, Kleiner DE, Fioravanti S, Walker M et al (2016) A pilot study of AMP-224, a PD-L2 Fc fusion protein, in combination with stereotactic body radiation therapy (SBRT) in patients with metastatic colorectal cancer. J Clin Oncol 34(Suppl. 4):560. https://doi.org/10.1200/jco.2016.34.4_suppl.560
123. Segal NH, Kemeny NE, Cercek A, Reidy DL, Raasch PJ, Warren P et al (2016) Non-randomized phase II study to assess the efficacy of pembrolizumab (Pem) plus radiotherapy (RT) or ablation in mismatch repair proficient (pMMR) metastatic colorectal cancer (mCRC) patients. J Clin Oncol 34(Suppl. 15):3539. https://doi.org/10.1200/JCO.2016.34.15_suppl.3539
124. Pardee AD, Wesa AK, Storkus WJ (2009) Integrating costimulatory agonists to optimize immune-based cancer therapies. Immunotherapy 1(2):249–264. https://doi.org/10.2217/1750743x.1.2.249
125. Bansal-Pakala P, Halteman BS, Cheng MH, Croft M (2004) Costimulation of CD8 T cell responses by OX40. J Immunol (Baltimore, MD: 1950) 172(8):4821–4825. https://doi.org/10.4049/jimmunol.172.8.4821
126. Evans DE, Prell RA, Thalhofer CJ, Hurwitz AA, Weinberg AD (2001) Engagement of OX40 enhances antigen-specific CD4(+) T cell mobilization/memory development and humoral immunity: comparison of alphaOX-40 with alphaCTLA-4. J Immunol (Baltimore, MD: 1950) 167(12):6804–6811. https://doi.org/10.4049/jimmunol.167.12.6804
127. Curti BD, Kovacsovics-Bankowski M, Morris N, Walker E, Chisholm L, Floyd K et al (2013) OX40 is a potent immune-stimulating target in late-stage cancer patients. Cancer Res 73(24):7189–7198. https://doi.org/10.1158/0008-5472.can-12-4174
128. Emerson DA, Redmond WL (2018) Overcoming tumor-induced immune suppression: from relieving inhibition to providing costimulation with T cell agonists. BioDrugs 32(3):221–231. https://doi.org/10.1007/s40259-018-0277-2
129. Narumi K, Miyakawa R, Shibasaki C, Henmi M, Mizoguchi Y, Ueda R et al (2019) Local administration of GITR agonistic antibody induces a stronger antitumor immunity than systemic delivery. Sci Rep 9(1):5562. https://doi.org/10.1038/s41598-019-41724-x
130. Balmanoukian AS, Infante JR, Aljumaily R, Naing A, Chintakuntlawar AV, Rizvi NA et al (2020) Safety and clinical activity of MEDI1873, a Novel GITR agonist, in advanced solid tumors. Clin Cancer Res 26(23):6196–6203. https://doi.org/10.1158/1078-0432.ccr-20-0452
131. Etxeberria I, Glez-Vaz J, Teijeira Á, Melero I (2020) New emerging targets in cancer immunotherapy: CD137/4-1BB costimulatory axis. ESMO Open 4(Suppl. 3). https://doi.org/10.1136/esmoopen-2020-000733

132. Curran MA, Kim M, Montalvo W, Al-Shamkhani A, Allison JP (2011) Combination CTLA-4 blockade and 4-1BB activation enhances tumor rejection by increasing T-cell infiltration, proliferation, and cytokine production. PLoS One 6(4):e19499. https://doi.org/10.1371/journal.pone.0019499
133. Sinicrope FA, Ou F-S, Zemla T, Nixon AB, Mody K, Levasseur A et al (2019) Randomized trial of standard chemotherapy alone or combined with atezolizumab as adjuvant therapy for patients with stage III colon cancer and deficient mismatch repair (ATOMIC, Alliance A021502). J Clin Oncol 37(Suppl. 15):e15169. https://doi.org/10.1200/JCO.2019.37.15_suppl.e15169

Immunotherapy of Rectal Cancer

Thibaud Koessler and Francesco Sclafani

Contents

Abstract

Rectal cancer (RC) is responsible for the death of 300'000 patients per year in the world. Compared to other part of the large intestine, RC is the least immunosensitive part with the lowest MSI-H and CMS1 frequency. RC is frequently treated with neo-adjuvant radiotherapy (RT), chemoradiotherapy and more recently with total neoadjuvant therapy before surgery. Evidence is mounting that modification of the tumor microenvironment can be achieved by chemotherapy, RT, and/or targeted agents some specifically inducing T cell trafficking to the tumor or upregulating of signals (e.g., IFN-γ, IL-1, and IL-6) that promote

T. Koessler (✉)
Oncology Department, University Hospital Geneva, Geneva, Switzerland

Swiss Cancer Center Leman, Geneva, Switzerland
e-mail: Thibaud.Kossler@hcuge.ch

F. Sclafani
Gastrointestinal Unit, Department of Medical Oncology, Institut Jules Bordet, Brussels, Belgium

Cancer Immunotherapy (2021)

https://doi.org/10.1007/13905_2021_7,
Published Online: 25 August 2021

the recruitment of dendritic cells. These early observations paved the way for combining immune check point inhibition with standard neo-adjuvant care. Despite interesting translational research results, early clinical results do not currently show a substantial effect of this combination.

Keywords

Immunotherapy · Short course radiotherapy · Chemoradiotherapy · Watch and wait · MSS · MSI-H/dMMR · Pathological complete response

1 Introduction

Colorectal cancer (CRC) is the fourth most common cancer worldwide, contributing to over two million new cases and one million cancer-related deaths in 2018 [1, 2]. Of these, one-third is represented by rectal cancer (RC) [3]. Incidence rates of CRC have been steadily rising, particularly in developing countries, probably due to the westernization of lifestyle conditions and consequent exposure to risk factors (e.g., obesity, alcohol, and limited physical activity) [4]. Despite the fact that the term CRC has long been used to identify tumors of the large intestine, growing evidence suggests that colon cancer (CC) and RC are distinct tumor entities [5]. Differences exist in terms of embryonic origin, anatomic location, microbiota, macroscopic, histopathological appearance, molecular characteristics, and patient management [6]. This chapter will discuss the rational and early results of immunotherapy in localized rectal cancer. Impact of immunotherapy in metastatic rectal cancer is discussed elsewhere.

2 Biology of Rectal Cancer

The genetic make-up of RC is different from the one of CC. In RC, *TP53* and *APC* mutations are more common compare to CC; on the opposite *BRAF*, *PIK3CA*, *CTNNB1*, *ATM*, *PTEN*, *BRCA1* mutations are less frequent in RC. Mismatch repair gene deficiency (dMMR) is also less frequent in RC (0.7%) compare to left-sided CC (4.6%) and right-sided CC (22.3%). On the opposite, HER-2 amplification evaluated by chromogenic in situ hybridization was more frequent in RC (5.4%) compared to left CC (2.8%) and right CC (1.3%). Tumor mutation load in MMR proficient tumors is comparable in all three localizations with an average of 5.7 mutations/MB (megabase) [7]. In 2015, the Consensus Molecular Subtypes (CMS) of colorectal cancer was published. It used gene expression to determine four different CMS. Each CMS had specific features: CMS1 (Immune, 14%), hypermutated, microsatellite unstable, strong immune activation; CMS2 (Canonical, 37%), epithelial, chromosomally unstable, marked WNT and MYC signaling activation; CMS3 (Metabolic, 13%), epithelial, metabolic dysregulation; and CMS4 (Mesenchymal, 23%), prominent transforming growth factor β activation, stromal invasion, and angiogenesis. Interestingly, principal component analysis (PCA) revealed no clear differences between rectal and colon cancers, and samples were combined for the final analysis [8]. However, using the same CMS classification Loree et al. showed subtle but significant differences when the large bowel was split into nine different parts. CMS1 frequency decreases going distally (4% in RC) while CMS2 increases (56% in RC). CMS3 shows a gradual decrease moving distally (13% in RC) and CMS4 stays stable along the colon and rectum (27% in RC) [9]. All these data suggest that immunotherapy could be a useful treatment for only a small proportion or RC patients (i.e., those who have MSI-H or possibly CMS4 tumors, which account for 1% and 4%, respectively, of the entire RC population), making RC the least immune sensitive part of the GI track.

On top of a different biology, treatments for localized RC differ greatly from those for localized CC with the use of neoadjuvant radiotherapy (RT), chemoradiotherapy (CRT) or, more recently, total neoadjuvant therapy (TNT), followed by surgery. A bulk of pre-clinical work showed that modification of the tumor microenvironment (TME) can be achieved by chemotherapy, RT, and/or targeted agents [10]. Recent evidence suggests that ionizing radiation can induce important immunomodulatory effects that may stimulate an *in situ* vaccine phenomenon by reconditioning the TME and inducing T cell trafficking to the tumor [11]. Upon irradiation, cancer cells undergo immunogenic cell death that is associated with the release of damage associated molecular patterns (DAMPs), accumulation of cytosolic DNA, and upregulation of signals (e.g., IFN-γ, IL-1, and IL-6) that promote the recruitment of dendritic cells, and expression of immunomodulatory genes including antigen presentation genes [12, 13]. Mice models also demonstrated that dose is important in remodeling the TME; with high dose irradiation (e.g., 6 Gy × 3) or low doses (e.g., 0.5–1 Gy) polarizing macrophage (M) into M2 phenotype with pro-tumoral activity while moderate doses (e.g., 2 Gy) shifting them toward M1 phenotype with anti-tumoral activity [14]. Indeed, retrospective analyses showed that long course RT (1.8 Gy × 25) or short course RT (scRT, 5 Gy × 5) have different impact on the TME with scRT decreasing $CD8^+/FoxP3^+$ tumor infiltrating lymphocytes in the stroma while the ratio $CD8^+/FoxP3^+$ remains constant in the tumor with both modalities [15].

3 Completed Clinical Trials of Immunotherapy for Rectal Cancer

Only four trials (VOLTAGE [NCT02948348], NRG-GI002 [NCT02921256], [NCT04231552], and [NCT03503630]) have reported so far on the value of adding immunotherapy to the neoadjuvant treatment of RC. The first two trials used chemoRT, while the last two used scRT. Furthermore trials using scRT combined immunotherapy with chemotherapy—either CAPOX [NCT04231552] or mFOLFOX-6 [NCT03503630] for two to six cycles before surgery.

VOLTAGE is a phase I/II trial in which patients were treated with long course chemoradiotherapy (chemoRT) followed by nivolumab monotherapy and subsequent radical surgery. The trial enrolled patients with cT3–4 and cN0 or cN+ RC, treated with chemoRT (Capecitabine + 50.4 Gy) followed by five injections of nivolumab (240 mg every 2 weeks). Surgery was planned 2 weeks after the last nivolumab injection. Patients had radiologic and endoscopic assessments after chemoRT, after three nivolumab injections and before surgery. The primary outcome measure for the phase I part was dose-limiting toxicity, while that for the phase II part was pathological complete response (pCR). A total of 39 patients were recruited (37 MSS and 2 MSI-H, median tumor mutation burden 0.99 mutation/Mbp). No DLT was observed during the phase I, while grade 3/4 toxicities in the whole cohort occurred in 7.7% of cases (3 patients), and two immune related adverse events were observed in 2 patients (grade 3 myasthenia and grade 2 interstitial nephritis). A pCR was observed in 30% and 100% of patients with MSS and MSI-H tumors, respectively (11). The neoadjuvant rectal score (NAR) score, another indicator of tumor response to treatment, was 9.4 in the MSS cohort and 0.9 in the MSI-H cohort. In an exploratory analysis, PD-L1 expression (≥1%—present in 9/37 patients) on tumor cells before chemoRT was associated with pCR (67% versus 17%, *P*-Value: 0.009). CD8 and effector regulatory T cells (eTreg) were quantified by flow cytometry. Likewise for PD-L1, a CD8/eTreg ratio of ≥2.5—present in 9/37 patients—was associated with pCR (78% versus 13%, *P*-Value: 0.003). Notably, all patients with a high CD8/eTreg ratio and PD-L1 positive tumors (5/37) had pCR. Among other biomarkers, KI-67$^+$CD8$^+$ T Cell, PD-1$^+$CD8$^+$ T Cell, and CTLA-4$^+$CD8$^+$ T Cell in pre-chemoRT biopsy were all significantly (*P*-Value <0.05) associated with major tumor regression. Bearing in mind the small numbers, a numerical association was also found between CMS and major tumor regression. This was more commonly observed among patients with CMS1 and CMS3 tumors ($n = 2/2$, 100%, and $n = 4/6$, 60%, respectively) than among those with CMS2 and CMS4 tumors ($n = 3/7$, 43% and $n = 2/7$, 29%, respectively) [16].

NRG-GI002 is a phase II clinical trial platform investigating a number of experimental TNT strategies in locally advanced RC. This trial accrues very high-risk stage II and III RC defined as bulky (cT4), cN2, distal or in need of an abdominal perineal resection. In the immunotherapy arm, patients were treated with eight cycles of FOLFOX followed by chemoRT (45 Gy in 25 fractions over 5 weeks followed by 5.4 Gy boost in 3 fractions associated with capecitabine 850 mg/m^2 PO BID) plus pembrolizumab (200 mg IV every 3 weeks) on day 1 of RT for six doses total. Surgery was performed 8–12 weeks following the last dose of RT. The primary objective was a 4.7 points decrease in the NAR score in the immunotherapy arm compared to a control arm of standard FOLFOX followed by chemoRT. A total of 185 patients were accrued (95 in the control arm and 90 in the experimental arm). Immunotherapy did not affect treatment compliance with similar proportion of patients in arm completing induction chemotherapy, chemoRT, and undergoing surgery. Patients in the control arm had a mean NAR score of 14.08 compared to 11.53 for those in the pembrolizumab arm (*P*-Value: 0.26) making it a negative trial. pCR was similar in both arms (29.4% and 31.9%, *P*-Value: 0.75) as well as R0 resection (89.4% and 94%, *P*-Value: 0.36) [17].

NCT04231552 is a phase II clinical trial in which patients with T3–T4 N0 or T1–4 N+ rectal cancer were treated with scRT (5 × 5 Gy) followed 1 week later by two cycles of CAPOX chemotherapy (oxaliplatin 130 mg/m^2 and capecitabine 1000 mg/m^2 bid day 1 to 14) associated with two cycles of camrelizumab (anti-PD-1) 200 mg followed one week later by radical surgery. The primary outcome was pCR. Thirty patients were enrolled, 26 out of 30 had stage III, 28 had MSS rectal cancer, and 21 had a positive CRM. All patients received scRT, while only 27 had chemotherapy and surgery. R0 resection rate was 100% and pCR 48% with 13 out of 27 showing no tumor cell left. The treatment related adverse event ≥3 was 23% and consisted of neutrophil count decrease (13%), anemia (10%), and white blood cell count decrease (3%). *Post*-surgery complication consisted of 1 bleeding and three patients with infection (11%) [20].

In NCT03503630, patient with stage II and III rectal cancer (cT2 N1–3, cT3 N0–3, or cT4a N0–3), underwent scRT (5 × 5 Gy) followed by six cycles of mFOLFOX-6 (oxaliplatin 85 mg/m^2, leucovorin 400 mg/m^2, and 48-h infusion of fluorouracil 2400 mg/m^2) with avelumab: 10 mg/kg. Patients underwent TME, 3 4 weeks after the last cycle. Primary endpoint was pCR. Thirteen patients were recruited all MSS with 12 having stage III and 3 with positive CRM. All patients received scRT and the six chemotherapy cycles although one patient progressed and dropped out before surgery. Following TME, three patients (25%) had pCR. A total of three adverse events, grade 3 were documented: small intestinal obstruction, one case of *salmonella* colitis, and one case of acute kidney injury [21].

The available evidence on immunotherapy in the setting of localized RC is still scarce with pCR ranging from 25% to 48%. The few MSI-H patients recruited in these four trials, as expected, display a higher pCR (≈60%) than the MSS population. Importantly, there is no safety signal precluding large randomized trial to take place. However, based on the above reported results, immune checkpoint inhibitors cannot be considered as a standard of care in the treatment of these patients. While anti-PD-1 compounds seem to add little value to TNT, the promising rate of pCR from the VOLTAGE and NCT04231552 trials needs confirmation in large studies. Of course, long-term results from these trials, especially with regard to the recurrence free survival and overall survival data from NRG-GI002, are eagerly awaited as a late benefit for immunotherapy-treated patients cannot be excluded.

4 Ongoing Clinical Trials of Immunotherapy for Rectal Cancer

No less than 30 trials, totalizing about 1700 patients are currently on their way. All investigate the added value of anti-PD-1 or anti-PD-L1 inhibitors to standard of care. These trials are briefly reported in Table 1. Two-thirds are using a chemoRT back bone, nine are using scRT, and a third have a TNT design adding chemotherapy before or after radiotherapy. Most are using pCR as primary outcome measure. The only biomarker driven trials are seven trials addressing the place of immunotherapy within the population of dMMR/MSI-H RC patients but

Table 1 Ongoing trials in localized rectal cancer combining immunotherapy and standard of care

NCT number	Phase	Clinical stage	Microsatellite status	Arm	Neoadjuvant treatment sequence: *Pre*-radiotherapy treatment	Radiotherapy treatment	*Post*-radiotherapy treatment	Time to surgery	Adjuvant treatment	Nb of patients	Primary outcome
Short course radiotherapy trials											
NCT04663763	II	T3–4 and/or N+	MSS	A		scRT (5× 5 Gy)	4 cycles of CAPOX and anti-PD-1 antibody (Sintilimab)	1 week after the end of neoadjuvant therapy	4 cycles of CAPOX	32	pCR rate
			MSI-H	B		scRT (5× 5 Gy)	4 cycles of CAPOX and PD-1 antibody (Sintilimab)	1 week after the end of neoadjuvant therapy	4 cycles of CAPOX	8	pCR rate
NCT04518280	II R*	T3–4 and/or N+	MSS	A	2 cycles of CAPOX and anti-PD-1 antibody (Toripalimab)	scRT (5× 5 Gy)	4 cycles of CAPOX and anti-PD-1 antibody (Toripalimab)	2–4 weeks after the end of neoadjuvant therapy		65	pCR rate
				B		scRT (5× 5 Gy)	6 cycles of CAPOX and anti-PD-1 antibody (Toripalimab)	2–4 weeks after the end of neoadjuvant therapy		65	pCR rate
NCT04558684	II	>T2N0 or low T2N0				scRT (5× 5 Gy)	6 cycles of CAPOX and anti-PD-1 antibody (Camrelizumab)	8 (±4) weeks after the end of neoadjuvant therapy		30	cCR rate

NCT04621370 PRIME-RT study	II R*	cT3b+, N+, EMVI+		A	Anti-PD-L1 antibody (Durvalumab) week prior radiotherapy	scRT (5× 5 Gy)	6 cycles of FOLFOX and anti-PD-L1 antibody (Durvalumab)	3–5 weeks after the end of neoadjuvant therapy		24	pCR rate
				B	Anti-PD-L1 antibody (Durvalumab) week prior radiotherapy	Capecitabine radiosensitized NACRT (50 Gy)	4 cycles of FOLFOX and anti-PD-L1 antibody (Durvalumab)	3–5 weeks after the end of neoadjuvant therapy		24	pCR rate
NCT04109755 PEMREC study	II	cT3–T4 N0 or cT any and N1–2	MSS			scRT (5× 5 Gy) with anti-PD-1 antibody (Pembrolizumab)	3 cycles of anti-PD-1 antibody (Pembrolizumab)	3 weeks after the end of neoadjuvant therapy		25	TRG
NCT04231552	II	cT3–4 or N+				scRT (5× 5 Gy)	2 cycles of CAPOX and anti-PD-1 antibody (Camrelizumab)			30	pCR rate
NCT03503630	II	cT2 N1–3, cT3 N0–3				scRT (5× 5 Gy)	6 cycles of FOLFOX and anti-PD-L1 antibody (COMPOUND 2055269)	2–3 weeks after the end of neoadjuvant therapy		44	pCR
NCT04503694 REGINA study	II	Intermediate risk MRI-defined rectal cancer			Two cycles anti-PD-1 antibody (Nivolumab) + regorafenib	scRT (5× 5 Gy)	Three cycles anti-PD-1 antibody (Nivolumab) + regorafenib	7–8 weeks after the end of scRT therapy		60	pCR

(continued)

Table 1 (continued)

NCT number	Phase	Clinical stage	Microsatellite status	Arm	Neoadjuvant treatment sequence: *Pre*-radiotherapy treatment	Radiotherapy treatment	*Post*-radiotherapy treatment	Time to surgery	Adjuvant treatment	Nb of patients	Primary outcome
NCT04636008	Ib	≥cT2	MSI-H/ dMMR			scRT (5× 5 Gy)	3 cycles of anti-PD-1 antibody (Sintilimab)	1–2 weeks after the end of neoadjuvant therapy		20	TRAE rate
Long course chemoradiotherapy trials											
NCT04411537	II	T3–4 and/or N+	MSS		2 cycles of anti-PD-1 antibody	Capecitabine plus irinotecan radiosensitized NACRT (50 Gy)	3 cycles of anti-PD-1 antibody	1–2 weeks after the end of neoadjuvant therapy	6 cycles of XELOX	50	pCR rate
NCT04411524	II	T3–4 and/or N+	MSI-H		2 cycles of anti-PD-1 antibody	Capecitabine plus irinotecan radiosensitized NACRT (50 Gy)	3 cycles of anti-PD-1 antibody	1–2 weeks after the end of neoadjuvant therapy	6 cycles of XELOX	50	pCR rate
NCT03854799 AVANA study	II	cN+, cT4, high risk cT3				Capecitabine radiosensitized NACRT (50.4 Gy) with anti-PD-L1 antibody (Avelumab)		8–10 weeks after the end of neoadjuvant therapy		101	pCR rate
NCT04357587	II	Stage II or stage III or oligometastatic	dMMR			Capecitabine radiosensitized NACRT (50 Gy) with PD-1 antibody (Pembrolizumab)	1 cycle of anti-PD-1 antibody (Pembrolizumab)			10	Rate of AE Feasability
NCT03921684	II	T3–4 N0 or TX N+				Capecitabine radiosensitized NACRT (50.4 Gy)	6 cycles of FOLFOX and anti-PD-1 antibody (nivolumab)	4 weeks after the end of neoadjuvant therapy		29	pCR rate TRAE

NCT02921256	II	Stage II or stage III		C	8 cycles of FOLFOX	Capecitabine radiosensitized NACRT (50 Gy) with anti-PD-1 antibody (Pembrolizumab)	5 cycles of anti-PD-1 antibody (Pembrolizumab)			>100	Change in NAR score
NCT03127007 R-IMMUNE study	Ib/II R*	Stage II or stage III		A		5-FU radiosensitized NACRT (50 Gy) with anti-PD-L1 antibody (Atezolizumab)	3 cycles of anti-PD-L1 antibody (Atezolizumab)	3 weeks after the end of neoadjuvant therapy		54	pCR rate AE rate
				B		5-FU radiosensitized NACRT (50 Gy)		10 weeks after the end of neoadjuvant therapy			
NCT04443543	II	T2–4 and/or N+	MSS	A		Capecitabine plus irinotecan radiosensitized NACRT (50 Gy)	XELIRI or FOLFIRINOX adaptive number of cycles and regimen	No surgery for those in cCR		222	cCR rate
			MSI-H/ dMMR	B		Capecitabine plus irinotecan radiosensitized NACRT (50 Gy)	3 cycles of anti-PD-1 antibody (Tislelizumab)	No surgery for those in cCR			cCR rate
NCT04017455 TARZAN study	II	Intermediate risk rectal cancer or low risk distal rectal cancer				Radiotherapy	3 cycles of anti-VEGF antibody (bevacizumab) combined with anti-PD-L1 antibody (atezolizumab)	3 weeks after the end of neoadjuvant therapy		38	cCR rate ncCR rate

(continued)

Table 1 (continued)

NCT number	Phase	Clinical stage	Microsatellite status	Arm	Neoadjuvant treatment sequence			Time to surgery	Adjuvant treatment	Nb of patients	Primary outcome
					Pre-radiotherapy treatment	Radiotherapy treatment	*Post*-radiotherapy treatment				
NCT04124601 CHINOREC Study	II R*			A		Capecitabine radiosensitized NACRT (50 Gy)				80	TRAE rate
				B		Capecitabine radiosensitized NACRT (50 Gy)	Anti-CTLA-4 antibody (Ipilimumab) on day 7 and anti-PD-1 antibody (Nivolumab) on day 14, 28 and 42)				
NCT04293419 DUREC study	II	High risk MRI-defined rectal cancer			6 cycles of FOLFOX + Four cycles anti-PD-L1 (Durvalumab)	Capecitabine radiosensitized NACRT (50.4 Gy) + anti-PD-L1 (Durvalumab)	2 cycles anti-PD-L1 (Durvalumab)	2–6 weeks after the end of neoadjuvant therapy		58	pCR rate
NCT03102047 FR-2 study	II	Stage II–IV rectal cancer	MSS			Capecitabine radiosensitized NACRT (50.4 Gy)	4 cycles anti-PD-L1 (Durvalumab)	1–4 weeks after the end of neoadjuvant therapy		47	NAR
NCT02948348 VOLTAGE trial	Ib/II	T3 and T4, N any				Capecitabine radiosensitized NACRT (50.4 Gy)	Five cycles anti-PD-1 antibody (Nivolumab)	2 weeks after the end of neoadjuvant therapy		50	pCR rate
NCT03299660	II	T3bN1-N2M0, T3c/dN0-N2M0, T4N0-N2M0				Capecitabine/5FU radiosensitized NACRT (50.4 Gy)	4 cycles of anti-PD-L1 antibody (Avelumab)	8–10 weeks after the end of neoadjuvant therapy		45	pCR rate

NCT04083365 PANDORA study	II	cT3/4N0/M0 or Tx N1–2/M0				Capecitabine radiosensitized NACRT (50.4 Gy)	3 cycles of anti-PD-L1 antibody (Avelumab)	1–2 weeks after the end of neoadjuvant therapy		60	pCR rate
No radiotherapy and no surgery											
NCT04643041 BASKET study	II	TxNxM0	MSI-H/dMMR		6 cycles of anti-PD-1 antibody	No radiotherapy		No surgery		47	1 year DFS rate
No anti-PD1 or CTL-4 immunotherapies											
NCT03300544	I	cT3–4, N+			4 injections of T-VEC with 2 cycle of FOLFOX	Capecitabine radiosensitized NACRT (50.4 Gy)		8–12 weeks after the end of neoadjuvant therapy		21	DLT
NCT02688712 ExIST Study	II	Stage II or stage III			TGFβ Type I Receptor Inhibitor (LY2157299) for 15 days	Capecitabine radiosensitized NACRT (50.4 Gy) with (LY2157299) 15 days after start		6–10 weeks after the end of neoadjuvant therapy		50	pCR rate
NCT04130854 INNATE study	II R*	cT4 or within 3 mm of MR fascia		A		CD-40 agonist antibody with scRT (5× 5 Gy)	6 cycles of FOLFOX and CD-40 agonist antibody (APX005M)			58	pCR rate
				B		scRT (5× 5 Gy)	6 cycles of FOLFOX				
NCT03916510 CEDAR study	I	cT3mrf+ or N+ or low tumors			3 enadenotucirev loading doses in weeks 1–2	Capecitabine radiosensitized NACRT (50.4 Gy) ± enadenotucirev	±Enadenotucirev			30	DLT MRI-TRG

(continued)

Table 1 (continued)

NCT number	Phase	Clinical stage	Microsatellite status	Arm	Neoadjuvant treatment sequence			Time to surgery	Adjuvant treatment	Nb of patients	Primary outcome
					Pre-radiotherapy treatment	Radiotherapy treatment	*Post*-radiotherapy treatment				
NCT04304209	II R*	cT3–4N0M0 or cTxN+M0	dMMR or MSI-H	A	4 cycles of anti-PD-1 antibody (Sintilimab)	No Radiotherapy	Four cycles of anti-PD-1 antibody (Sintilimab) ± CAPEOX chemotherapy	Surgery or watch and wait		195	pCR
			pMMR/ MSS/MSI-L	B1	4 cycles of anti-PD-1 antibody (Sintilimab)	Capecitabine radiosensitized NACRT (50.4 Gy) + CAPEOX		Surgery or watch and wait			
				B2		Capecitabine radiosensitized NACRT (50.4 Gy) + CAPEOX		Surgery or watch and wait			

scRT short course radiotherapy (5× 5 Gy), *pCR* pathological complete response, *TME* total mesorectal excision, *NACRT* neoadjuvant chemoradiotherapy, *IMRT DT* 50 Gy/25 Fractions, *cCR* clinical complete response, *AE* adverse event, *TRAE* treatment related adverse event, *NAR* neoadjuvant rectal cancer, *TRG* Tumor Regression Grade, *ncCR* near-complete response rate, *DLT* dose-limiting toxicities, *R** randomized only two of those incorporate a watch and wait arm (NCT04643041 and NCT04304209).

5 Conclusion

Localized RC provides the perfect setting to study the promising interactions between immunotherapy and RT or chemoRT. However, the NRG-GI002 negative results should come as a reminder that a successful interaction will only come with the deep understanding of the TME contexture and the study of the dynamic changes during neoadjuvant treatment. As previously seen, these changes depend on the RT dose and fractionation and undoubtedly whether chemotherapy is used as a radio-sensitizer or as a systemic treatment.

It should also be considered that the interactions between immunotherapy and the TME may depend on practical factors such as the timing of the immunotherapy administration. Indeed, in their murine model, Dovedi et al. showed that anti-PD1 antibody should be administered simultaneously with RT instead of 7 days later in order to enhance the positive effect of such combinations [18]. On the contrary, CTLA-4 inhibition was more effective when given 7 days prior to RT compared to day 1 and 5 after RT [19], a difference that may be explained by the different mechanisms of action of these two immunotherapies.

Most investigators seem to have forgotten that immunotherapy is a targeted therapy and as such rely on biomarkers. The few trials investigating the addition of immunotherapy in MSI-H RC could pave the way to practices such as organ preservation at least for a subset of patients. It will certainly be worth studying if patients harboring CMS1 gene expression profile could benefit from immunotherapy.

Finally, other immunotherapy-based combinations could be worth investigating in specific molecular subgroups such as patients with HER-2 positive tumors (following the results of the PANTHERA trial, NCT02901301) or those with *BRAF* mutated tumors (in line with the interest for the investigation of encorafenib, cetuximab, and nivolumab in MSS metastatic colorectal cancer).

Compliance with Ethical Standards

Disclosure T.K discloses consulting or advisory role for MSD, BMS, Lilly, Roche, Boeringer Ingelheim and Servier. F.S discloses consulting role for Amal therapeutics, bayer; research funding: Amgen (inst), AstraZeneca (inst), Bayer (inst), BMS (inst), Roche (inst), Sanofi (inst); travel grants : Bayer and Lilly.

References

1. Bray F, Ferlay J, Soerjomataram I, Siegel RL, Torre LA, Jemal A (2018) Global cancer statistics 2018: GLOBOCAN estimates of incidence and mortality worldwide for 36 cancers in 185 countries. CA Cancer J Clin 68:394–424. https://doi.org/10.3322/caac.21492
2. Arnold M, Sierra MS, Laversanne M, Soerjomataram I, Jemal A, Bray F (2017) Global patterns and trends in colorectal cancer incidence and mortality. Gut 66:683–691. https://doi.org/10.1136/gutjnl-2015-310912

3. https://gco.iarc.fr/
4. Rawla P, Sunkara T, Barsouk A (2019) Epidemiology of colorectal cancer: incidence, mortality, survival, and risk factors. Prz Gastroenterol 14:89–103. https://doi.org/10.5114/pg.2018.81072
5. Patel M, McSorley ST, Park JH, Roxburgh CSD, Edwards J, Horgan PG, McMillan DC (2018) The relationship between right-sided tumour location, tumour microenvironment, systemic inflammation, adjuvant therapy and survival in patients undergoing surgery for colon and rectal cancer. Br J Cancer 118:705–712. https://doi.org/10.1038/bjc.2017.441
6. Paschke S, Jafarov S, Staib L, Kreuser ED, Maulbecker-Armstrong C, Roitman M, Holm T, Harris CC, Link KH, Kornmann M (2018) Are colon and rectal cancer two different tumor entities? A proposal to abandon the term colorectal cancer. Int J Mol Sci 19:2577. https://doi.org/10.3390/ijms19092577
7. Salem ME, Weinberg BA, Xiu J, El-Deiry WS, Hwang JJ, Gatalica Z, Philip PA, Shields AF, Lenz H-J, Marshall JL (2017) Comparative molecular analyses of left-sided colon, right-sided colon, and rectal cancers. Oncotarget 8:86356–86368
8. Guinney J, Dienstmann R, Wang X, de Reynies A, Schlicker A, Soneson C, Marisa L, Roepman P, Nyamundanda G, Angelino P et al (2015) The consensus molecular subtypes of colorectal cancer. Nat Med 21:1350–1356. https://doi.org/10.1038/nm.3967
9. Loree JM, Pereira AAL, Lam M, Willauer AN, Raghav K, Dasari A, Morris VK, Advani S, Menter DG, Eng C et al (2018) Classifying colorectal cancer by tumor location rather than sidedness highlights a continuum in mutation profiles and consensus molecular subtypes. Clin Cancer Res 24:1062–1072. https://doi.org/10.1158/1078-0432.CCR-17-2484
10. van den Ende T, van den Boorn HG, Hoonhout NM, van Etten-Jamaludin FS, Meijer SL, Derks S, de Gruijl TD, Bijlsma MF, van Oijen MGH, van Laarhoven HWM (2020) Priming the tumor immune microenvironment with chemo(radio)therapy: a systematic review across tumor types. Biochim Biophys Acta Rev Cancer 1874:188386. https://doi.org/10.1016/j.bbcan.2020.188386
11. Lhuillier C, Rudqvist NP, Elemento O, Formenti SC, Demaria S (2019) Radiation therapy and anti-tumor immunity: exposing immunogenic mutations to the immune system. Genome Med 11:40. https://doi.org/10.1186/s13073-019-0653-7
12. Wang Y, Deng W, Li N, Neri S, Sharma A, Jiang W, Lin SH (2018) Combining immunotherapy and radiotherapy for cancer treatment: current challenges and future directions. Front Pharmacol 9:185. https://doi.org/10.3389/fphar.2018.00185
13. Prise KM, Schettino G, Folkard M, Held KD (2005) New insights on cell death from radiation exposure. Lancet Oncol 6:520–528. https://doi.org/10.1016/S1470-2045(05)70246-1
14. Genard G, Lucas S, Michiels C (2017) Reprogramming of tumor-associated macrophages with anticancer therapies: radiotherapy versus chemo and immunotherapies. Front Immunol 8:828. https://doi.org/10.3389/fimmu.2017.00828
15. Mirjolet C, Charon-Barra C, Ladoire S, Arbez-Gindre F, Bertaut A, Ghiringhelli F, Leroux A, Peiffert D, Borg C, Bosset JF et al (2018) Tumor lymphocyte immune response to preoperative radiotherapy in locally advanced rectal cancer: the LYMPHOREC study. Oncoimmunology 7:e1396402. https://doi.org/10.1080/2162402X.2017.1396402
16. Inamori K, Togashi Y, Bando H, Tsukada Y, Fukuoka S, Suzuki A et al. Translational research of VOLTAGE-A: efficacy predictors of preoperative chemoradiotherapy and consolidation nivolumab in patients with both microsatellite stable and microsatellite instability-high locally advanced rectal cancer. https://ascopubs.org/doi/abs/10.1200/JCO.2021.39.3_suppl.100
17. Rahma OE, Yothers G, Hong TS, McGory Russell M, You YN, Parker W et al NRG-GI002: a phase II clinical trial platform using total neoadjuvant therapy (TNT) in locally advanced rectal cancer (LARC)—Pembrolizumab experimental arm (EA) primary results. https://ascopubs.org/doi/abs/10.1200/JCO.2021.39.3_suppl.8
18. Dovedi SJ, Adlard AL, Lipowska-Bhalla G, McKenna C, Jones S, Cheadle EJ, Stratford IJ, Poon E, Morrow M, Stewart R et al (2014) Acquired resistance to fractionated radiotherapy can be overcome by concurrent PD-L1 blockade. Cancer Res 74:5458–5468. https://doi.org/10.1158/0008-5472.CAN-14-1258

19. Young KH, Baird JR, Savage T, Cottam B, Friedman D, Bambina S, Messenheimer DJ, Fox B, Newell P, Bahjat KS et al (2016) Optimizing timing of immunotherapy improves control of tumors by hypofractionated radiation therapy. PLoS One 11:e0157164. https://doi.org/10.1371/journal.pone.0157164
20. Lin Z, Cai M, Zhang P, Li X, Cai K, Nie X, Tao X et al. Short-course radiotherapy and subsequent CAPOX plus camrelizumab followed by delayed surgery for locally advanced rectal cancer: short-term results of a phase II trial. https://ascopubs.org/doi/abs/10.1200/JCO.2021.39.3_suppl.63
21. Shamseddine A, Zeidan YH, El Husseini Z, Kreidieh M, Al Darazi M, Turfa R et al (2020) Efficacy and safety-in analysis of short-course radiation followed by mFOLFOX-6 plus avelumab for locally advanced rectal adenocarcinoma. Radiat Oncol 15(1):233. https://doi.org/10.1186/s13014-020-01673-6

Perspective on Immunotherapy of Colon Cancer: Challenges for the Future

Elisa Fontana

Contents

Abstract

Immune checkpoint inhibitors (ICIs) are highly effective drugs and established standard of care options for several tumour types, for example, melanoma, lung cancer, renal and urothelial cancers. In colorectal cancer (CRC), most tumours are immunogenically cold, as demonstrated in several negative clinical trials with ICIs. ICIs are only available for patients with metastatic dMMR/microsatellite unstable tumours: these represent 5% of metastatic CRC and are characterized by a high tumour mutational burden. Although the benefit of ICIs is durable in responding patients, primary and secondary resistance are frequently observed. Multiple biomarkers of response and resistance have been characterized; however, their implementation into clinical practice is technically challenging and undermined by the high heterogeneity of this disease. Combination therapies with dual immune checkpoint blockade, with chemotherapy or targeted agents in different molecular subtypes are under evaluation in clinical trials in the attempt to overcome resistance to ICIs in both dMMR/microsatellite unstable and stable tumours.

Keywords

Colorectal cancer · Immune checkpoint inhibitors · Microsatellite instability · Biomarkers · Tumour heterogeneity · Circulating tumour DNA

E. Fontana (✉)
Drug Development Unit, Sarah Cannon Research Institute UK, London, UK
e-mail: Elisa.Fontana@hcahealthcare.co.uk

Cancer Immunotherapy (2022)
https://doi.org/10.1007/13905_2022_16,
Published Online: 13 October 2022

In the last decade, immune checkpoint inhibitors (ICIs) have been a game-changer in many cancers, especially in those with high tumour mutation burden (TMB). While in melanoma and lung cancers the high TMB is a result of driver carcinogenic events induced by ultraviolet (UV) radiations or smoking, in CRC the high TMB is a result of defects in the DNA repair machinery (mismatch repair deficient tumours, dMMR) or DNA synthesis (polymerase epsilon or delta, POLE and POLD) [1]. This explains why only a small proportion of CRC cancers (dMMR or POLE/POLD mutant) benefits from ICIs, while the vast majority (microsatellite stable tumours, MSS) do not.

Recently, ICIs became standard treatment option in previously untreated metastatic dMMR/microsatellite instability high (MSI-H) CRC. However, up to 30% of these cancers demonstrate primary resistance to ICIs and another 15% progress within one year [2].

Biologically speaking, intrinsic/de novo resistance has been frequently associated with defects in antigen presentation, as example in case of biallelic loss of beta-2-microglibulin (B2M), Human Leukocyte Antigen (HLA) gene copy number alterations and loss of heterozygosity and with Wnt pathway activation. These events lead to lack of T-lymphocytes infiltration, phenomenon also known as immune exclusion, with consequent ICIs refractoriness [3, 4].

Tumour volume and its consequent metabolism may also play an important role in ICIs response. A proteogenomic study identified how hypoxia in tumours with high volume may induce a reduced T-lymphocyte infiltration due to the inhibiting effect of lactate produced by glycolysis [5].

Technically speaking, accurate identification of dMMR/MSI-H CRCs is crucial since misdiagnosis of MSS tumours can contribute to the observed lack of ICIs benefit. A post hoc analysis of 38 prospectively identified dMMR/MSI-H patients for ICIs therapy demonstrated that up to 10% of CRC samples were misdiagnosed; the 90% positive predictive value of MSI assessed by immunohistochemistry (IHC) or dMMR status assessed using polymerase chain reaction (PCR) and pentaplex markers was confirmed in a retrospective cohort of 93 samples [6]. Importantly, both IHC and PCR testing methods are recommended to confirm dMMR/MSI-H status prior to ICIs treatment.

With increasing usage of ICIs in dMMR/MSI-H CRCs, it is expected that mechanisms of secondary resistance to ICIs after initial response will be further elucidated with significant impact on the design of post-ICIs strategies. The intrinsic genomic instability associated with dMMR status is a dynamic process continuously inducing new gene alterations, which can ultimately lead to ICI acquired resistance and further immune escape. Multiple acquired alterations in Wnt, TGF beta, Janus kinases gene pathways, and Major Histocompatibility Complex (MHC) class I molecules have been characterized under the pressure of ICI therapy in different cancer types including CRC [7]. Notably, most of these pathways are actionable, leading to the development of combination strategies in clinical trials in ICI-pre-treated patients.

Further combination strategies with or without chemotherapy (extensively discussed in the previous chapter) are under evaluation in MSS CRCs. These tumours are immunogenically cold and frequently driven by oncogenic mutations, as example KRAS, which have very limited immunogenic activity, explaining why immune evasion can easily happen [8]. Recently, Liao et al. demonstrated how oncogenic KRAS mutations in MSS CRC repress the expression of interferon regulatory factor 2 (IRF2) and upregulation of CXCL-3, with consequent increased infiltration of myeloid-derived suppressor cells (MDSC), creating an immune suppressive tumour microenvironment and de novo resistance to ICIs [9]. Targeting the IRF2-CXCL-3 axis may represent a further strategy to overcome ICI resistance in KRAS mutant MSS CRCs. Similarly, the *BRAF V600E* mutation, other crucial oncogenic driver in CRC, produces neopeptides with very weak affinity for HLA molecules with consequent lack of exposure on the cell surface favouring immune evasion [10]. Evidence from preclinical models demonstrated increased T-cell infiltration after *BRAF* pathway blockade and a synergistic effect between BRAF-MEK inhibitors and anti-PD1 agents [11]. Clinical trials testing these combinations are ongoing (NCT04044430 and NCT03668431).

Although multiple mechanisms and biomarkers of response and resistance to ICIs have been elucidated in *post hoc* translational analyses, their prospective identification for treatment personalization is challenging in routine clinical practice. Pathways analyses frequently require transcriptomic data or multiplex IHC/immunofluorescence technologies which are expensive and with long turnaround time for clinical applicability. Similarly, tumour mutational burden, emerging biomarker for ICI, has been initially discovered and assessed with whole exome sequencing; however, due to high costs and turnaround time of this methodology, sequencing of different targeted panels is currently more frequently deployed [12]. This led to challenging analytical and clinical validation of TMB as biomarker, with standardization and optimization of relevant cut-offs for benefit prediction still to be fully defined, especially in the context of a highly heterogeneous disease like CRC. Liquid biopsies have been successfully deployed in the detection of minimal residual disease in adjuvant setting, in the early identification of drug response and resistance and in optimization of re-challenge strategies [13]. Whether circulating tumour DNA plays a role in ICIs benefit prediction and immunotherapy, personalization requires further evaluation. Both dMMR/MSI-H and TMB can be evaluated using ctDNA; their dynamic changes under ICIs pressure have been effectively measured in melanoma and gastric cancer and correlated with response and resistance, opening a possible application in CRC [14, 15].

Liquid biomarkers may help overcoming the sampling errors associated with tissue biomarkers in presence of tumour heterogeneity and possible differences between the primary tumour and metastatic sites. The natural tumour evolution in CRC has been demonstrated to be punctuated: in this evolutionary model a high number of genomic aberrations occur in a short time frame and at a very early stage with a small number of dominant clones expanding. This leads to high intratumoural heterogeneity at baseline with expansion of stable clones that minimally modify during cancer progression [16, 17]. This explains the high biomarker concordance between primary and metastatic sites, giving clinicians the option to test the *RAS/BRAF* status for treatment decisions either on primary tumour or metastatic sites.

This may not be the case for future immune biomarkers, due to mechanisms of immune escape influencing the homing of metastatic clones in different organs with consequent diverse immune phenotype based on organ-specific microenvironment. As example, HLA class I loss of expression have been reported in the majority of dMMR/MSI-H primary tumours, explaining their immunogenic character and low tendency to metastasize. Conversely, HLA class I loss is very rarely found in liver metastases, independently of their MMR status [18]. Together with the known immunosuppressive hepatic microenvironment maintained by cytokines like TGF-beta and IL-10, different molecular immune biomarkers may be expected in primary and metastatic sites with possible limited activity of ICIs in liver metastases requiring different combination approaches [19].

Another emerging challenge for ICIs therapy in CRC is represented by the increasing incidence of early-onset (EO) CRC, especially in Western Countries [20]. Environmental and lifestyle changes, including obesity, high red or processed meat intake, and lack of physical activity are possible causes of the shift in disease burden. Ethnicity and genetic predisposition to specific iatrogenic environmental substances may also play a role in the differential pattern of disease incidence in different geographical areas. The vast majority of these tumours seems to be sporadic; only 20% of cases are possibly associated with Lynch syndrome and consequent dMMR/MSI-H status, which has been historically observed in older population with right-sided tumours and peritoneal metastases [21]. Hence, these new cancer entities are expected to be immunogenically cold and possibly presenting an inflammatory phenotype, as more frequently found in older populations exposed to chronic low levels of inflammatory insults (immune ageing or inflammaging phenomenon) [22]. Recent evidence pointed at the innate immune system, in particular the complement system, as substantial difference between EO-CRC and older patients, opening the possibility to tackle these cancers by adding complement inhibitors to standard chemo- or immunotherapy [23].

In conclusion, immunotherapy is now a fundamental treatment option for a small proportion of metastatic CRC patients. Ongoing clinical trials are trying to address how to effectively expand the activity of immunotherapy to the majority of CRC patients, especially to those with MSS tumours. Future research should focus on overcoming de novo and acquired resistance to ICIs and how to prospectively identify patients requiring monotherapies or combinations of agents for precision and personalized immunotherapy.

Compliance with Ethical Standards

Disclosure of Interests Elisa Fontana is an employee of Hospital Corporation of America (HCA) International.

Studies Involving Humans *Ethical approval*: This article does not contain any studies with human participants performed by any of the authors.

Studies Involving Animals *Ethical approval*: This article does not contain any studies with animals performed by any of the authors.

References

1. Galuppini F, Dal Pozzo CA, Deckert J, Loupakis F, Fassan M, Baffa R (2019) Tumor mutation burden: from comprehensive mutational screening to the clinic. Cancer Cell Int 19(1):209
2. André T, Shiu KK, Kim TW, Jensen BV, Jensen LH, Punt C, Smith D, Garcia-Carbonero R, Benavides M, Gibbs P, de la Fouchardiere C (2020) Pembrolizumab in microsatellite-instability–high advanced colorectal cancer. N Engl J Med 383(23):2207–2218
3. Gurjao C, Liu D, Hofree M, AlDubayan SH, Wakiro I, Su MJ, Felt K, Gjini E, Brais LK, Rotem A, Rosenthal MH (2019) Intrinsic resistance to immune checkpoint blockade in a mismatch repair–deficient colorectal cancer. Cancer Immunol Res 7(8):1230–1236
4. Grasso CS, Giannakis M, Wells DK, Hamada T, Mu XJ, Quist M, Nowak JA, Nishihara R, Qian ZR, Inamura K, Morikawa T (2018) Genetic mechanisms of immune evasion in colorectal cancer. Cancer Discov 8(6):730–749
5. Vasaikar S, Huang C, Wang X, Petyuk VA, Savage SR, Wen B, Dou Y, Zhang Y, Shi Z, Arshad OA, Gritsenko MA (2019) Proteogenomic analysis of human colon cancer reveals new therapeutic opportunities. Cell 177(4):1035–1049
6. Cohen R, Hain E, Buhard O, Guilloux A, Bardier A, Kaci R, Bertheau P, Renaud F, Bibeau F, Fléjou JF, André T (2019) Association of primary resistance to immune checkpoint inhibitors in metastatic colorectal cancer with misdiagnosis of microsatellite instability or mismatch repair deficiency status. JAMA Oncol 5(4):551–555
7. Sahin IH, Akce M, Alese O, Shaib W, Lesinski GB, El-Rayes B, Wu C (2019) Immune checkpoint inhibitors for the treatment of MSI-H/MMR-D colorectal cancer and a perspective on resistance mechanisms. Br J Cancer 121(10):809–818
8. Tran E, Robbins PF, Lu YC, Prickett TD, Gartner JJ, Jia L, Pasetto A, Zheng Z, Ray S, Groh EM, Kriley IR (2016) T-cell transfer therapy targeting mutant KRAS in cancer. N Engl J Med 375(23):2255–2262
9. Liao W, Overman MJ, Boutin AT, Shang X, Zhao D, Dey P, Li J, Wang G, Lan Z, Li J, Tang M (2019) KRAS-IRF2 axis drives immune suppression and immune therapy resistance in colorectal cancer. Cancer Cell 35(4):559–572
10. Claeys A, Luijts T, Marchal K, Van den Eynden J (2021) Low immunogenicity of common cancer hot spot mutations resulting in false immunogenic selection signals. PLoS Genet 17(2):e1009368
11. Corcoran R, Giannakis M, Allen J, Chen J, Pelka K, Chao S, Meyerhardt J, Enzinger A, Enzinger P, McCleary N, Yugelun M (2020) SO-26 Clinical efficacy of combined BRAF, MEK, and PD-1 inhibition in BRAFV600E colorectal cancer patients. Ann Oncol 31:S226–S227
12. Meléndez B, Van Campenhout C, Rorive S, Remmelink M, Salmon I, D'Haene N (2018) Methods of measurement for tumor mutational burden in tumor tissue. Transl Lung Cancer Res 7(6):661
13. Wills B, Gorse E, Lee V (2018) Role of liquid biopsies in colorectal cancer. Curr Probl Cancer 42(6):593–600
14. Riaz N, Havel JJ, Makarov V, Desrichard A, Urba WJ, Sims JS, Hodi FS, Martín-Algarra S, Mandal R, Sharfman WH, Bhatia S (2017) Tumor and microenvironment evolution during immunotherapy with nivolumab. Cell 171(4):934–949
15. Kwon M, An M, Klempner SJ, Lee H, Kim KM, Sa JK, Cho HJ, Hong JY, Lee T, Min YW, Kim TJ (2021) Determinants of response and intrinsic resistance to PD-1 blockade in microsatellite instability-high gastric cancer. Cancer Discov 11(9):2168–2185
16. Davis A, Gao R, Navin N (2017) Tumor evolution: linear, branching, neutral or punctuated? Biochim Biophys Acta (BBA)-Rev Cancer 1867(2):151–161
17. Sottoriva A, Kang H, Ma Z, Graham TA, Salomon MP, Zhao J, Marjoram P, Siegmund K, Press MF, Shibata D, Curtis C (2015) A Big Bang model of human colorectal tumor growth. Nat Genet 47(3):209–216
18. Ijsselsteijn ME, Petitprez F, Lacroix L, Ruano D, van der Breggen R, Julie C, Morreau H, Sautès-Fridman C, Fridman WH (2019) Revisiting immune escape in colorectal cancer in the era of immunotherapy. Br J Cancer 120(8):815–818

19. Robinson MW, Harmon C, O'Farrelly C (2016) Liver immunology and its role in inflammation and homeostasis. Cell Mol Immunol 13(3):267–276
20. Siegel RL, Miller KD, Jemal A (2017) Colorectal cancer mortality rates in adults aged 20–54 years in the United States, 1970–2014. JAMA 318(6):572–574
21. Campos FG (2017) Colorectal cancer in young adults: a difficult challenge. World J Gastroenterol 23(28):5041
22. Oh SJ, Lee JK, Shin OS (2019) Aging and the immune system: the impact of immunosenescence on viral infection, immunity and vaccine immunogenicity. Immune Netw 19(6):e37
23. Gardner IH, Siddharthan R, Watson K, Dewey E, Ruhl R, Khou S, Guan X, Xia Z, Tsikitis VL, Anand S (2021) A distinct innate immune signature of early onset colorectal cancer. Immunohorizons 5(6):489–499

Part V

HCC

Immune Strategies for Gastrointestinal Cancer: HCC

Danny N. Khalil, Imane El Dika, Hassan Azhari, James J. Harding, Eileen M. O'Reilly, and Ghassan K. Abou-Alfa

Contents

Abstract

While important progress has been made to control the main risk factors for hepatocellular carcinoma, it remains a common malignancy throughout the world and the most common primary liver cancer.

Consistent with an improved understanding of the pathophysiology and immunobiology of the disease, there are now more therapeutic options available to patients. While single-agent PD-1 axis blockade has failed to improve overall survival in this cancer, anti-PD 1 in combination with other immune checkpoint inhibitors, or with multitargeted tyrosine kinase inhibitors, and antiangiogenic therapies, provides a strong rationale for a multitargeted approach. Much work

D. N. Khalil · I. El Dika · H. Azhari · J. J. Harding · E. M. O'Reilly · G. K. Abou-Alfa (✉)
Memorial Sloan Kettering Cancer Center, New York, NY, USA

Weill Medical College at Cornell University, New York, NY, USA
e-mail: abou-alg@mskcc.org

Cancer Immunotherapy (2023)
https://doi.org/10.1007/13905_2021_13,
Published Online: 04 March 2023

remains to determine how to optimally use combination therapy and how treatment can be tailored to patients' unique biology. Important studies are underway to clarify the relationship between HCC etiology, immunobiology, and intrinsic signaling pathways. Here we review ongoing work in the field together with the epidemiology, risk factors, and current therapies for HCC.

Keywords
Hepatocellular carcinoma · Immunobiology · Immunotherapy

Epidemiology with Immune Perspective (HA)

Primary liver cancer constitutes the seventh most common cause of cancer worldwide and the second most common cause of cancer mortality with the highest incidence rates in Asia and Africa [1]. Hepatocellular carcinoma (HCC) accounts for around 75% of all liver cancers and has shown evidence of decrease in incidence over time in areas with high incidence, such as Japan and South Korea, and increase in low-incidence areas, such as the United States and much of Europe [2, 3]. In 2018, the estimated global incidence rate of HCC was 9.3 per 100,000 person years with a high mortality rate of 8.5 per 100,000 person years [1].

Older age correlates directly with the incidence of HCC in most populations, although the median age of diagnosis varies significantly between countries. For example, in the United States, HCC has a median age of diagnosis of 60–64 years in men and 65–69 years in women [4]. In many African countries on the other hand, the median age of diagnosis is 46 years [5]. Incidence rates among men are also 2–4 times higher than in women in most countries [2]. Racial and ethnic factors also influence the incidence in a fashion that relates to the known risk factors for HCC [4].

Hepatitis B virus (HBV) and hepatitis C virus (HCV) infections remain the most prevalent risk factors leading to the development of HCC worldwide [6]. These are followed by alcohol, metabolic syndrome, and nonalcoholic steatohepatitis as increasingly prominent risk factors for HCC predicted to become more prevalent with the expected decline in the prevalence of HBV and HCV infections as effective vaccines and treatment become more available [7–9]. HCC is most commonly associated with cirrhosis, a finding that also influences available treatment options [10]. Cirrhosis itself is the final and irreversible stage of liver fibrosis, often a product of chronic inflammation caused by one of the risk factors mentioned. Chronically inflamed livers exhibit changes in gene expression as well as de novo somatic mutations that lead to immune dysregulation and predispose to oncogenic transformation and development of HCC [11]. The inflammation also leads to a state of immune dysfunction that provides a favorable environment for neoplasia [12]. This inflammatory process leads to DNA damage, hepatocellular necrosis, regenerative nodular formation, dysplastic nodules, and eventually carcinoma [13]. In addition, the liver is a unique organ with dual blood supply of arterial and portal venous sources which exposes it to gut pathogens that it has developed immune tolerogenicity to adapt to [14, 15]. The liver is also heavily laden with various immune cells including Kupffer cells, liver sinusoidal endothelial cells (LSECs), natural killer (NK) cells, and innate T cells [16]. This makes HCC an immunogenic liver lesion that expresses tumor-associated antigens as well as neoantigens resulting from specific gene mutations [17].

Drug development for HCC has been a challenging task, with a very limited number of therapies showing promise [18]. This has led to an understandable interest in exploring immunotherapy as an option for HCC treatment, especially with what we know about the immunogenicity of this neoplasm [19].

1 Introduction

Historically, the treatment of cancer has largely been driven by histology. For systemic disease, this has produced a treatment landscape, dominated by cytotoxic chemotherapy, in which the tissue of origin determines the choice of regimen. However, unlike for most cancers, cytotoxic chemotherapy has not been associated with an improvement in the overall survival for HCC. Tyrosine kinase inhibitors (TKIs), generally with broad specificity, and the VEGFR2 blocking monoclonal antibody (mAb) ramucirumab have more recently been associated with modest improvements in overall survival [20]. In 2020, the combination of PD-L1 and VEGF blockade (two distinct mechanisms, each with an important impact on antitumor immunity) joined other standard-of-care TKI therapies in the first-line setting for advanced HCC based on a significant improvement in landmark survival [21]. This raises the question of whether historic approaches to tumor classification and treatment are best suited to understand pathophysiology and treatment of HCC. As we enter a new era in the treatment of this disease, the role of the immune response to this cancer is likely to increase in importance.

PD-1 axis blockade has had a profound impact on the treatment of a host of solid and liquid malignancies since this approach was shown to be effective for the treatment of melanoma [22]. In the years that followed, there was significant anticipation that HCC would be included in the growing category of cancers that benefit from immune checkpoint blockade. Indeed, blockade of PD-1 alone was associated with a promising response rate in advanced HCC of 14%, but ultimately failed to show improvement in the overall survival [23]. It was not until PD-L1 and VEGF blockade were used in combination that an improved overall survival was achieved with immunotherapy in HCC [21]. This suggests that a complete understanding of the HCC biology and treatment will require a more nuanced understanding of the liver's unique immunobiology.

2 Hepatic Immunobiology

Evolution has conferred the liver with the complex capacity to discriminate among the innumerable foreign dietary and microbial molecules that enter the portal circulation from the digestive tract. Among these foreign molecules are highly inflammatory pattern recognition receptor (PRR) agonists such as lipopolysaccharide [24] which normally serve to initiate both an innate and adaptive immune response. It is in the context of perpetual exposure to these factors that the liver must achieve at least three important goals. First, it must prevent microbes and inflammatory microbial products from transitioning from the portal circulation to the central vein and thus the systemic circulation. Second, it must protect specific hepatocytes, particularly those lining the central vein that often serve critical metabolic functions (via the expression of glutamine synthetase and other metabolic enzymes), from apoptosis secondary to an antimicrobial immune response [25]. Third, and perhaps most important from an oncology perspective, the hepatic immune system must diminish the potential to respond to benign dietary and microbial antigens that would otherwise initiate a systemic inflammatory response.

The first two tasks are primarily achieved within the hepatic sinusoids. These sinusoids represent unique immune microenvironments separating the portal circulation from the systemic circulation. They are lined by liver sinusoidal endothelial cells (LSECs), and are surveyed by specialized macrophages known as Kupffer cells as well as resident memory T cells and natural killer T (NKT) cells. It is now clear from murine models that the LSECs serve to sense microbial products and initiate immune signaling through the MYD88 adaptor protein. The LSECs then modify the extracellular matrix (ECM) to trap and enrich key chemokines such as C-X-C motif ligand 9 (CXCL9) in the periportal region. This, in turn, recruits immune cells expressing corresponding receptors, such as C-X-C motif receptor 3 (CXCR3), including Kupffer cells, NKT cells, and resident memory T cells. This results in the immune cells becoming poised to eliminate inflammatory molecules and microbes before they approach the central vein and enter the systemic circulation [25].

The third key task, that of diminishing the antigen-specific adaptive immune response to antigens that appear benign, is largely achieved by antigen-presenting cells (APCs) including dendritic cells (DCs). APCs normally require two signals (known as signal 1 and 2) to initiate a T-cell response to a given antigen. Signal 1 occurs when the T-cell receptor binds a cognate peptide presented on a major histocompatibility complex (MHC) molecule on the surface of an APC. Signal 2 occurs when another stimulatory interaction takes place between the T cell and the APC—classically, this is the interaction between CD28 on T cells and CD80/CD86 on APCs. Both are required to prime an antigen-specific T cell which exists at baseline in an inactivated state. Crucially, when signal 1 occurs in the absence of signal 2, the T cell which recognizes the presented antigen is deleted, becomes anergic, or becomes suppressive [26, 27]. Thus, the absence of signal 2 diminishes the possibility of response to a given antigen. This form of T-cell inhibition is particularly active in the hepatic microenvironment where APCs are maintained in a tolerogenic state, by immunosuppressive mediators such as TGF-beta, in which signal 2 does not readily occur [28].

3 Implications for HCC Classification and Treatment

The three tasks of the hepatic immune system described above suggest a new way of considering the setting in which HCC arises, and potentially a new way of categorizing HCC that could have implications for treatment.

It has recently been found that disruption of the spatial distribution of hepatic immune cells results in damage to hepatocytes that are otherwise protected from immune-mediated lysis [25]. Furthermore, unlike other forms of spatial redistribution in the liver such as metabolic zonation driven by the Wnt/beta-catenin pathway [29, 30], immune cell spatial distribution is largely determined by the microbiota [25]. This suggests that the impact of the microbiota on the prevention and treatment of HCC should be revisited with special attention to how the microbiota affect the relationship between hepatocytes, HCC, and hepatic immunity.

Lastly, the role of APCs as particularly important for the treatment of HCC appears to be of growing importance. For example, dual CTLA-4 and PD-1 checkpoint blockade, which strengthens T-cell priming by APCs and T cells' capacity to lyse tumor cells, has demonstrated a compelling 32% investigator-assessed objective response rate [31]. APCs that confer only signal 1 and not signal 2 may be eliminating the potential to respond to HCC antigens inside and outside of the liver by functionally eliminating HCC-antigen-specific T cells, even in the context of immune checkpoint blockade, as appears to be the case in other malignancies [32]. This may explain the failure of PD-1 blockade as monotherapy to improve the overall survival in HCC [23] as PD-1 blockade works primarily through tumor-specific T cells that have previously been primed by APCs [33]. It is noteworthy that the combination of atezolizumab and bevacizumab may overcome the obstacle due to the ability of bevacizumab to augment APC activation [34] and thus reverse the tolerogenic state of APCs which prevails in the liver at baseline. This also implies that a host of other immunotherapies that target innate immune cells, including APCs, may have a role in HCC treatment, potentially in combination with immune checkpoint blockade [35]. Along these lines, approaches that inhibit cytokines which maintain APCs in a tolerogenic state (e.g., TGF beta) are being actively investigated [36].

4 Immunotherapy and HCC

4.1 Immune Checkpoint Blockade as Monotherapy

With the better understanding of the liver immunobiology as described in this chapter and following the success stories of immunotherapy in other solid tumors, several immune checkpoint inhibitors were and are being explored in HCC. This started early on with the anti-CTLA-4 monoclonal antibody tremelimumab [37]. The drug showed antitumor activity in patients with advanced HCC and HCV-related cirrhosis who progressed on sorafenib. Three out of 17 patients (17.6%) achieved a partial response (PR) and 10 patients (58.8%) had stable disease (SD). Durvalumab, a human IgG1 monoclonal antibody of PD-L1, was also looked at as a single agent in the earlier phases [38]. Of 19 patients with HCC, there were no responders as per RECIST1.1. Single agent nivolumab, another PD-1 antibody, showed promising signals of activity in a phase 1/2 study [39]. Nivolumab showed an objective response rate (ORR) of 20% (95% CI: 15–26) in the dose-expansion phase. Median OS was 15 months (95% CI 9.6–20.2). Responses were noted irrespective of etiology, tumor PD-L1 expression, and prior sorafenib exposure. Based on this study, nivolumab was granted conditional FDA approval as a second-line treatment for advanced and metastatic HCC. However, when nivolumab was compared to sorafenib in a randomized phase 3 study, it failed to show an improvement in survival against the standard-of-care treatment. The results of CheckMate 459 study (NCT02576509) were recently reported [40]. Median OS was 16·4 months (95% CI 13·9–18·4) with nivolumab and 14·7 months (11·9–17·2) with sorafenib (HR 0·85 [95% CI 0·72–1·02]; p = 0·075). Among patients with HCV and HBV etiology, a suggested difference in median OS was irrelevant, despite a numerically longer period with nivolumab versus sorafenib, 17.5 vs. 12.7 months (HR 0.72, 95% CI 0.51–1.02) for HCV and 16.1 vs. 10.4 months (HR 0.79, 95% CI 0.59–1.07) for HBV, respectively. Pembrolizumab was also granted accelerated FDA approval in patients with disease progression after sorafenib based on results from a nonrandomized, open-label, phase 2 trial [41]. ORR, which was the study's primary endpoint, was observed in 17% of patients (95% CI 11–26), with 1 (1%) complete response and 17 (16%) partial responses. Median PFS was 4.9 months and median OS was 12.9 months. This is despite pembrolizumab undergoing further assessment in a phase 3, randomized, double-blind trial versus placebo as a second-line treatment in patients with HCC [23]. This study did not meet its co-primary endpoints of OS and PFS. The study enrolled 413 patients. Median OS was 13.9 months (95% CI 11.6 to 16.0 months) for pembrolizumab versus 10.6 months (95% CI 8.3–13.5 months) for placebo (HR, 0.781; 95% CI 0.611–0.998; *P* = 0.0238). Median PFS for pembrolizumab was 3.0 months (95% CI 2.8–4.1 months) versus 2.8 months (95% CI, 1.6–3.0 months) at the final analysis (HR 0.718; 95% CI 0.570–0.904; *P* = 0.0022). Tislelizumab is a PD-1 monoclonal antibody which was engineered to minimize binding to macrophages and hence decrease immune inhibitory effects. In a phase 1/2 study which included 18 patients with previously treated HCC, ORR was 17% and median PFS was 4 months (95% CI 2.1-NE) [42]. Results from a global phase 2 study were recently reported. The study enrolled 249 patients with previously treated HCC. ORR was 13.8% and median OS reached 13.2 months (95% CI 10.8–15) [43]. The drug was granted approval in China based on these results and is currently being compared to sorafenib in a large global randomized study with a plan to randomize 640 patients (RATIONALE-301).

These results indicated that single-agent immune checkpoint blockade has limited activity in patients with advanced HCC as depicted above. APCs that confer only signal 1 and not signal 2 may be eliminating the potential to respond to HCC antigens inside and outside of the liver by functionally eliminating HCC-antigen-specific T cells, even in the context of single-agent immune checkpoint blockade as with pembrolizumab and nivolumab.

4.2 Immunotherapy-Based Combinations

Thus, combination therapies evolved rapidly and continue to be evaluated extensively in HCC, mainly antiangiogenic therapy plus checkpoint inhibitors, TKI plus checkpoint inhibitors, and combinations of checkpoint inhibitors.

4.2.1 Anti-VEGF plus Checkpoint Inhibitors

One rationale behind this combination is that proangiogenic factors have immunosuppressive activity [44], and by inhibiting angiogenesis, immune checkpoint blockade can be potentiated. Vascular endothelium plays a direct role in antigen recognition through interaction between endothelium and immune cells [45]. Blockade of the vascular endothelial growth factor and its receptor (VEGF/VEGFR) axis and the resulting induced hypoxia could potentiate the effects of immunomodulators such as PD-1/PDL-1 inhibitors.

Atezolizumab and Bevacizumab Combination

The combination of the PDL-1 inhibitor atezolizumab plus bevacizumab showed tolerable toxicity and an impressive ORR of 62% in a phase 1 study. These results prompted the phase 3 trial of the combination compared to single agent sorafenib in untreated patients with locally advanced or metastatic HCC (IMbrave150) [21]. The study accrued 501 patients. The combination of atezolizumab plus bevacizumab showed improvement in OS and PFS, the two co-primary endpoints of the study, compared to sorafenib. After a median follow-up of 8.6 months at the time of study report, median OS for sorafenib was 13.2 months and not yet reached for the combination, and HR was 0.58 (95% CI 0.42–0.79; $P < 0.001$). PFS was improved from 4.3 months for sorafenib to 6.8 months for atezolizumab and bevacizumab combination (HR = 0.59; CI 0.47–0.76; $P < 0.001$). ORR was 27.3% vs. 11.9% in sorafenib ($P < 0.001$). Patient-reported outcomes demonstrated a delayed time to deterioration of quality of life with atezolizumab-bevacizumab combination (11.2 months) compared to sorafenib (3.2 months) (HR 0.63; 95% CI, 0.46–0.85). In view of the previous experience of single agent bevacizumab and the concern for potential bleeding [46], all subjects underwent screening and treatment of esophageal varices before initiating therapy, within 6 months of enrollment. Antidrug antibodies (ADAs) can decrease the amount of drug available; the effect of ADA on antitumor activity and clinical outcomes of immunotherapy are not entirely understood [47]. The rate of ADA positivity varies significantly between studied agents, from 1.5%

with pembrolizumab to as high as 54% for atezolizumab interestingly. The IMbrave 150 study investigators conducted an exploratory analysis to determine the clinical consequences of ADA status in the study population (Peter Galle et al., AACR, 2021). The incidence of treatment-emergent atezolizumab ADAs was 29.6% (94/318) among patients with available ADA status. PFS benefit and ORR were similar with atezolizumab + bevacizumab over sorafenib regardless of the ADA status. OS-adjusted modeling analyses showed that patients with ADA+ status had a similar OS (HR 0.96; 95% CI: 0.62, 1.48), whereas those with ADA− status had an improved OS (HR 0.55; 95% CI: 0.41, 0.75) with atezolizumab + bevacizumab vs. sorafenib. Prospective data is needed to better evaluate the clinical implications of ADA.

4.2.2 TKI and Checkpoint Inhibitor

Sorafenib, lenvatinib, and cabozantinib are tyrosine kinase inhibitors shown to exert an immune modulation effect in preclinical and clinical data. In order to potentiate the role of immunotherapy in HCC, several checkpoint inhibitors were combined with these agents.

Pembrolizumab and Lenvatinib

Pembrolizumab and lenvatinib combination was studied initially in an open-label, phase 1b trial [48]. The trial started with a dose escalation/dose-limiting toxicity (DLT) phase to assess for safety and tolerability. The dose expansion primary endpoints were ORR and PFS. The combination therapy was well tolerated, with no DLT observed. The ORR was 46.0% (95% CI, 36.0% to 56.3%) per mRECIST. Median PFS was 9.3 months per mRECIST and 8.6 months per RECIST v1.1. Median OS was 22 months. Grade $\geq$ 3 treatment-related adverse events were observed in 67% of the patients. These promising results led to the phase 3 trial LEAP-002 (NCT03713593) where patients with HCC are randomized to receive the combination compared to lenvatinib alone as a frontline treatment. The results are still awaited.

Ipilimumab and Nivolumab with Cabozantinib

CheckMate 040, the multi-arm phase 1/2 study, tested the efficacy of ipilimumab in combination with nivolumab and cabozantinib (triplet therapy) in both sorafenib-naïve and sorafenib-treated advanced HCC compared to the combination of nivolumab and cabozantinib alone [31]. Preliminary results demonstrated an ORR of 26% in the triplet vs. 17% in the nivolumab and cabozantinib combination. Grade 3 and 4 treatment-related adverse events were more common in patients receiving the triplet therapy (71%) compared to those receiving the combination therapy (42%).

Pembrolizumab and Regorafenib

A phase Ib study evaluated this combination as a first-line treatment in patients with advanced HCC [49]. Three different doses of regorafenib are explored, 80 mg, 120 mg, and 160 mg, in addition to a fixed dose of pembrolizumab 200 mg every 3 weeks. Twenty-nine patients were treated at the 120 mg dose level. No unexpected safety issues were noted. Of 23 evaluable patients, 7 had partial responses (30%) and 14 had stable disease (61%).

Atezolizumab and Lenvatinib or Sorafenib

A phase 3, open-label, randomized study was designed to evaluate the combination of atezolizumab plus lenvatinib or sorafenib versus lenvatinib or sorafenib alone, as a second-line treatment in patients who have progressed following atezolizumab and bevacizumab (ClinicalTrials.gov Identifier: NCT04770896). The role of continuing the same checkpoint blockade strategy beyond primary progression is questionable as the understanding of mechanisms and types of PDL-1 inhibitor resistance remains a work in progress.

4.2.3 Combinations of Checkpoint Inhibitors

Preclinical data has shown that blocking both PD-L1 and anti-CTLA-4 pathways enhances antitumor activity. Concurrent targeting of different immune checkpoint pathways improved outcomes in various solid tumors and this approach is being extensively evaluated in HCC.

Durvalumab and Tremelimumab

Results from a phase 1/2 trial combining anti-PD-L1 and anti-CTLA-4 antibodies established an acceptable toxicity profile and promising efficacy [50]. 332 patients were enrolled, and four regimens were evaluated: durvalumab and tremelimumab as monotherapy, and two different dosing of the two drugs. Median OS reached 18.7 months (10.8-not reached) for tremelimumab 300 mg/durvalumab group, 11.3 months (8.4–14.6) for tremelimumab 75 mg/durvalumab combination, 11.7 months (8.5–16.9) for durvalumab monotherapy, and 17.1 months (10.9-not reached) for tremelimumab monotherapy. The highest ORR was for the tremelimumab 300 mg/durvalumab combination which reached 24%. Grade 3 or 4 treatment-related adverse events were 35.1%, 24.4%, 17.8%, and 42%, for each of the study arms, respectively. Updated results after adding the single-dose tremelimumab/durvalumab combination cohort showed an ORR that reached 30% and OS of 22 months. The pharmacodynamic analysis showed that single-dose tremelimumab 300 mg and durvalumab was associated with an increase in Ki-67- and CD-8-positive cells. These are activated immune cells which may explain the favorable antitumor activity observed [50]. A phase 3 open-label, multicenter, randomized study is evaluating the combination of CTLA-4 and PD-1 checkpoint blockade in HCC-HIMALAYA (NCT03298451). Patients are randomized to receive durvalumab monotherapy versus durvalumab and tremelimumab combination, versus sorafenib. The study is looking at OS as the primary endpoint, and PFS and ORR as secondary endpoints. The study aimed to enroll 1310 patients across the world.

In a recent press release, the study was announced positive, with the combination showing statistically significant and clinically meaningful improvement in OS. The results will be presented at the Gastrointestinal Cancer Symposium in January 2022 [51].

Ipilimumab and Nivolumab

Nivolumab at 3 mg/kg and ipilimumab at 1 mg/kg for 4 dose combinations was evaluated in one of the CheckMate 040 multicohort studies [31]. Patients were randomized 1:1:1 to either nivolumab 1 mg/kg plus ipilimumab 3 mg/kg for 4 doses followed by nivolumab 240 mg every 2 weeks (A); nivolumab 3 mg/kg plus ipilimumab 1 mg/kg for 4 doses followed by nivolumab 240 mg every 2 weeks (B); or nivolumab 3 mg/kg every 2 weeks plus ipilimumab 1 mg/kg every 6 weeks (C). 148 patients were evaluated. ORR was 32% (95% CI, 20–47%) in arm A, 27% (95% CI, 15–41%) in arm B, and 29% (95% CI, 17–43%) in arm C. Any-grade treatment-related adverse events were higher in arm A, 46 of 49 patients (94%), compared to 35 of 49 patients (71%) in arm B, and 38 of 48 patients (79%) in arm C. The types of events were similar across arms, and in patients with and without HBV or HCV infection. Arm A had higher rates of immune-mediated adverse events and immune-mediated adverse events leading to discontinuation compared with arms B and C. One grade 5 serious treatment-related adverse event (pneumonitis) occurred in arm A.

Table 1 summarizes immunotherapy-based clinical trials reported to date.

Table 1 Summary of immunotherapy trials in HCC reported to date

Clinicaltrial.gov	Agent	Line of therapy	Target	Phase	Results
NCT02576509 (CheckMate-459)	Nivolumab vs sorafenib	First line	PD-1 vs. TKI	Phase 3	OS 16.4 vs. 14.8 months $P = 0.0522$ HR 0.85 (95% CI 0.72–1.00) [40]
NCT02702401 (KEYNOTE-240)	Pembrolizumab vs. BSC	Second line	PD-1	Phase 3	OS 13.9 vs. 10.6 months HR 0.781 (95% CI 0.611–0.998) $P = 0.0238$ PFS 3.0 vs. 2.8 months HR 0.718 (95% CI 0.570–0.904) $P = 0.0022$ [23]
NCT03434379 (IMbrave)	Atezolizumab plus bevacizumab vs. sorafenib	First line	PD-L1/ VEGFR vs. TKI	Phase 3	OS 19.2 vs. 13.4 months $P = 0.0009$ [21]
NCT01658878 CheckMate-040	Ipilimumab and nivolumab	Second line	PD-L1 and CTLA-4 combination	Phase 1/2	ORR 32% [31]
NCT03006926	Pembrolizumab and lenvatinib	First line	PD-L1 and TKI	Phase 1b	Median OS 22 months; ORR 46% [48]
NCT02519348	Durvalumab and tremelimumab	First line	PD-L1 and CTLA-4 combination	Phase 2	Median OS 18.7 months; ORR 22.7% [50]

5 Locoregional Therapies and Immune System

An area of great interest is the combination of local regional therapies (i.e., ablation, embolization with or without chemotherapy, and radioembolization) with immune checkpoint blockade at earlier stages of disease. Our group was keen on looking into that perspective from the start when initial tremelimumab data surfaced. The underlying hypothesis is that local tumor destruction by various methods has the potential to transform relatively immunologically inert tumors to immune-active tumors which will be more responsive to immune checkpoint blockade. Embolization procedures when paired with chemotherapy or radiotherapeutics have been shown to have direct effects on the local immune microenvironment. Anthracyclines enhance APC activity and have the potential to sensitize HCC to NK cell killing in preclinical models [52]. The hypoxia response, a consequence of regional therapy with transarterial embolization, also modulates the expression of critical immunotherapy targets in the tumor microenvironment [53, 54]. For example, hypoxia leads to hypoxia-inducible factor 1-α-dependent upregulation of PD-L1 in myeloid-derived suppressor cells (MDSC). MDSC activity is suppressed by applying PD-L1 blockade [55]. Regional therapy in HCC has been shown to alter cytokine profiles [56], CD4+/CD8+ T-cell subset populations, and T-cell activation [57]. The kinetics of these changes last for hours (as is the case with IL-6/IL-8/TNF-α surge post-embolization) to months (as in the case of expansion and activation of T-cell subsets). In one study, expansion and activation of tumor-specific CD4+ T cells against three AFP epitopes occurred following embolization [57]. Importantly, heightened levels of AFP-specific CD4+ T cells following treatment were associated with more than 50% tumor necrosis and improved clinical outcome.

Given these, the above clinical data of how different methods of local tumor destruction and their timing can augment or be augmented by checkpoint blockade is reasonable. A phase 1 study recently assessed the safety and efficacy of tremelimumab with subtotal radiofrequency ablation or chemoablation in 32 patients with advanced HCC [58, 59]. This study found that the combination was safe with an objective response rate of 26.3% (95% CI: 9.1–51.2%)—comparing favorably to historic studies of tremelimumab in a similar advanced patient population [40]. On-treatment biopsies revealed an accumulation of tumoral CD8+ T cells in long-term responders. Interestingly, although an increase in cytotoxic immune effectors was noted in PBMCs over treatment, embolization procedures did not impact the peripheral immune response [59]. Another ongoing pilot study has evaluated nivolumab at various time points related to deb-TACE in liver-limited HCC confirming safety of this combination [60]. These data have served to support several ongoing phase 3 studies aimed to determine the relative contribution of immunotherapy to embolization for liver-limited HCC (i.e., Checkmate 74W NCT04340193; Emerald-1 NCT03778957; LEAP-012 NCT04246177).

6 Conclusion

The treatment of HCC is evolving rapidly. Tyrosine kinase targeting (including FGF axis inhibition) is playing a growing role, and now immunotherapy is as well [48]. This raises new possibilities for combination therapies and it also means that clinicians and researchers need to take into account the unique immunobiology of the liver as novel treatments are explored. Such an understanding may open the door to new classes of immunotherapy that are uniquely suited to treat HCC.

Compliance with Ethical Standards

This work was performed in compliance with ethical standards.

References

1. Bray F et al (2018) Global cancer statistics 2018: GLOBOCAN estimates of incidence and mortality worldwide for 36 cancers in 185 countries. CA Cancer J Clin 68:394–424
2. Petrick JL et al (2020) International trends in hepatocellular carcinoma incidence, 1978–2012. Int J Cancer 147:317–330
3. Valery PC et al (2018) Projections of primary liver cancer to 2030 in 30 countries worldwide. Hepatology 67:600–611
4. Surveillance, Epidemiology, and End Results (SEER) Program (www.seer.cancer.gov) SEER*Stat Database: Incidence—SEER 9 Regs Research Data, Nov 2018 Sub (1975–2016)—Linked To County Attributes—Total U.S., 1969–2017 Counties, National Cancer Institute, DCCPS, Surveillance Research Program, released April 2019, based on the November 2018 submission; 2019. http://www.seer.cancer.gov.
5. Yang JD et al (2017) Characteristics, management, and outcomes of patients with hepatocellular carcinoma in Africa: a multicountry observational study from the Africa Liver Cancer Consortium. Lancet Gastroenterol Hepatol 2:103–111
6. McGlynn KA, Petrick JL, El-Serag HB (2021) Epidemiology of hepatocellular carcinoma. Hepatology 73(Suppl. 1):4–13
7. El-Serag HB, Kanwal F (2014) Epidemiology of hepatocellular carcinoma in the United States: where are we? Where do we go? Hepatology 60:1767–1775
8. Bagnardi V et al (2015) Alcohol consumption and site-specific cancer risk: a comprehensive dose-response meta-analysis. Br J Cancer 112:580–593
9. Jinjuvadia R, Patel S, Liangpunsakul S (2014) The association between metabolic syndrome and hepatocellular carcinoma: systemic review and meta-analysis. J Clin Gastroenterol 48:172–177
10. Heimbach JK et al (2018) AASLD guidelines for the treatment of hepatocellular carcinoma. Hepatology 67:358–380
11. Flecken T et al (2014) Immunodominance and functional alterations of tumor-associated antigen-specific CD8+ T-cell responses in hepatocellular carcinoma. Hepatology 59:1415–1426
12. Albillos A, Lario M, Álvarez-Mon M (2014) Cirrhosis-associated immune dysfunction: distinctive features and clinical relevance. J Hepatol 61:1385–1396
13. Severi T, van Malenstein H, Verslype C, van Pelt JF (2010) Tumor initiation and progression in hepatocellular carcinoma: risk factors, classification, and therapeutic targets. Acta Pharmacol Sin 31:1409–1420
14. Thomson AW, Knolle PA (2010) Antigen-presenting cell function in the tolerogenic liver environment. Nat Rev Immunol 10:753–766
15. Bowen DG et al (2004) The site of primary T cell activation is a determinant of the balance between intrahepatic tolerance and immunity. J Clin Invest 114:701–712

16. Jenne CN, Kubes P (2013) Immune surveillance by the liver. Nat Immunol 14:996–1006
17. Prieto J, Melero I, Sangro B (2015) Immunological landscape and immunotherapy of hepatocellular carcinoma. Nat Rev Gastroenterol Hepatol 12:681–700
18. Abou-Alfa GK, Venook AP (2013) The antiangiogenic ceiling in hepatocellular carcinoma: does it exist and has it been reached? Lancet Oncol 14:e283–e288
19. Harding JJ, El Dika I, Abou-Alfa GK (2016) Immunotherapy in hepatocellular carcinoma: primed to make a difference? Cancer 122:367–377
20. El Dika I, Khalil DN, Abou-Alfa GK (2019) Immune checkpoint inhibitors for hepatocellular carcinoma. Cancer 125:3312–3319
21. Finn RS et al (2020) Atezolizumab plus Bevacizumab in unresectable hepatocellular carcinoma. N Engl J Med 382:1894–1905
22. Robert C et al (2015) Nivolumab in previously untreated melanoma without BRAF mutation. N Engl J Med 372:320–330
23. Finn RS et al (2020) Pembrolizumab as second-line therapy in patients with advanced hepatocellular carcinoma in KEYNOTE-240: a randomized, double-blind phase III trial. J Clin Oncol 38:193–202
24. Roh JS, Sohn DH (2018) Damage-associated molecular patterns in inflammatory diseases. Immune Netw 18:e27
25. Gola A et al (2021) Commensal-driven immune zonation of the liver promotes host defence. Nature 589:131–136
26. Yamazaki S et al (2003) Direct expansion of functional CD25+ CD4+ regulatory T cells by antigen-processing dendritic cells. J Exp Med 198:235–247
27. Idoyaga J et al (2013) Specialized role of migratory dendritic cells in peripheral tolerance induction. J Clin Invest 123:844–854
28. Karimi MH, Geramizadeh B, Malek-Hosseini SA (2015) Tolerance induction in liver. Int J Organ Transplant Med 6:45–54
29. Burke ZD et al (2009) Liver zonation occurs through a beta-catenin-dependent, c-Myc-independent mechanism. Gastroenterology 136:2316–2324. e1
30. Shiojiri N et al (1995) Heterogeneous hepatocellular expression of glutamine synthetase in developing mouse liver and in testicular transplants of fetal liver. Lab Investig 72:740–747
31. Yau T et al (2020) Efficacy and safety of nivolumab plus ipilimumab in patients with advanced hepatocellular carcinoma previously treated with sorafenib: the checkmate 040 randomized clinical trial. JAMA Oncol 6:e204564
32. Yu J et al (2021) Liver metastasis restrains immunotherapy efficacy via macrophage-mediated T cell elimination. Nat Med 27:152–164
33. Khalil DN, Smith EL, Brentjens RJ, Wolchok JD (2016) The future of cancer treatment: immunomodulation, CARs and combination immunotherapy. Nat Rev Clin Oncol 13:273–290
34. Alfaro C et al (2009) Influence of bevacizumab, sunitinib and sorafenib as single agents or in combination on the inhibitory effects of VEGF on human dendritic cell differentiation from monocytes. Br J Cancer 100:1111–1119
35. Khalil DN et al (2019) In situ vaccination with defined factors overcomes T cell exhaustion in distant tumors. J Clin Invest 129:3435–3447
36. Kelley RK et al (2019) A Phase 2 Study of Galunisertib (TGF-**β**1 receptor Type I inhibitor) and sorafenib in patients with advanced hepatocellular carcinoma. Clin Transl Gastroenterol 10:e00056
37. Merle P (2021) The new immuno-oncology-based therapies and their perspectives in hepatocellular carcinoma. Cancers (Basel) 13
38. Segal NH et al (2014) Preliminary data from a multi-arm expansion study of MEDI4736, an anti-PD-L1 antibody. J Clin Oncol 32(5s):abstr 3002
39. El-Khoueiry AB et al (2017) Nivolumab in patients with advanced hepatocellular carcinoma (CheckMate 040): an open-label, non-comparative, phase 1/2 dose escalation and expansion trial. Lancet 389:2492–2502
40. Yau T, Park J-W, Finn RS, Cheng A-L, Mathurin P, Edeline J et al (2021) Nivolumab versus sorafenib in advanced hepatocellular carcinoma (CheckMate 459): a randomised, multicentre, open-label, phase 3 trial. Lancet Oncol

41. Zhu AX et al (2018) Pembrolizumab in patients with advanced hepatocellular carcinoma previously treated with sorafenib (KEYNOTE-224): a non-randomised, open-label phase 2 trial. Lancet Oncol 19:940–952
42. Shen L et al (2020) Tislelizumab in Chinese patients with advanced solid tumors: an open-label, non-comparative, phase 1/2 study. J Immunother Cancer 8
43. Ducreux M, Abou-Alfa G, Ren Z, Edeline J, Li Z, Assenat E, Rimassa L, Blanc J, Ross P, Fang W, Hu S (2021) O-1 Results from a global phase 2 study of tislelizumab, an investigational PD-1 antibody, in patients with unresectable hepatocellular carcinoma. Ann Oncol 32:S217
44. Osada T et al (2008) The effect of anti-VEGF therapy on immature myeloid cell and dendritic cells in cancer patients. Cancer Immunol Immunother 57:1115–1124
45. Geppert TD, Lipsky PE (1985) Antigen presentation by interferon-gamma-treated endothelial cells and fibroblasts: differential ability to function as antigen-presenting cells despite comparable Ia expression. J Immunol 135:3750–3762
46. Pazo Cid RA, Esquerdo G, Puertolas T, Calderero V, Gil I, Lao J, Millastre E, Alvarez-Alejandro M, Madani J, Anton A (2010) Bevacizumab (BVZ) as second-line treatment after sorafenib (SFB) progression in patients (pts) with advanced hepatocellular carcinoma (HCC). J Clin Oncol 28(15_suppl):e14619–e14619
47. de Spéville BD, Moreno V (2021) Antidrug antibodies and drug development: challenges in the immunotherapy era. Clin Cancer Res 27:2669–2671
48. Finn RS et al (2020) Phase Ib study of lenvatinib plus pembrolizumab in patients with unresectable hepatocellular carcinoma. J Clin Oncol 38:2960–2970
49. El-Khoueiry AB, Kim RD, Harris WP, Sung MW, Waldschmidt D, Iqbal S, Zhang X, Nakajima K, Galle PR (2020) Phase Ib study of regorafenib (REG) plus pembrolizumab (PEMBRO) for first-line treatment of advanced hepatocellular carcinoma (HCC). J Clin Oncol 38(4)
50. Kelley RK, Sangro B, Harris W, Ikeda M, Okusaka T, Kang YK, Qin S, Tai DW, Lim HY, Yau T, Yong WP, Cheng AL, Gasbarrini A, Damian S, Bruix J, Borad M, Bendell J, Kim TY, Standifer N, He P, Makowsky M, Negro A, Kudo M, Abou-Alfa GK (2021) Safety, efficacy, and pharmacodynamics of tremelimumab plus durvalumab for patients with unresectable hepatocellular carcinoma: randomized expansion of a phase I/II study. J Clin Oncol 39(27):2991–3001. https://doi.org/10.1200/JCO.20.03555. Epub 2021 Jul 22. PMID: 34292792; PMCID: PMC8445563
51. Abou-Alfa GK, Chan SL, Kudo M, Lau G, Kelley RK, Furuse J, et al (2022) Phase 3 randomized, open-label, multicenter study of tremelimumab (T) and durvalumab (D) as first-line therapy in patients (pts) with unresectable hepatocellular carcinoma (uHCC): HIMALAYA. J Clin Oncol 40(4_suppl):379–379. https://doi.org/10.1200/JCO.2022.40.4_suppl.379
52. Kohga K et al (2009) Anticancer chemotherapy inhibits MHC class I-related chain a ectodomain shedding by downregulating ADAM10 expression in hepatocellular carcinoma. Cancer Res 69:8050–8057
53. Palazón A et al (2012) The HIF-1α hypoxia response in tumor-infiltrating T lymphocytes induces functional CD137 (4-1BB) for immunotherapy. Cancer Discov 2:608–623
54. Labiano S, Palazon A, Melero I (2015) Immune response regulation in the tumor microenvironment by hypoxia. Semin Oncol 42:378–386
55. Noman MZ, Desantis G, Janji B, Hasmim M, Karray S, Dessen P, Bronte V, Chouaib S (2014) PD-L1 is a novel direct target of HIF-1α, and its blockade under hypoxia enhanced MDSC-mediated T cell activation. J Exp Med 211(5):781–790
56. Ikei S et al (1992) Changes in IL-6, IL-8, C-reactive protein and pancreatic secretory trypsin inhibitor after transcatheter arterial chemo-embolization therapy for hepato-cellular carcinoma. Cytokine 4:581–584
57. Ayaru L et al (2007) Unmasking of alpha-fetoprotein-specific CD4(+) T cell responses in hepatocellular carcinoma patients undergoing embolization. J Immunol 178:1914–1922
58. Duffy AG et al (2017) Tremelimumab in combination with ablation in patients with advanced hepatocellular carcinoma. J Hepatol 66:545–551
59. Agdashian D et al (2019) The effect of anti-CTLA4 treatment on peripheral and intra-tumoral T cells in patients with hepatocellular carcinoma. Cancer Immunol Immunother 68:599–608
60. Harding JJ et al (2020) Nivolumab (NIVO) and drug eluting bead transarterial chemoembolization (deb-TACE): preliminary results from a phase I study of patients (pts) with liver limited hepatocellular carcinoma (HCC). J Clin Oncol 38(4s):abstr 525

Immunotherapy in GI Cancers: Hepatocellular Carcinoma: Perspective

Friedrich Foerster and Peter Robert Galle

Contents

Abstract

Cancer immunotherapy has finally entered the realm of hepatocellular carcinoma (HCC). The first immune checkpoint inhibitor (ICI) containing systemic treatment to be ever approved for HCC in the first-line setting is the combination of atezolizumab and bevacizumab which has produced previously unseen clinical outcomes in the advanced stage in the IMbrave150 trial. The relevance of these results for the field of HCC research can hardly be overstated. We contemplate in this perspective three key questions which arise from this success: (1) Which groups of HCC patients do or do not benefit from checkpoint inhibition? (2) Is immunotherapy effective at earlier HCC stages? 3. What immunotherapies beyond PD1/PD-L1/CTLA4 inhibition are effective? We summarize the current evidence regarding biomarkers for response prediction, give an overview of the currently ongoing clinical trials testing immunotherapeutic agents in earlier HCC stages, and highlight novel immune interventions for HCC which go beyond the established ICIs. In light of our understanding of the pathogenesis of HCC and emerging data from immunotherapeutic trials, it appears likely that the combination of atezolizumab and bevacizumab represents just the beginning of a much larger development that will fundamentally change the treatment and improve the outcome of patients with HCC.

F. Foerster (✉) · P. R. Galle
First Department of Medicine, University Medical Center of the Johannes Gutenberg University Mainz, Mainz, Germany
e-mail: Friedrich.Foerster@unimedizin-mainz.de

Cancer Immunotherapy (2022)
https://doi.org/10.1007/13905_2021_14,
Published Online: 19 March 2022

Keywords

Clinical trials · Hepatocellular carcinoma · Immunotherapy · Liver cirrhosis · systemic treatment · Tumour microenvironment

The remarkable efficacy of checkpoint inhibitors in entities such as lung cancer and melanoma has raised the question whether cancer immunotherapy could also be similarly effective in treating patients with HCC. As Ghassan Abou-Alfa and colleagues have elaborated in the previous chapter, this question has been at least partially answered with a "yes" by a series of large state-of-the-art clinical trials. It is all but certain that cancer immunotherapy will have its place in the treatment algorithm of HCC in the future (Fig. 1). However, against initial expectations based on promising data from phase 2 trials [1, 2], the PD1 inhibitors nivolumab and pembrolizumab failed to meet their primary endpoints in the subsequent phase 3 trials [3, 4]. In contrast, the combination of atezolizumab, a PD-L1 inhibitor, and bevacizumab, a VEGF inhibitor, succeeded in demonstrating superior efficacy in comparison to sorafenib in unresectable HCC and has become the new standard of care for this disease stage replacing sorafenib which has held this position for over a decade. While this combination can be regarded as a game changer, several contestants for first-line therapy are in the works. The combinations of cabozantinib and atezolizumab (COSMIC-312; NCT03755791) [5], lenvatinib and pembrolizumab (LEAP-002; NCT03713593) [6], durvalumab and tremelimumab (HIMALAYA; NCT03298451) [7], nivolumab and ipilimumab (CheckMate 9DW; NCT04039607), as well as camrelizumab (SHR-1210) and apatinib (rivoceranib) (NCT03764293) are all being evaluated in phase 3 trials with results being expected as early as 2021. Monotherapy with tislelizumab is also being tested (RATIONALE-301;

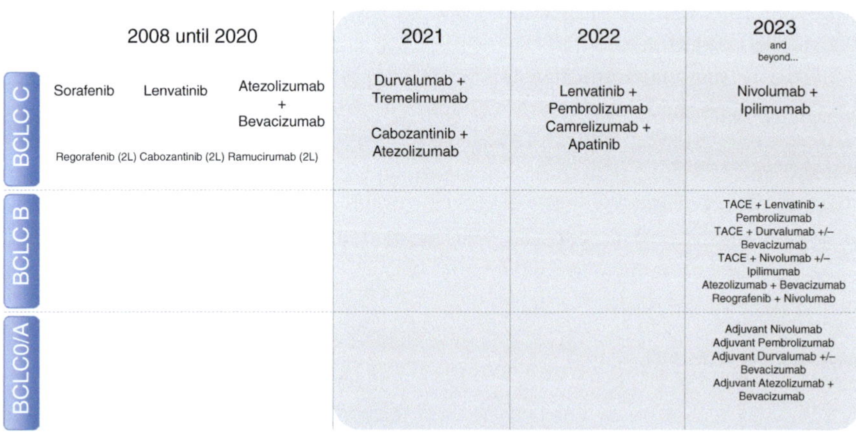

Fig. 1 Historic and expected years of publication of results from past positive and ongoing phase 3 trials in HCC

NCT03412773) [8]. Further checkpoint inhibitor-containing combination therapies are at an earlier stage of clinical development such as the combination of regorafenib and nivolumab (phase 2; NCT04170556 and NCT04310709), regorafenib and pembrolizumab (NCT03347292; phase 1b), cabozantinib and pembrolizumab (NCT04442581; phase 2), regorafenib and tislelizumab (phase 2; NCT04183088), and sitravatinib and tislelizumab (phase 2; NCT03941873).

From today's point of view, it seems likely that there will be several approved first-line combination therapies containing at least one immunotherapeutic agent. With these combination therapies for advanced HCC on the horizon, the three most pressing questions regarding immunotherapy of HCC, which need to be addressed in the coming years, are the following:

1. Which groups of HCC patients do or do not benefit from checkpoint inhibition?
2. Is immunotherapy effective at earlier HCC stages?
3. What immunotherapies beyond PD1/PD-L1/CTLA4 inhibition are effective in treating HCC?

Regarding the first question, it is well established that HCC is a highly heterogeneous disease which is also reflected in the immune contexture of tumours. The composition of the immune contexture alone has prognostic relevance [9–11]. Consequently, immunophenotypic classifications of HCC have been suggested [10, 12]. So far, it is unknown whether any of the proposed immune signatures or classifications has the potential to predict response to immunotherapy. However, first proofs-of-concept have been reported: WNT/CTNNB1 mutations have been linked to resistance against checkpoint inhibition [13, 14]. Furthermore, an interferon-γ-related gene signature has been shown to predict response to pembrolizumab [15], but this has not been demonstrated for HCC. Recently, two meta-analyses have demonstrated that checkpoint inhibition appears to provide greater benefit to patients with viral than non-viral HCC suggesting that particularly patients with non-alcoholic fatty liver disease (NAFLD) and non-alcoholic steatohepatitis (NASH) as underlying aetiologies benefit less [16, 17]. An underlying mechanism may be the accumulation of exhausted CD8+ PD1+ T cells which cause both tissue damage and impaired immune surveillance in NASH livers [17]. All in all, it seems clear that the immune contexture plays a key role in the efficacy of checkpoint inhibitors. In light of the fact that not all patients respond to checkpoint inhibitor-containing regimens and that some experience severe, irreversible side effects, it is highly desirable to develop biomarkers which predict response to various HCC treatments. This would allow to stratify patients and select the most effective treatment for them reducing potential harm from individually ineffective regimens.

As for the second question, the combination of atezolizumab and bevacizumab is so far the first and only immunotherapy with a proven benefit in HCC, and this benefit has been demonstrated only in unresectable HCC, i.e., BCLC B and C stages (>80% of patients had BCLC C stage in the IMbrave150 trial). Therefore, it is currently unknown whether immunotherapy has efficacy in earlier stages. Since the proportion of patients with BCLC B stage was fairly small in the IMbrave150 trial

(~15%), it is not possible to draw a final conclusion regarding the efficacy of atezolizumab and bevacizumab in this patient group, particularly in comparison to treatment with TACE, the current standard of care. Two large trials comparing systemic treatment with TACE in intermediate HCC will start in 2021: One will evaluate the combination of atezolizumab and bevacizumab (ABC-HCC; NCT04803994), and the other will assess the combination of regorafenib and nivolumab (RENOTACE; NCT04777851). Both will hopefully provide insights whether systemic treatment is effective in the BCLC B stage. Other trials testing different systemic treatments against TACE in this setting may follow in the coming years.

Furthermore, it is equally unknown whether the addition of systemic immunotherapy to locoregional treatments or surgery will be beneficial. In this respect, the addition of lenvatinib and pembrolizumab (LEAP-012; NCT04246177) [18], of durvalumab with or without bevacizumab (EMERALD-1; NCT03778957), and of nivolumab with or without ipilimumab (CheckMate 74 W; NCT04340193) to TACE in comparison to TACE alone is currently tested in phase 3 trials. As adjuvant treatments after curative hepatic resection or ablation, nivolumab (CheckMate 9DX; NCT03383458) [19], pembrolizumab (KEYNOTE-937; NCT03867084) [20], atezolizumab and bevacizumab (IMbrave050; NCT04102098) [21], and durvalumab with or without bevacizumab after curative hepatic resection or ablation (EMERALD-2; NCT03847428) [22] are also currently evaluated in phase 3 studies.

In the neoadjuvant setting, the following agents are being tested: nivolumab before electroporation (NIVOLEP; NCT03630640; phase 2), the combination of cabozantinib and nivolumab before hepatic resection (NCT03299946; phase 1b), pembrolizumab before ablation or resection (NCT03337841; phase 2), and the combination of lenvatinib and pembrolizumab before liver transplantation (PLENTY202001; NCT04425226). It will be exciting to see which of these novel concepts will finally mature into clinical practice.

However, the third question is the most intriguing one: What immunotherapies beyond PD1/PD-L1/CTLA4 inhibition are effective in HCC? As mentioned before, it is evident that there are different subgroups of patients with HCC, e.g., those who respond to checkpoint inhibition and those who do not. There are three key tumour properties which can be exploited by different immune interventions (Fig. 2): the presence or absence of (a) effector immune cells (NK and T cells), (b) antigen presentation by the tumour, and (c) an immunosuppressive tumour microenvironment (generated and maintained among others by tumour-associated macrophages and myeloid-derived suppressor cells). These three properties help explain conceptually why a patient will or will not respond to a certain type of immunotherapy. For example, a patient whose tumour is not infiltrated by effector immune cells will not benefit from checkpoint inhibition. In contrast, this patient will require a treatment such as adoptive transfer of NK or T cells to boost infiltration of the tumour by effector cells.

Alas, most of the immune interventions beyond checkpoint inhibition are still at a preclinical or early clinical stage. At ClinicalTrials.gov, there are currently six phase 1 studies with glypican 3 (GPC3)-targeted CAR-T cells registered (NCT04121273; NCT04506983; NCT03198546; NCT02905188; NCT03884751;

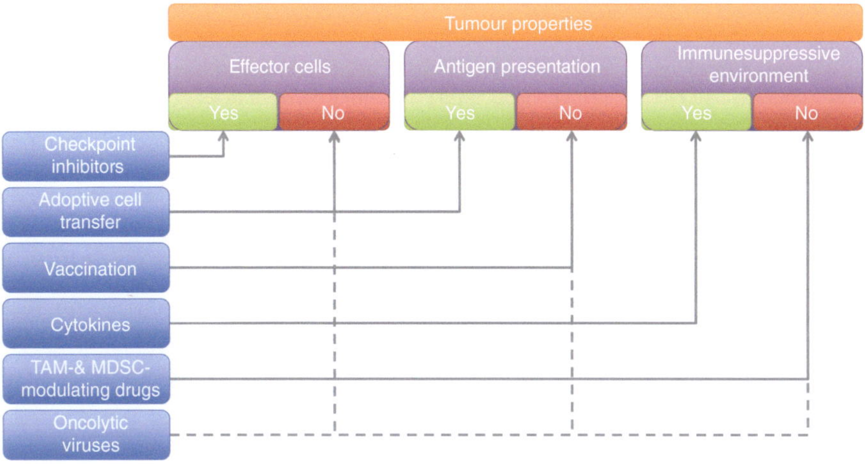

Fig. 2 A framework for future immune interventions as treatment for HCC

NCT03980288). One phase 2 study is comparing treatment with invariant NKT cells and TACE with TACE alone (NCT04011033). Furthermore, FT500, an allogeneic NK cell line, and FATE-NK100, which are donor-derived NK cells, are being tested in HCC among other entities in phase 1 trials (NCT03319459; NCT04106167; NCT03841110). Having failed as a second-line monotherapy in advanced HCC in the TRAVERSE phase 2b trial [23], pexastimogene devacirepvec (Pexa-Vec), an oncolytic virus, is currently being evaluated in combination with nivolumab in a phase 1/2a trial (NCT03071094). It is noteworthy that enrolment in the PHOCUS trial (NCT02562755; phase 3) [24], which tested the combination of Pexa-Vec and sorafenib, was stopped prematurely due to an apparent lack of benefit after a planned interim futility analysis. This exemplifies the odds of failure for these immune interventions at such an early developmental stage.

The success of atezolizumab and bevacizumab in advanced HCC heralds a new era of systemic treatment for HCC. It seems probable that several other combination therapies will follow. In the short to midterm, the most prevalent approach will be the combination of a tyrosine kinase inhibitor with a checkpoint inhibitor. It will be highly informative to learn how these will compare to atezolizumab and bevacizumab. In the long term, other immune interventions such as CAR-T or CAR-NK cells will expand the armamentarium for HCC. In addition, systemic treatment will probably not be bound to the realm of advanced HCC any longer but extend to earlier disease stages. It remains to be seen whether it will complement or replace modalities such as TACE in the intermediate stage. Moreover, neoadjuvant and adjuvant treatments in the context of surgery and ablation may define the future standard of care. In summary, the relevance of immunotherapy for the management of HCC cannot be fully assessed today. It seems likely that the arrival of atezolizumab and bevacizumab is just the beginning of a much larger development.

Compliance with Ethical Standards

Disclosure of Interests: FF reports receiving consulting and lecture fees from Roche and lecture fees from Lilly and Pfizer. PRG reports receiving consulting and lecture fees from Adaptimmune, AstraZeneca, Bayer, BMS, Eisai, Ipsen, Lilly, MSD, Roche, and Sirtex.

References

1. El-Khoueiry AB, Sangro B, Yau T, Crocenzi TS, Kudo M, Hsu C et al (2017) Nivolumab in patients with advanced hepatocellular carcinoma (CheckMate 040): an open-label, non-comparative, phase 1/2 dose escalation and expansion trial. Lancet 389(10088):2492–2502. https://doi.org/10.1016/s0140-6736(17)31046-2
2. Zhu AX, Finn RS, Edeline J, Cattan S, Ogasawara S, Palmer D et al (2018) Pembrolizumab in patients with advanced hepatocellular carcinoma previously treated with sorafenib (KEYNOTE-224): a non-randomised, open-label phase 2 trial. Lancet Oncol 19(7):940–952. https://doi.org/10.1016/s1470-2045(18)30351-6
3. Finn RS, Ryoo BY, Merle P, Kudo M, Bouattour M, Lim HY et al (2020) Pembrolizumab as second-line therapy in patients with advanced hepatocellular carcinoma in KEYNOTE-240: a randomized, double-blind, Phase III Trial. J Clin Oncol 38(3):193–202. https://doi.org/10.1200/JCO.19.01307
4. Yau T, Park JW, Finn RS, Cheng AL, Mathurin P, Edeline J et al (2019) CheckMate 459: a randomized, multi-center phase III study of nivolumab (NIVO) vs sorafenib (SOR) as first-line (1L) treatment in patients (pts) with advanced hepatocellular carcinoma (aHCC). Ann Oncol 30:v874–v8v5. https://doi.org/10.1093/annonc/mdz394.029
5. Rimassa L, Cheng A, Braiteh F, Benzaghou F, Hazra S, Borgman A et al (2019) Phase 3 (COSMIC-312) study of cabozantinib in combination with atezolizumab vs sorafenib in patients with advanced hepatocellular carcinoma (aHCC) who have not received previous systemic anticancer therapy. Ann Oncol 30:iv65–iiv6. https://doi.org/10.1093/annonc/mdz155.237
6. Josep ML, Masatoshi K, Ann-Lii C, Richard SF, Peter RG, Shuichi K et al (2019) Lenvatinib (len) plus pembrolizumab (pembro) for the first-line treatment of patients (pts) with advanced hepatocellular carcinoma (HCC): Phase 3 LEAP-002 study. J Clin Oncol 37(Suppl. 15):TPS4152. https://doi.org/10.1200/JCO.2019.37.15_suppl.TPS4152%U
7. Ghassan KA-A, Stephen Lam C, Junji F, Peter RG, Robin Kate K, Shukui Q et al (2018) A randomized, multicenter phase 3 study of durvalumab (D) and tremelimumab (T) as first-line treatment in patients with unresectable hepatocellular carcinoma (HCC): HIMALAYA study. J Clin Oncol 36(Suppl. 15):TPS4144. https://doi.org/10.1200/JCO.2018.36.15_suppl.TPS4144
8. Qin S, Finn RS, Kudo M, Meyer T, Vogel A, Ducreux M et al (2019) RATIONALE 301 study: tislelizumab versus sorafenib as first-line treatment for unresectable hepatocellular carcinoma. Future Oncol 15(16):1811–1822. https://doi.org/10.2217/fon-2019-0097
9. Foerster F, Hess M, Gerhold-Ay A, Marquardt JU, Becker D, Galle PR et al (2018) The immune contexture of hepatocellular carcinoma predicts clinical outcome. Sci Rep 8(1):5351. https://doi.org/10.1038/s41598-018-21937-2
10. Sia D, Jiao Y, Martinez-Quetglas I, Kuchuk O, Villacorta-Martin C, Castro de Moura M et al (2017) Identification of an immune-specific class of hepatocellular carcinoma, based on molecular features. Gastroenterology 153(3):812–826. https://doi.org/10.1053/j.gastro.2017.06.007
11. Kurebayashi Y, Ojima H, Tsujikawa H, Kubota N, Maehara J, Abe Y et al (2018) Landscape of immune microenvironment in hepatocellular carcinoma and its additional impact on histological and molecular classification. Hepatology 68(3):1025–1041. https://doi.org/10.1002/hep.29904

12. Zhang Q, Lou Y, Yang J, Wang J, Feng J, Zhao Y et al (2019) Integrated multiomic analysis reveals comprehensive tumour heterogeneity and novel immunophenotypic classification in hepatocellular carcinomas. Gut 68(11):2019–2031. https://doi.org/10.1136/gutjnl-2019-318912
13. Harding JJ, Nandakumar S, Armenia J, Khalil DN, Albano M, Ly M et al (2019) Prospective genotyping of hepatocellular carcinoma: clinical implications of next-generation sequencing for matching patients to targeted and immune therapies. Clin Cancer Res 25(7):2116–2126. https://doi.org/10.1158/1078-0432.CCR-18-2293
14. Pinyol R, Sia D, Llovet JM (2019) Immune exclusion-Wnt/CTNNB1 class predicts resistance to immunotherapies in HCC. Clin Cancer Res 25(7):2021–2023. https://doi.org/10.1158/1078-0432.CCR-18-3778
15. Ayers M, Lunceford J, Nebozhyn M, Murphy E, Loboda A, Kaufman DR et al (2017) IFN-gamma-related mRNA profile predicts clinical response to PD-1 blockade. J Clin Invest 127(8):2930–2940. https://doi.org/10.1172/JCI91190
16. Haber PK, Puigvehi M, Castet F, Lourdusamy V, Montal R, Tabrizian P et al (2021) Evidence-based management of HCC: systematic review and meta-analysis of randomized controlled trials (2002–2020). Gastroenterology. https://doi.org/10.1053/j.gastro.2021.06.008
17. Pfister D, Nunez NG, Pinyol R, Govaere O, Pinter M, Szydlowska M et al (2021) NASH limits anti-tumour surveillance in immunotherapy-treated HCC. Nature 592(7854):450–456. https://doi.org/10.1038/s41586-021-03362-0
18. Llovet JM, El-Khoueiry AB, Vogel A, Madoff DC, Finn RS, Ogasawara S et al (2020) 1016TiP LEAP-012 trial in progress: Pembrolizumab plus lenvatinib and transarterial chemoembolization (TACE) in patients with intermediate-stage hepatocellular carcinoma (HCC) not amenable to curative treatment. Ann Oncol 31:S702–S7S3. https://doi.org/10.1016/j.annonc.2020.08.1132
19. Exposito MJ, Akce M, Alvarez J, Assenat E, Balart L, Baron A et al (2019) Abstract No. 526 CheckMate-9DX: phase 3, randomized, double-blind study of adjuvant nivolumab vs placebo for patients with hepatocellular carcinoma (HCC) at high risk of recurrence after curative resection or ablation. J Vasc Interv Radiol 30(3):S227–S2S8. https://doi.org/10.1016/j.jvir.2018.12.607
20. Zhu A, Kudo M, Vogel A, Yau T, Zhou J, Kim E et al (2020) Abstract CT284: Phase 3 KEYNOTE-937: adjuvant pembrolizumab versus placebo in patients with hepatocellular carcinoma and complete radiologic response after surgical resection or local ablation. Cancer Res 80(Suppl. 16):CT284. https://doi.org/10.1158/1538-7445.Am2020-ct284
21. Hack SP, Spahn J, Chen M, Cheng AL, Kaseb A, Kudo M et al (2020) IMbrave 050: a Phase III trial of atezolizumab plus bevacizumab in high-risk hepatocellular carcinoma after curative resection or ablation. Future Oncol 16(15):975–989. https://doi.org/10.2217/fon-2020-0162
22. Knox J, Cheng A, Cleary S, Galle P, Kokudo N, Lencioni R et al (2019) A phase 3 study of durvalumab with or without bevacizumab as adjuvant therapy in patients with hepatocellular carcinoma at high risk of recurrence after curative hepatic resection or ablation: EMERALD-2. Ann Oncol 30:iv59–iv60. https://doi.org/10.1093/annonc/mdz155.216
23. Moehler M, Heo J, Lee HC, Tak WY, Chao Y, Paik SW et al (2019) Vaccinia-based oncolytic immunotherapy Pexastimogene Devacirepvec in patients with advanced hepatocellular carcinoma after sorafenib failure: a randomized multicenter Phase IIb trial (TRAVERSE). Onco Targets Ther 8(8):1615817. https://doi.org/10.1080/2162402X.2019.1615817
24. Ghassan KA-A, Peter RG, Yee C, Karen TB, Jeong H, Mitesh JB et al (2016) PHOCUS: A phase 3 randomized, open-label study comparing the oncolytic immunotherapy Pexa-Vec followed by sorafenib (SOR) vs SOR in patients with advanced hepatocellular carcinoma (HCC) without prior systemic therapy. J Clin Oncol 34(Suppl. 15):TPS4146. https://doi.org/10.1200/JCO.2016.34.15_suppl.TPS4146%U

Part VI

Biliary Tract

Immunotherapy of Biliary Tract Cancer

Joachim C. Mertens and Ralph Fritsch

Contents

Abstract

The immune landscape in CCA has become a mayor focus of interest as new targeted therapies are becoming an important component of CCA treatment. Distict immune cell population such as TAMS, TANS and MDSC have been identified in the CCA microenvironment and tumor promoting effects have been

J. C. Mertens (✉)
Digestive Diseases Institute, GastroZentrum Hirslanden, Zürich, Switzerland
e-mail: Joachim.Mertens@gastrozentrum.ch

R. Fritsch
Universtity Hospital Zurich, Zürich, Switzerland

Cancer Immunotherapy (2023)
https://doi.org/10.1007/13905_2022_35,
Published Online: 11 July 2023

described. Recent trials have shown very promising results for immune targeted therapies in combination with current standard of care, improving response rates and overall survival. This chapter will give an overview of current knowledge on the immune environment as well as evolving immune targeted therapies.

Keywords
CTL4 · dMMR · FGFR2 · HRD · IDH · Immune Landscape · Immunotherapy Microenvironment · Molecular Subgroups · PD1 · PDL1 · T-cell therapies

1 Biliary Tract Cancer

Cholangiocarcinoma (CCA) is a highly desmoplastic cancer that contains large amounts of extracellular matrix and nonmalignant cells besides the actual cancer cells. As many solid tumors, CCA can indeed be seen as a complex tissue composed of cancer cells and nonmalignant stroma cells in their ECM [1, 2]. Besides mesenchymal fibroblastic cells, the tumor microenvironment contains an abundance of infiltrating immune cells, such as tumor-associated macrophages, lymphocytes, and neutrophils. It has become clear that this tumor-reactive stroma and the contained immune cell populations play an important and potentially tumor-promoting role. CCA often develops as a complication of chronic inflammatory conditions and has for decades been described as a "stroma-rich" tumor, with a characteristic and extensive microenvironment surrounding small clusters of cancer cells.

2 Microenvironment and Immune Landscape in Biliary Tract Cancer

To evade immune surveillance and circumvent killing by cytotoxic lymphocytes, malignant cells alter their environment in an immunosuppressive way to become more immunologically tolerant. Cancer cells are in close cell-cell interaction with tumor-infiltrating immune cells from the innate and adaptive immune system, resulting in immunosuppression and eventually tumor progression. The proposed role of different immune cell populations in CCA is summarized in Table 1.

Table 1 Immune cells in cholangiocarcinoma and their proposed role

Immune cell type	Role in cholangiocarcinoma
TAMs	• Stimulation of angiogenesis by VEGF secretion • Immunosuppressive IL-10 secretion and T cell suppression • ECM remodeling by MPP9 secretion
TANs	• Recruitment of immunoregulatory and -suppressive cells
MDSCs	• Immunosuppressive regulation of other immune cells such as inhibition of T and NK cells
DCs	• Possible inhibition of tumor growth via recruitment and activation of lymphocytes
NKs	• Tumor cell cytotoxicity
TILs	• Tumor cell inhibition

2.1 Cell Populations of the Innate Immune Response

Tumor-associated macrophages (TAMs) are pro-tumorigenic M2-like macrophages that become alternatively activated and exert immunosuppressive effects by ECM remodeling, promotion of angiogenesis, and inhibition of T cell proliferation and activity. M2 macrophages are recruited into the tumor microenvironment mainly by monocyte chemoattractant protein 1 (MCP1), also named CCL2 [3]. In CCA, the number of M2-like phenotype TAM has been reported to correspond with poor prognosis and metastasis [4]. TAMs produce a number of signaling molecules with potentially tumor-promoting effects such as angiogenesis (VEGFA), ECM remodeling (TGF-β, MMP9), antigen presentation, and immunomodulation (IL-10) [5]. TAMs were demonstrated to be the main producer of MMP9 in CCA, and the number of MMP9-secreting TAMs has been significantly correlated with patient survival [6].

Tumor-associated neutrophils (TANs) are attracted into the CCA microenvironment mainly by CXCL5, a chemoattractant derived from stromal cells of the TME as well as cancer cells [7]. TANs themselves express CCL2 and CCL17. These molecules in turn recruit further immune cells such as TAMs and Tregs to the TME. As for previously discussed cell types, the number of TANs in CCA has been associated with poor prognosis [8].

Myeloid-derived suppressor cells (MDSCs), a subtype of immature myeloid cells, exhibit a potent immunosuppressive effect [9]. The exact definition of MDSC is still subject to discussion, as they are closely related to neutrophils and might even represent a specialized subtype of neutrophil lymphocytes [10]. Given their strong immunosuppressive activities, MDSCs regulate the function of other immune cells and can be found in increased numbers in the cancer TME. MDSC can inhibit cytotoxic T cells and NK cells in an antigen-independent as well as -dependent manner. MDSC recruitment via CCL2/MCP1 secretion in CCA results in immunosuppression and tumor-promoting inflammatory activity [11]. Still, the role of MDSC in CCA development and progression is widely unknown, and further studies are needed.

Dendritic cells (DCs) represent a heterogeneous group of specialized antigen-presenting cells, with the unique capability to initiate the adaptive immune response. This initiation of the innate immune system, namely naïve T cells, is achieved by presentation of immunogenetic peptides on antigen-presenting major histocompatibility complex (MHC) class I and II molecules [12]. Through this mechanism, the cellular immune response induced by DC involves CD4+ T helper as well as cytolytic CD8+ T cells.

In the TME, DCs downregulate their MHC class II molecules in a TGF-b-dependent manner, reducing their capability to activate cytotoxic T cells [13]. In CCA, the number of mature DCs along the invasive margin has been shown to correlate significantly with the number of CD8-positive or CD4-positive T cells within the tumor, supporting their presumed role in increasing CD8- and CD4-positive cell infiltration into cancers [14]. Moreover, increased numbers of mature DCs have been correlated with reduced incidence of lymph node metastasis and better overall outcome in CCA patients [14]. Aspartate-β-hydroxylase is a highly expressed tumor-associated cell surface protein. Therapeutic DCs loaded with this particular antigen have been reported to induce antigen-specific immunity and cytotoxic activity against tumor cells and inhibit tumor growth in a syngeneic rat model of CCA [15].

Besides the aforementioned immune cells, the liver contains large numbers of *natural killer* (NK) cells, important regulators of immune tolerance [16]. Genetic variants of NKG2D, an NK cell receptor, have been associated with the development of CCA in PSC patients [17]. In vitro studies, cultivating CCA cells with cytokine-activated killer cells (acNK and T cells) combined with cetuximab, have been shown to enhance cytotoxic effects [18]. Furthermore, infusion of ex vivo-expanded human NK cells into nude mice bearing experimental HuCCT-1 CCAs did result in significant inhibition of tumor growth [19].

2.2 Components of the Adaptive Immune Response

Tumor-infiltrating lymphocytes (TILs) are a diverse group of immune cells that are recruited into the TME from the bloodstream with the potential to directly eliminate cancer cells. This group includes CD8+ cytotoxic T cells, CD4+ T helper cells, Foxp3+ regulatory T cells, and B lymphocytes.

Patients suffering from biliary tract cancers that contained higher numbers of tumor-infiltrating CD4+, CD8+, and FoxP3+ T lymphocytes had a significantly better overall survival [20]. While these cells of the adaptive immune response decrease in number as CCAs progress, over 50% of CCAs remain positive for CD4+ and CD8+ TILs [20], with the number of TILs positively associated with improved overall patient survival [21, 22]. Within the tumor tissue, different TILs are differentially distributed. CD8+ TILs are located predominantly within the tumor node, while CD4+ TILs are found more frequently in the peritumoral area [23].

FoxP3-positive regulatory T cells have been described to promote antigen tolerance and immunosuppression in various malignancies. In CCA, FoxP3 expression has been correlated with worse prognosis [24].

Adoptive T cell cancer therapy as an approach to increase the number of activated cytotoxic T lymphocytes within the TME is being investigated in clinical trials and also in biliary tract cancers [25].

Finally, while B cells only represent a minor proportion of TILs in CCA, their presence has been associated with a more favorable prognosis [20].

3 Molecular Subgroups of Biliary Tract Carcinoma in the Context of Immunotherapy

3.1 Targetable Molecular Alterations in Biliary Tract Carcinoma

Biliary tract carcinomas (BTCs) represent a clinically and genetically heterogeneous group of malignancies arising from the biliary epithelium. All four anatomical subgroups of BTCs (intrahepatic, iCC; perihilar, pCC; distal extrahepatic, eCC; gallbladder, GBC) in principle show overlapping genetic features; however, the prevalence of individual molecular alterations varies significantly between these groups (Fig. 1, modified from [26]). iCCs show the highest abundance of targetable genetic alterations, while hitherto undruggable driver alterations are more common in pCC/eCC and GBC. For precision treatment, the currently most relevant alterations in BTCs are fibroblast growth factor receptor 2 (*FGFR*2) alterations (oncogenic fusions and mutations), as well as isocitrate dehydrogenase 1 (*IDH1*) mutations, for both of which targeted agents have been approved based on pivotal phase II and III trial evidence [27]. Moreover, several smaller molecular subgroups of BTC including tumors harboring BRAF-V600E, *ERBB2(HER2)* amplifications, or mutations or mismatch repair deficiency (dMMR) are therapeutically highly relevant. eCC/pCCs more frequently harbor non-targetable alterations, including mutated *KRAS* (30–45%) and *TP53* (30–50%) [28]. Gallbladder cancers relatively frequently harbor *HER2* amplifications or HER2/HER3 mutation amplifications as potentially molecularly targetable alterations [29] (Fig. 1).

Whether certain molecular alterations or different anatomical locations of BTC are associated with distinct immune profiles and different sensitivities towards immunotherapeutic agents remains currently under investigation [30–32]. A large body of preclinical and translational data points to a link between defined molecular alterations and immune biomarkers including PD-L1 expression [33], immune cell infiltrate [20, 34], and tumor mutational burden (TMB) [35, 36]. Consequently, several clinical trials are currently studying the effect of anti-PD1/PD-L1 checkpoint inhibitors (CPIs) in combination with molecularly targeted agents in specific molecular subgroups including tumors with FGFR2 fusions and rearrangements (ADVANCE phase 2 trial, EudraCT 2020–004938-38) and in tumors with homologous recombination deficiency (HRD) (NCT04298021, NCT04306367, NCT03991832, NCT03639935) [35]. Of note, immunotherapy is now the standard of care for BTCs with mismatch repair deficiency (dMMR), based on their highly immunogenic phenotype and exquisite response to anti-PD1 immune checkpoint inhibitors (CPIs) [37].

3.2 *FGFR2* Alterations

Up to 20% of ICCs harbor oncogenic *FGFR* alterations, most commonly oncogenic fusions [38], but also activating mutations or gene amplifications [39, 40]. Aberrations in FGFR signaling promote tumor cell survival, proliferation, and invasion in BTC [41]. Tumors exhibiting *FGFR2* fusions show high response rates to selective FGFR inhibitors such as erdafitinib, pemigatinib, and infigratinib [42–46]. In a recently published phase II trial (FIGHT-202), pemigatinib led to an objective response rate of 35.5% in patients with pretreated advanced FGFR2 rearrangement-positive BTCs. Both pemigatinib and more recently infigratinib obtained FDA approval for pretreated BTCs with *FGFR2* fusions or rearrangements. Both agents are moreover being compared to first-line chemotherapy with cisplatin and gemcitabine in ongoing phase III (NCT03656536, NCT03773302) [47]. The immune

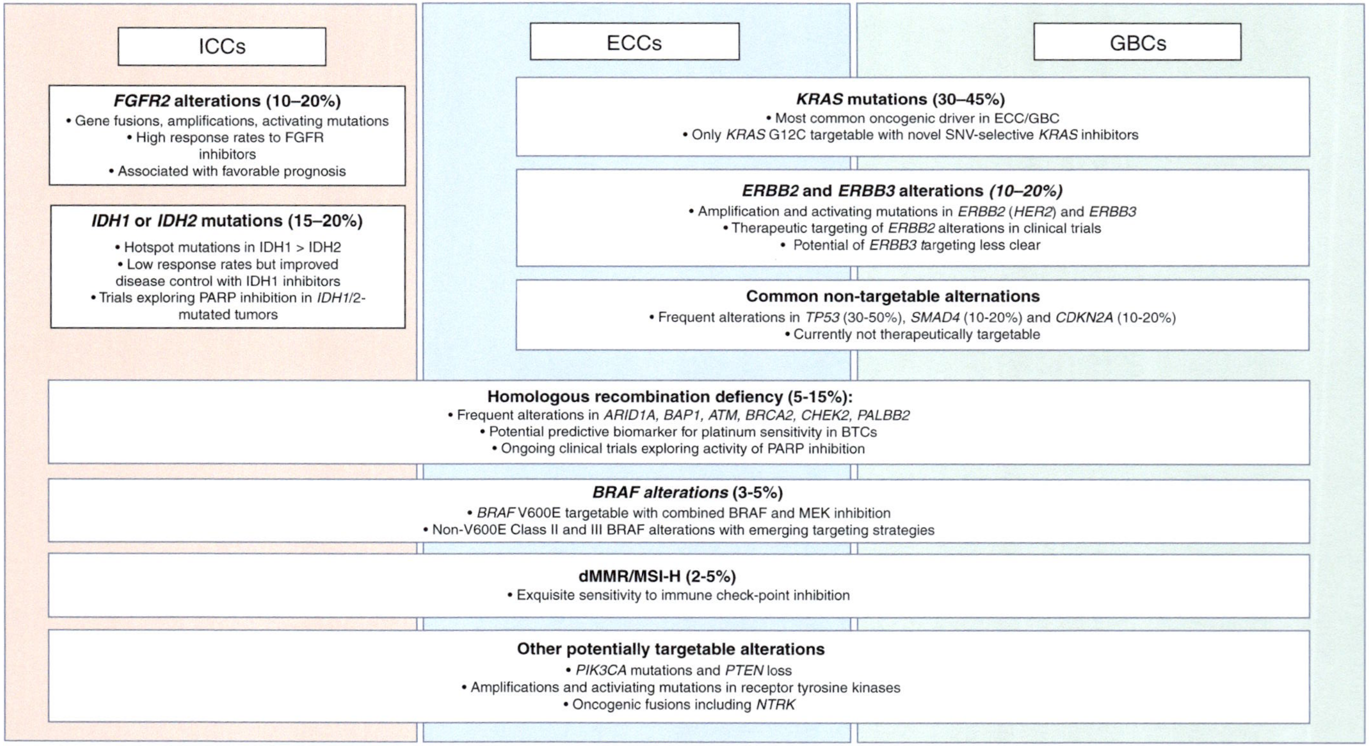

Fig. 1 Genomic alterations in biliary tract carcinomas. Prevalence of targetable genetic alterations varies significantly between iCCs, eCCs, and GBCs, with the highest frequency of *FGFR2* and *IDH1/IDH2* alterations found in iCCs. *dMMR/MSI-H* mismatch repair-deficient/microsatellite instability-high, *eCCs* extrahepatic cholangiocarcinomas (including perihilar), *GBCs* gallbladder cancers, *HRD* homologous recombination deficiency, *iCCs* intrahepatic cholangiocarcinomas, *SNV* single nucleotide variant. (Figure modified from [26])

landscape of FGFR2-driven BTCs has been studied in more detail recently, demonstrating a positive association between inhibition of FGFR signaling and increased T cell infiltration in FGFR-driven BTCs [32]. The combination of pemigatinib and pembrolizumab has been assessed in a phase II study in refractory solid cancers including a cohort of FGFR-altered tumors [48]. Ongoing trials are exploring the potential of combining FGFR inhibitors with anti-PD1 CPIs (EudraCT 2020–004938-38).

3.3 IDH1/IDH2 Mutations

IDH1 alterations are found in up to 20% of ICCs [49–52]. *IDH1/2* hotspot mutations are neomorphic, leading to accumulation of D-2-hydroxyglutarate, an oncogenic metabolite causing epigenetic changes and cellular dedifferentiation [53]. The selective IDH1 inhibitor ivosidenib showed significant improvement in PFS in a phase III study as compared to placebo in pretreated *IDH1*-mutated advanced BTCs and has been recently FDA approved for this indication [54, 55]. Enasidenib (AG-221) is a selective IDH2 inhibitor, currently being evaluated for BTCs harboring IDH2 hotspot mutations [56]. Characteristically, disease stabilization is the predominant outcome of treatment with IDH inhibitor in ICCs, with very low objective response rates. The connection between IDH1 or IDH2 mutations and immunogenicity is not well established. However, increasing evidence suggests that IDH1/2 alterations can induce a state of functional homologous recombination deficiency (HRD), also termed functional BRCAness [57, 58]. BTCs with HRD however appear vulnerable to combined inhibition of PARP and immune checkpoint blockade [33, 59], a hypothesis currently evaluated in at least two ongoing clinical trials (NCT03991832, NCT03878095).

3.4 Homologous Recombination Deficiency (HRD)

Five to fifteen percent of BTCs harbor defects within the DNA homologous recombination repair (HRR) pathway, leading to homologous recombination repair deficiency (HRD). Most frequent molecular alterations leading to HRD in BTCs are *ARID1A*, *BAP1*, *ATM*, *BRCA2*, *CHEK2*, and *PALB2* genes [60]. In general, tumors exhibiting HRD show high sensitivity to platinum chemotherapeutic agents and vulnerability to PARP inhibitors. Consequently, several trials study the potential of PARP inhibition in HRD-BTCs [61]. Notably, tumors with HRD have also appeared to be more immunogenic than tumor with intact HRR [62], and combining PARP inhibitor with CPIs has shown promise in a number of early-phase clinical trials for breast, ovarian, and prostate cancers, with many ongoing trials further exploring potential synergy between PARP and CPIs in solid tumors [63] including trials for advanced BTC (NCT03639935).

3.5 Mismatch Repair Deficiency (dMMR/MSI-H)

Roughly 2–4% of iCCs, and up to 5% of GBCs and eCCs, show mismatch repair deficiency/high microsatellite instability (dMMR/MSI-H) and are therefore highly responsive to CPIs [37, 64]. Within the landmark KEYNOTE-158 trial, dMMR/MSI-H cohort, 22 patients with mismatch repair-deficient BTCs were treated with pembrolizumab after failure of prior therapy, reaching an impressive ORR of 40.9% and a median OS of 24.3 months [31]. Immunotherapy with pembrolizumab is the standard of care for pretreated dMMR/MSI-H BTCs and approved by the FDA (site/tissue agnostic approval for pembrolizumab for pretreated cMMR/MSI-H tumors).

3.6 Other Targetable Molecular Subgroups of BTC

Three to five percent of BTCs, mainly iCCs, harbor *BRAF* alterations, most commonly the BRAF-V600E mutation, leading to high objective response rates to synergistic BRAF and MEK inhibition [65]. Moreover, a relevant subset of BTCs harbor alterations in *HER2* or *HER3* receptor tyrosine kinases. Targeting strategies *HER2*-amplified BTCs are emerging [26, 66], while the role of *HER2* and *HER3* mutations as therapeutic targets in BTC is currently less clear. The impact of BRAF mutations or HER2/HER3 alterations on immunogenicity and response to immunotherapy in BTC has not been fully elucidated. However, the impact of BRAF-V600E on immunotherapy responses has been studied extensively for melanoma [67] (no clear impact) and colorectal cancer (CRC). In a subset of CRCs, BRAF-V600E induced acquired dMMR/MSI-H status [68], an association less well studied for BTCs. For HER2-positive gastric cancer, strong synergy appears to emerge for anti-HER2 and anti-PD1 therapy [69], a feature yet to be explored for HER2-positive BTCs.

4 Immunotherapy for BTCs: Reported Clinical Outcomes

4.1 Anti-PD1/PD-L1 Immune Checkpoint Inhibitor Monotherapy

The efficacy of anti-PD1/PD-L1 CPI monotherapy for pretreated BTCs has been evaluated in several phase I and phase II trails (Table 2).

Twenty-three patients with BTC were evaluated in the phase I KEYNOTE-028 trial, assessing safety and efficacy of pembrolizumab in refractory solid tumors with a PD-L1 tumor cell expression of >1% (Table 2). 13% of the included BTC patients showed an objective tumor response, with a global disease control rate (DCR) of 26% [70]. The phase II KEYNOTE-158 trial assessed the activity of pembrolizumab in distinct cohorts of solid tumors, including 104 patients with BTCs. ORRs for BTCs reported by this trial were 5.8% and DCR 22.1%. Median PFS and OS for BTCs were 2 and 7.4 months, respectively [70, 71]. Notably, median duration of

Table 2 Anti-PD-1/PD-L1 alone or in combination with anti-CTLA-4

Study	Phase	*n*	Treatment line	Anti-PD-1/PD-L1	Anti-CTLA4	ORR (%)	mPFS (m)	mOS (m)
NCT02054806 (KEYNOTE-028)	1	23	2 or >	Pembrolizumab	–	13	1.8	5.7
NCT02628067 (KEYNOTE-158)	2	104	2 or >	Pembrolizumab	–	5.8	2.0	7.4
NCT02829918	2	54	2 or >	Nivolumab	–	11	4.0	14.2
NCT02923934 (CA209-538)	2	39	2 or >	Nivolumab	Ipilimumab	24	2.9	5.7
NCT01938612	1	42	2 or >	Durvalumab		4.7	1.5	8.1
NCT01938612	1	65	2 or >	Durvalumab	Tremelimumab	10.7	1.6	10.1

Abbreviations: *n* number of evaluated patients, *ORR* objective response rate, *m* months, *mOS* median overall survival, *mPFS* median progression-free survival response (DR) was not reached in either trial, indicating that, despite overall low response rates, some responders achieved long-term disease control. The subgroup of patients with high TMB (defined as ≥10 mutations/megabase) exhibited a global ORR of 29%, as compared to 6% in the cohort with a TMB of less than 10 [72]. Post hoc analysis of the trial showed positive correlation of tumor responses with high levels of tumor mutational burden (TMB) and inflammatory markers such as PD-L1 CPS or T cell inflamed gene expression profile (GEP) [70, 73].

Nivolumab monotherapy was assessed in a phase II trial including 54 patients with refractory BTCs. The ORR, primary endpoint of the study, was 11% assessed by an independent review, and the DCR was 50%. Median PFS and OS were 3.68 and 14.24 months, respectively [74].

4.2 Anti-PD1/PD-L1 Plus Anti-CTLA-4 Combination Regimens

Combinations of anti-PD1/PD-L1 and anti-CTLA-4 CPIs have been evaluated in a few reported phase I and phase II trials (Table 3).

The phase II study CA 209-538 evaluated the combination of nivolumab and ipilimumab in refractory rare cancers including 39 patients with advanced pretreated BTCs (Table 3). The treatment schedule consisted of the anti-PD-1 antibody nivolumab 3 mg/kg and the anti-CTLA-4 antibody ipilimumab 1 mg/kg administered every 3 weeks for four cycles followed by nivolumab monotherapy 3 mg/kg every 2 weeks. The ORR in the biliary cohort was 24%, with a DCR of 45%. At time point of data analysis, the median response duration was not reached, the median PFS was 2.9, and OS was 5.7 months. Interestingly, all the responders had MSI-stable tumors [75].

A phase I study evaluated anti-PD-L1 antibody durvalumab alone or in combination with anti-CTLA-4 antibody tremelimumab for pretreated BTC in Asia [76]. Reported response rates were 2/42 and 5/65 for durvalumab and durvalumab plus tremelimumab, respectively, with DCRs of 16.7% and 32.2%. Tumor microsatellite status and other biomarkers have not been reported.

Taken together, anti-PD1/PD-L1 monotherapy in an unselected patient population induced overall low response rates in BTC, with some correlation with biomarkers TMB and PD-L1 suggested in post hoc analyses. Nivolumab plus ipilimumab showed somewhat more encouraging response rates at the expense of—by cross comparison—higher toxicity compared to anti-PD1/PD-L1 monotherapy.

4.3 Immune Checkpoint Inhibitors in Combination with Chemotherapy

Treatment standard for unresectable and metastatic BTCs is first-line chemotherapy with gemcitabine and cisplatin based on the pivotal ABC02 trial [77]. Several smaller trials have therefore evaluated the safety and feasibility of combining standard chemotherapy with immunotherapeutic agents (Table 2), with several larger trials currently ongoing.

Table 3 Combination treatment anti-PD1/PD-L1/CTLA4 with chemotherapy

Study	Phase	*n*	Treatment line	CPIs	Chemotherapy	ORR (%)	mPFS (m)	mOS (m)
JapiCCTI-153098	1	39	1	Nivolumab	Cisplatin/gemcitabine	36.7	4.2	15.4
NCT03796429	2	50	1	Toripalimab	Cisplatin/S1	27.1	7.0	16.0
NCT03046862	1	45	1	Durvalumab	Cisplatin/gemcitabine	73.4	11.0	18.1
NCT03046862	1	46	1	Durvalumab + tremelimumab	Cisplatin/gemcitabine	73.3	11.9	20.7

Abbreviations: *n* number of evaluated patients, *CPIs* immune checkpoint inhibitors, *ORR* objective response rate, *m* months, *mOS* median overall survival, *mPFS* median progression-free survival

The combination of nivolumab with the ABC02 regimen was assessed in a phase I study in Japan. Thirty patients received the triple combination without unexpected toxicity. ORR was 36.7%, median PFS and OS were 4.2 and 15.4 months, respectively [78].

The anti-PD-1 antibody toripalimab, combined with first-line cisplatin plus the oral fluoropyrimidine S1, was assessed in a monocentric phase II study conducted in China. Reported ORR was 27.1%, PFS 7.0 months, and OS 16.0 months [79, 80].

A Korean phase II study evaluated the triple and quadruple combinations of gemcitabine, cisplatin, and durvalumab, with or without tremelimumab, reporting an impressive ORR of approximately 73% and nearly 100% DCR for either arm. Median PFS and OS were 11.0 and 18.1 months for the triple and 11.9 and 20.7 months for the quadruple combination [81]. A separate biomarker cohort receiving the quadruple combination showed no clear correlation between survival endpoints and pretreatment PD-L1 status, TMB, or other biomarkers.

The results of the recent Topaz-1 trial provide further support for the strategy of combining standard-of-care chemotherapy with checkpoint inhibitors. The study enrolled almost 700 patients that were assigned 1:1 to Gem/Cis plus placebo or Gem/Cis plus durvalumab. With a HR for overall survival of 0.8 and an estimated OS rate of 25% at 24 months, the durvalumab treatment group had a significantly better outcome than the placebo group with an estimated 24-month OS of 10%. Accordingly, the progression-free survival HR was 0.75 for the durvalumab group and ORR 27% versus 19%. There was no difference in the safety profile of the two treatment arms [82].

Taken together, combining CPIs with chemotherapy for the first-line treatment of advanced BTCs is likely to become the mainstay of therapy given the convincing results of the Topaz-1 trial, the first successful trial of a CPI-containing regime in CCA.

4.4 Anti-PD1/PD-L1 Immune Checkpoint Inhibitors in Combination with Small-Molecule Inhibitors

Synergies between anti-PD1/PD-L1 CPIs and molecularly targeted agents have been emerging from preclinical work as well as clinical trials, most prominently for anti-VEGF/VEGFR targeting agents [83], leading to several FDA approvals for hepatocellular carcinoma [84] and other tumor entities [85].

For BTC, the combination of several anti-VEGF targeting small tyrosine kinase inhibitors is currently under clinical investigation with encouraging reported results (Table 4).

The combination of multi-tyrosine kinase inhibitor lenvatinib (12 mg/day) and pembrolizumab (200 mg every 3 weeks) was first evaluated for pretreated BTC in a Chinese investigator-initiated phase II study [86], reporting an ORR of 25%, with a DCR of 78.1%. 59.3% of patients exhibited grade 3 AEs, most frequently fatigue, hypertension, and increased aminotransferase levels [86].

Table 4 Combination treatment anti-PD1/PD-L1 with small-molecule inhibitors

Study	Phase	*n*	Treatment line	CPIs	Small molecule	ORR (%)	mPFS (m)	mOS (m)
NCT03895970	2	32	>1	Pembrolizumab	Lenvatinib	25	4.9	11.0
NCT03797326 (LEAP-005)	2	31	2	Pembrolizumab	Lenvatinib	10	6.1	8.6
NCT034759539 (REGOMUNE)	1/2	29	>1	Avelumab	Regorafenib	13.8	2.5	11.9
NCT03201458	2	38	2/3	Atezolizumab	Cobimetinib	3.2	3.7	–

Abbreviations: *n* number of evaluated patients, *CPIs* immune checkpoint inhibitors, *ORR* objective response rate, *m* months, *mOS* median overall survival, *mPFS* median progression-free survival

Lenvatinib plus pembrolizumab is currently also evaluated in the international phase II multi-cohort LEAP005 study. In this trial, pembrolizumab is given at 200 mg every 3 weeks and lenvatinib at 20 mg/day in patients with advanced BTCs who have progressed after one previous treatment line. The preliminary analysis at a median follow-up of 9.5 months revealed an ORR of 10%, with further 58% of patients remaining in stable disease (SD). The median PFS and OS of the cohort were 6.1 (95% CI, 2.1–6.4) and 8.6 (95% CI, 5.6 to NR) months, respectively [87].

The phase I/II REGOMUNE trial studied the combination of multi-kinase inhibitor regorafenib and anti-PD-L1 antibody avelumab. Thirty-four patients were enrolled with pretreated BTCs. Twenty-nine patients underwent at least one radiographic assessment, with partial response (PR) and SD in 4 (13.8%) and 11 (37.9%) patients, respectively. Median PFS was 2.5 months and median OS 11.9. Dose adjustments or treatment interruptions due to AEs were performed in 85.3% of patients [88].

A small randomized phase II study compared the combination of the anti-PD-L1 antibody atezolizumab plus the MEK inhibitor cobimetinib to the monotherapy with atezolizumab in BTCs progressing during or after previous treatment. The median PFS was 3.65 months for the combination and 1.87 months for the monotherapy ($p = 0.027$); ORR for the combination arm was 3.2% [89].

In summary, combining small-molecule kinase inhibitors, in particular the VEGFR-targeting agents lenvatinib and regorafenib, with anti-PD1/PD-L1 CPIs has shown some potential for treating advanced BTCs. Further trial results and biomarker analyses are pending.

4.5 Novel Immunotherapeutic Agents Evaluated for BTCs

Bintrafusp alpha (M7824) is a bifunctional fusion protein containing the extracellular domain of TGF-β receptor II, aimed to trap TGF-β, linked to the heavy chains of an anti-PD-L1 antibody [90]. The drug safety and activity were assessed in pretreated patients with BTCs in a phase I study, showing an ORR of 20%, with a PFS of 2.5 and OS of 12.7 months at data analysis. Grade 3 adverse events (AEs) presented in 37% of patients, with 3 out of 30 patients experiencing grade 5 AEs [91]. A phase II trial is assessing the compound in patients with pretreated BTCs in monotherapy (NCT03833661), and a phase II/III trial in combination with cisplatin-gemcitabine as first-line treatment (NCT04066491).

4.6 T Cell Therapies, Tumor Vaccines, and Oncolytic Viruses

Cellular immunotherapies for BTC are still in early, mainly preclinical, stages of development. However, a very few first results of clinical studies have been reported.

A phase II study assessing the antitumor activity of infused autologous tumor-infiltrating lymphocytes, combined with high-dose IL-2 (aldesleukin) in pretreated BTCs, is currently ongoing (NCT03801083). In a previously published cohort, 36 patients with intrahepatic cholangiocarcinoma were postoperatively treated with autologous tumor lysate pulsed dendritic cells, as well as activated T cells. The outcome results were compared to an exclusively resected cohort of 26 patients, with PFS of 18.3 vs. 7.7 months ($p = 0.005$) and OS of 31.9 vs. 17.4 months ($p = 0.022$) [25, 92].

Safety and antitumor activity of chimeric antigen receptor (CAR) T cells have been assessed in nine patients with advanced Her2-positive BTCs in a phase I study. The conditioning was performed employing nab-paclitaxel and cyclophosphamide. The median PFS of the entire cohort, which also included two patients with pancreatic adenocarcinoma, was of 4.5 months [93].

Another CAR T phase I trial enrolled 19 patients with EGFR-positive refractory BTCs. One complete and 10 stable responses were observed, out of 17 radiographically assessed patients, with a median PFS of 4 months [94].

So far, little clinical success has been reported with tumor vaccines and oncolytic viruses across tumor entities with a few notable exceptions [95]. For BTC, a retrospective study reviewed a cohort of 65 refractory BTC patients treated with dendritic cells pulsed with WT1 and/or MUC1 tumor antigens. Median OS from DC immunotherapy treatment start was 7.2 months [96]. A phase I/II trial is assessing the safety and efficacy of LOAd703, an oncolytic adenovirus [97], in refractory solid tumors, including BTCs. Other oncolytic virus-base therapies are currently in preclinical development [98].

5 Summary and Outlook

The fundamental scientific and clinical advances of molecular oncology, along with the availability of many novel therapeutic agents, are rapidly changing the way we stratify and treat patients with advanced-stage BTCs. After decades of incremental advances, precision oncology is now driving long-awaited progress against these difficult-to-treat tumors.

Immunotherapeutic agents have been tested for BTCs in phase I and phase II trials yielding overall mixed results. CPIs are now the standard of care for dMMR/MSI-H BTCs. Moreover, a subset of BTCs with proficient mismatch repair (pMMR, MSS) appear susceptible to CPIs and combinations of CPIs with molecular targeted agents.

Further trial results and biomarker analyses are required to better identify BTC patients with potential benefit from immunotherapy. Moreover, results from trials combining CPIs with standard-of-care first-line chemotherapy are eagerly awaited. While more data are pending, we encourage our colleagues to enroll BTC patients in clinical trials wherever possible.

Compliance with Ethical Standards

Funding No funding was received for this work.

Disclosure of interests All authors declare they have no conflict of interest.

Ethical approval This article does not contain any studies with human participants or animals performed by any of the authors.

References

1. Quail DF, Joyce JA (2013) Microenvironmental regulation of tumor progression and metastasis. Nat Med 19:1423–1437
2. Greaves M, Maley CC (2012) Clonal evolution in cancer. Nature 481:306–313
3. Zhang J, Chen L, Xiao M, Wang C, Qin Z (2011) FSP1+ fibroblasts promote skin carcinogenesis by maintaining MCP-1-mediated macrophage infiltration and chronic inflammation. Am J Pathol 178:382–390
4. Thanee M et al (2015) Quantitative changes in tumor-associated M2 macrophages characterize cholangiocarcinoma and their association with metastasis. Asian Pac J Cancer Prev 16:3043–3050
5. Hasita H et al (2010) Significance of alternatively activated macrophages in patients with intrahepatic cholangiocarcinoma. Cancer Sci 101:1913–1919
6. Subimerb C et al (2010) Tissue invasive macrophage density is correlated with prognosis in cholangiocarcinoma. Mol Med Rep 3:597–605
7. Zhou SL et al (2014) CXCL5 contributes to tumor metastasis and recurrence of intrahepatic cholangiocarcinoma by recruiting infiltrative intratumoral neutrophils. Carcinogenesis 35:597–605
8. Shen M et al (2014) Tumor-associated neutrophils as a new prognostic factor in cancer: a systematic review and meta-analysis. PLoS One 9:e98259
9. Gabrilovich DI (2017) Myeloid-derived suppressor cells. Cancer Immunol Res 5:3–8
10. Shaul ME, Fridlender ZG (2019) Tumour-associated neutrophils in patients with cancer. Nat Rev Clin Oncol 16:601–620
11. Yang X et al (2016) FAP promotes immunosuppression by cancer-associated fibroblasts in the tumor microenvironment via STAT3-CCL2 signaling. Cancer Res 76:4124–4135
12. Patente TA et al (2018) Human dendritic cells: their heterogeneity and clinical application potential in cancer immunotherapy. Front Immunol 9:3176
13. Flavell RA, Sanjabi S, Wrzesinski SH, Licona-Limon P (2010) The polarization of immune cells in the tumour environment by TGFbeta. Nat Rev Immunol 10:554–567
14. Takagi S et al (2004) Dendritic cells, T-cell infiltration, and Grp94 expression in cholangiocellular carcinoma. Hum Pathol 35:881–886
15. Noda T, Shimoda M, Ortiz V, Sirica AE, Wands JR (2012) Immunization with aspartate-beta-hydroxylase-loaded dendritic cells produces antitumor effects in a rat model of intrahepatic cholangiocarcinoma. Hepatology 55:86–97
16. Mikulak J, Bruni E, Oriolo F, Di Vito C, Mavilio D (2019) Hepatic natural killer cells: organ-specific sentinels of liver immune homeostasis and physiopathology. Front Immunol 10:946
17. Melum E et al (2008) Cholangiocarcinoma in primary sclerosing cholangitis is associated with NKG2D polymorphisms. Hepatology 47:90–96
18. Morisaki T et al (2012) Combining cetuximab with killer lymphocytes synergistically inhibits human cholangiocarcinoma cells in vitro. Anticancer Res 32:2249–2256
19. Jung IH et al (2018) In vivo study of natural killer (NK) cell cytotoxicity against cholangiocarcinoma in a nude mouse model. In Vivo 32:771–781
20. Goeppert B et al (2013) Prognostic impact of tumour-infiltrating immune cells on biliary tract cancer. Br J Cancer 109:2665–2674
21. Oshikiri T et al (2003) Prognostic value of intratumoral CD8+ T lymphocyte in extrahepatic bile duct carcinoma as essential immune response. J Surg Oncol 84:224–228
22. Lim YJ et al (2015) High ratio of programmed cell death protein 1 (PD-1)(+)/CD8(+) tumor-infiltrating lymphocytes identifies a poor prognostic subset of extrahepatic bile duct cancer undergoing surgery plus adjuvant chemoradiotherapy. Radiother Oncol 117:165–170

23. Kasper HU, Drebber U, Stippel DL, Dienes HP, Gillessen A (2009) Liver tumor infiltrating lymphocytes: comparison of hepatocellular and cholangiolar carcinoma. World J Gastroenterol 15:5053–5057
24. Dunne RF et al (2016) Association of FoxP3 expression with worse outcomes in cholangiocarcinoma: evidence to support the use of immunotherapy. J Clin Oncol 34:e15631
25. Blair AB, Murphy A (2018) Immunotherapy as a treatment for biliary tract cancers: a review of approaches with an eye to the future. Curr Probl Cancer 42:49–58
26. Koeberle D, Fritsch R (2021) Targeting HER2 in biliary tract carcinomas: challenges and opportunities. Oncol Res Treat 44:1–3
27. Abou-Alfa GK et al (2020) Pemigatinib for previously treated, locally advanced or metastatic cholangiocarcinoma: a multicentre, open-label, phase 2 study. Lancet Oncol 21:671–684
28. Lowery MA et al (2018) Comprehensive molecular profiling of intrahepatic and extrahepatic cholangiocarcinomas: potential targets for intervention. Clin Cancer Res 24:4154–4161
29. Valle JW, Lamarca A, Goyal L, Barriuso J, Zhu AX (2017) New horizons for precision medicine in biliary tract cancers. Cancer Discov 7:943–962
30. Weinberg BA et al (2019) Molecular profiling of biliary cancers reveals distinct molecular alterations and potential therapeutic targets. J Gastrointest Oncol 10:652–662
31. Fontugne J et al (2017) PD-L1 expression in perihilar and intrahepatic cholangiocarcinoma. Oncotarget 8:24644–24651
32. Palakurthi S et al (2019) The combined effect of FGFR inhibition and PD-1 blockade promotes tumor-intrinsic induction of antitumor. Immunity 7:1457–1471
33. Mody K et al (2019) Patterns and genomic correlates of PD-L1 expression in patients with biliary tract cancers. J Gastrointest Oncol 2019(10):1099–1109
34. Fabris L et al (2019) The tumour microenvironment and immune milieu of cholangiocarcinoma. Liver Int 39:63–78
35. Neureiter D, Mayr C, Kiesslich T (2021) The challenges of combinatory immunotherapy for biliary tract cancer. Expert Opin Investig Drugs 30:591–594
36. Zhang R et al (2021) Comprehensive analysis of genomic mutation signature and tumor mutation burden for prognosis of intrahepatic cholangiocarcinoma. BMC Cancer 21:112
37. Le DT et al (2015) PD-1 blockade in tumors with mismatch-repair deficiency. N Engl J Med 372:2509–2520
38. Jain A et al (2018) Cholangiocarcinoma with FGFR genetic aberrations: a unique clinical phenotype. JCO Precis Oncol 2:1–12
39. Wu YM et al (2013) Identification of targetable FGFR gene fusions in diverse cancers. Cancer Discov 3:636–647
40. Goyal L et al (2017) Polyclonal secondary FGFR2 mutations drive acquired resistance to FGFR inhibition in patients with FGFR2 fusion-positive cholangiocarcinoma. Cancer Discov 7:252–263
41. Dienstmann R et al (2014) Genomic aberrations in the FGFR pathway: opportunities for targeted therapies in solid tumors. Ann Oncol 25:552–563
42. Krook MA et al (2020) Efficacy of FGFR inhibitors and combination therapies for acquired resistance in FGFR2-fusion cholangiocarcinoma. Mol Cancer Ther 19(3):847–857
43. Mahipal A, Tella SH, Kommalapati A, Anaya D, Kim R (2019) FGFR2 genomic aberrations: Achilles heel in the management of advanced cholangiocarcinoma. Cancer Treat Rev 78:1–7
44. Bahleda R et al (2019) Multicenter phase I study of erdafitinib (JNJ-42756493), oral pan-fibroblast growth factor receptor inhibitor, in patients with advanced or refractory solid tumors. Clin Cancer Res 25:4888–4897
45. Javle M et al (2018) Phase II study of BGJ398 in patients with FGFR-altered advanced cholangiocarcinoma. J Clin Oncol 36:276–282
46. Javle MM et al (2021) A phase II study of infigratinib in previously treated advanced/metastatic cholangiocarcinoma with FGFR gene fusions/alterations. J Clin Oncol 39:TPS356
47. Javle MM et al (2019) Infigratinib versus gemcitabine plus cisplatin multicenter, open-label, randomized, phase 3 study in patients with advanced cholangiocarcinoma with FGFR2 gene fusions/translocations: the PROOF trial. J Clin Oncol 37:TPS4155

48. Gutierrez M et al (2020) Safety and efficacy of pemigatinib plus pembrolizumab combination therapy in patients (pts) with advanced malignancies: results from FIGHT-101, an open-label phase I/II study. J Clin Oncol 38:3606
49. Saha SK et al (2014) Mutant IDH inhibits HNF-4alpha to block hepatocyte differentiation and promote biliary cancer. Nature 513:110–114
50. Farshidfar F et al (2017) Integrative genomic analysis of cholangiocarcinoma identifies distinct IDH-mutant molecular profiles. Cell Rep 18:2780–2794
51. Goyal L et al (2015) Prognosis and clinicopathologic features of patients with advanced stage isocitrate dehydrogenase (IDH) mutant and IDH wild-type intrahepatic cholangiocarcinoma. Oncologist 20:1019–1027
52. Saha SK et al (2016) Isocitrate dehydrogenase mutations confer dasatinib hypersensitivity and SRC dependence in intrahepatic cholangiocarcinoma. Cancer Discov 6:727–739
53. Dang L, Yen K, Attar EC (2016) IDH mutations in cancer and progress toward development of targeted therapeutics. Ann Oncol 27:599–608
54. Lowery MA et al (2017) ClarIDHy: a phase 3, multicenter, randomized, double-blind study of AG-120 vs placebo in patients with an advanced cholangiocarcinoma with an IDH1 mutation. J Clin Oncol 35:TPS4142
55. Lowery MA et al (2019) Safety and activity of ivosidenib in patients with IDH1-mutant advanced cholangiocarcinoma: a phase 1 study. Lancet Gastroenterol Hepatol 4:711–720
56. Rizzo A, Ricci AD, Brandi G (2021) IDH inhibitors in advanced cholangiocarcinoma: another arrow in the quiver? Cancer Treat Res Commun 27:100356
57. IDH-mutant tumors vulnerable to PARP inhibition (2017) Cancer Discov 7(4):OF4
58. Wang Y et al (2020) Targeting therapeutic vulnerabilities with PARP inhibition and radiation in IDH-mutant gliomas and cholangiocarcinomas. Sci Adv 6:eaaz3221
59. Hsiehchen D et al (2020) DNA repair gene mutations as predictors of immune checkpoint inhibitor response beyond tumor mutation burden. Cell Rep Med 1(3):100034
60. Heeke AL et al (2018) Prevalence of homologous recombination-related gene mutations across multiple cancer types. JCO Precis Oncol 2018:PO.17.00286. https://doi.org/10.1200/PO.1217.00286
61. Ricci AD et al (2020) PARP inhibitors in biliary tract cancer: a new kid on the block? Medicines (Basel) 7(9):54
62. van Wilpe S et al (2021) Homologous recombination repair deficiency and implications for tumor immunogenicity. Cancers 13:2249
63. Vikas P, Borcherding N, Chennamadhavuni A, Garje R (2020) Therapeutic potential of combining PARP inhibitor and immunotherapy in solid tumors. Front Oncol 10:570
64. Marabelle A et al (2020) Efficacy of pembrolizumab in patients with noncolorectal high microsatellite instability/mismatch repair-deficient cancer: results from the phase II KEYNOTE-158 study. J Clin Oncol 38:1–10
65. Subbiah V et al (2020) Dabrafenib plus trametinib in patients with BRAF(V600E)-mutated biliary tract cancer (ROAR): a phase 2, open-label, single-arm, multicentre basket trial. Lancet Oncol 21:1234–1243
66. Yarlagadda B, Kamatham V, Ritter A, Shahjehan F, Kasi PM (2019) Trastuzumab and pertuzumab in circulating tumor DNA ERBB2-amplified HER2-positive refractory cholangiocarcinoma. NPJ Precis Oncol 3:19
67. Puzanov I et al (2020) Association of BRAF V600E/K mutation status and prior BRAF/MEK inhibition with pembrolizumab outcomes in advanced melanoma: pooled analysis of 3 clinical trials. JAMA Oncol 6:1256–1264
68. Seppälä TT et al (2015) Combination of microsatellite instability and BRAF mutation status for subtyping colorectal cancer. Br J Cancer 112:1966–1975
69. Janjigian YY et al (2021) Pembrolizumab plus trastuzumab and chemotherapy for HER2+ metastatic gastric or gastroesophageal junction (G/GEJ) cancer: initial findings of the global phase 3 KEYNOTE-811 study. J Clin Oncol 39:4013–4013
70. Piha-Paul SA et al (2020) Efficacy and safety of pembrolizumab for the treatment of advanced biliary cancer: results from the KEYNOTE-158 and KEYNOTE-028 studies. Int J Cancer 147:2190–2198

71. Marabelle A et al (2019) Efficacy of pembrolizumab in patients with noncolorectal high microsatellite instability/mismatch repair–deficient cancer: results from the phase II KEYNOTE-158 study. J Clin Oncol 38:1–10
72. Marabelle A et al (2020) Association of tumour mutational burden with outcomes in patients with advanced solid tumours treated with pembrolizumab: prospective biomarker analysis of the multicohort, open-label, phase 2 KEYNOTE-158 study. Lancet Oncol 21:1353–1365
73. Ott PA et al (2019) T-cell-inflamed gene-expression profile, programmed death ligand 1 expression, and tumor mutational burden predict efficacy in patients treated with pembrolizumab across 20 cancers: KEYNOTE-028. J Clin Oncol 37:318–327
74. Kim RD et al (2020) A phase 2 multi-institutional study of nivolumab for patients with advanced refractory biliary tract cancer. JAMA Oncol 6:888–894
75. Klein O et al (2020) Evaluation of combination nivolumab and ipilimumab immunotherapy in patients with advanced biliary tract cancers: subgroup analysis of a phase 2 nonrandomized clinical trial. JAMA Oncol 6:1405–1409
76. Ioka T et al (2019) Evaluation of safety and tolerability of durvalumab (D) with or without tremelimumab (T) in patients (pts) with biliary tract cancer (BTC). J Clin Oncol 37:387–387
77. Valle J et al (2010) Cisplatin plus gemcitabine versus gemcitabine for biliary tract cancer. N Engl J Med 362:1273–1281
78. Ueno M et al (2019) Nivolumab alone or in combination with cisplatin plus gemcitabine in Japanese patients with unresectable or recurrent biliary tract cancer: a non-randomised, multicentre, open-label, phase 1 study. Lancet Gastroenterol Hepatol 4:611–621
79. Liu T et al (2020) 53P Toripalimab with chemotherapy as first-line treatment for advanced biliary tract tumors: a preliminary analysis of safety and efficacy of an open-label phase II clinical study. Ann Oncol 31:S261
80. Li W et al (2021) Toripalimab with chemotherapy as first-line treatment for advanced biliary tract tumors: update analytic results of an open-label phase II clinical study (JS001-ZS-BC001). J Clin Oncol 39:e16170
81. Oh D-Y et al (2020) Phase II study assessing tolerability, efficacy, and biomarkers for durvalumab (D) ± tremelimumab (T) and gemcitabine/cisplatin (GemCis) in chemo-naïve advanced biliary tract cancer (aBTC). J Clin Oncol 38:4520
82. Oh D-Y, He A, Qin S, Chen L-T, Okusaka T, Kim JW, Suksombooncharoen T, Lee M, Kitano M, Burris H, Bouattour M, Tanasanvimon S, McNamara M, Zaucha R, Avallone A, Tan B, Cundom J, Lee C-k, Valle J (2022) Durvalumab plus gemcitabine and cisplatin in advanced biliary tract cancer. NEJM Evid. 1(8). https://doi.org/10.1056/EVIDoa2200015
83. Lee WS, Yang H, Chon HJ, Kim C (2020) Combination of anti-angiogenic therapy and immune checkpoint blockade normalizes vascular-immune crosstalk to potentiate cancer immunity. Exp Mol Med 52:1475–1485
84. Finn RS et al (2020) Atezolizumab plus bevacizumab in unresectable hepatocellular carcinoma. N Engl J Med 382:1894–1905
85. Socinski MA et al (2018) Atezolizumab for first-line treatment of metastatic nonsquamous NSCLC. N Engl J Med 378:2288–2301
86. Lin J et al (2020) Pembrolizumab combined with lenvatinib as non-first-line therapy in patients with refractory biliary tract carcinoma. Hepatobiliary Surg Nutr 9:414–424
87. Villanueva L et al (2021) Lenvatinib plus pembrolizumab for patients with previously treated biliary tract cancers in the multicohort phase II LEAP-005 study. J Clin Oncol 39:321
88. Cousin S et al (2021) Regomune: a phase II study of regorafenib + avelumab in solid tumors—results of the biliary tract cancer (BTC) cohort. J Clin Oncol 39:4096
89. Yarchoan M et al (2020) Abstract CT043: A multicenter randomized phase 2 trial of atezolizumab as monotherapy or in combination with cobimetinib in biliary tract cancers (BTCs): a NCI Experimental Therapeutics Clinical Trials Network (ETCTN) study. Cancer Res 80:CT043
90. Lind H et al (2020) Dual targeting of TGF-β and PD-L1 via a bifunctional anti-PD-L1/TGF-βRII agent: status of preclinical and clinical advances. J Immunother Cancer 8:e000433

91. Yoo C et al (2020) Phase I study of bintrafusp alfa, a bifunctional fusion protein targeting TGF-β and PD-L1, in patients with pretreated biliary tract cancer. J Immunother Cancer 8:e000564
92. Shimizu K et al (2012) Clinical utilization of postoperative dendritic cell vaccine plus activated T-cell transfer in patients with intrahepatic cholangiocarcinoma. J Hepatobiliary Pancreat Sci 19:171–178
93. Feng K et al (2018) Phase I study of chimeric antigen receptor modified T cells in treating HER2-positive advanced biliary tract cancers and pancreatic cancers. Protein Cell 9:838–847
94. Guo Y et al (2018) Phase I study of chimeric antigen receptor-modified T cells in patients with EGFR-positive advanced biliary tract cancers. Clin Cancer Res 24:1277–1286
95. Dummer R et al (2019) One-year (yr) recurrence-free survival (RFS) from a randomized, open label phase II study of neoadjuvant (neo) talimogene laherparepvec (T-VEC) plus surgery (surgx) versus surgx for resectable stage IIIB-IVM1a melanoma (MEL). J Clin Oncol 37:9520–9520
96. Kobayashi M et al (2013) Dendritic cell-based immunotherapy targeting synthesized peptides for advanced biliary tract cancer. J Gastrointest Surg 17:1609–1617
97. Musher BL et al (2020) A phase I/II study combining a TMZ-CD40L/4-1BBL-armed oncolytic adenovirus and nab-paclitaxel/gemcitabine chemotherapy in advanced pancreatic cancer: an interim report. J Clin Oncol 38:716
98. Li Y et al (2020) Oncolytic virotherapy in hepato-bilio-pancreatic cancer: the key to breaking the log jam? Cancer Med 9:2943–2959

Perspective on Immunotherapy Use in Biliary Tract Cancer

Dinakshi Shah, Angela Lamarca, Mairéad G. McNamara, and Juan W. Valle

Contents

D. Shah
Department of Medical Oncology, The Christie NHS Foundation Trust, Manchester, UK
e-mail: dinakshi.shah@nhs.net

A. Lamarca
The Christie NHS Foundation Trust/Division of Cancer Sciences, Department of Medical Oncology, University of Manchester, Manchester, UK

M. G. McNamara · J. W. Valle (✉)
Division of Cancer Sciences, University of Manchester/Department of Medical Oncology, The Christie NHS Foundation Trust, Manchester, UK
e-mail: juan.valle@nhs.net

Cancer Immunotherapy (2022)
https://doi.org/10.1007/13905_2021_15,
Published Online: 19 March 2022

Abstract

Biliary tract cancers (BTC) are aggressive malignancies with a dismal prognosis. Given the modest benefit of standard-of-care chemotherapy for patients with advanced disease, novel treatments are needed. There is a well-established link between certain chronic inflammatory conditions and BTC. Enhancing the immune response offers the potential to improve the efficacy of therapies. Immune oncology (IO) has transformed treatment for several malignancies; however, the role of immunotherapy in BTC remains investigational. Promising results from early-phase studies of immunotherapy combined with chemotherapy warrant further evaluation. In this chapter, ongoing clinical trials of IO in BTC and perspectives for future study are explored.

Keywords

Biliary tract cancer · Chemotherapy · Immune checkpoint inhibitors · Immunotherapy · Microsatellite instability

1 Introduction

Biliary tract cancers (BTC) are heterogeneous and aggressive cancers, comprising intrahepatic, peri-hilar and distal bile duct cholangiocarcinoma and gallbladder carcinoma. These malignancies have a dismal prognosis, with a 5-year survival rate of 2% in the advanced setting [1].

Less than 20% of patients with BTC are eligible for surgery at diagnosis and many will have early recurrence following curative surgery and adjuvant chemotherapy. Most patients with BTC present with advanced disease and are treated with combination chemotherapy (currently, cisplatin and gemcitabine) as the standard of care, with a median overall survival of 11.7 months [2]. More than 50% of patients develop progression of disease within a year of treatment with first-line therapy and the efficacy of second-line chemotherapy is modest [1, 3]. Due to limited treatment options, there is a need for the development of new therapies.

Understanding the underlying immune processes in patients with BTC offers the potential for the development of immunomodulatory agents to enhance immune response. Immune oncology (IO) has revolutionised the management of several solid malignancies; however, the role of immunotherapy in BTC remains investigational. Results from early-phase studies of immune checkpoint inhibitors (ICIs) as monotherapy in unselected patients with BTC have thus far been disappointing. There has been an increased effort to develop novel approaches to enhance sensitivity and overcome resistance to checkpoint inhibition. In this chapter, ongoing clinical trials involving IO in BTC, as well as future perspectives, are discussed.

2 Monotherapy

Treatment with single-agent ICIs in patients with BTC has demonstrated limited efficacy in phase I and II studies. The KEYNOTE 028 (phase Ib) and KEYNOTE 158 (phase II) trials with pembrolizumab in advanced BTC demonstrated a median overall survival (OS) of 6.2 months and 7.4 months, respectively. Objective response rates have been between 5.8% and 13% when treated with either pembrolizumab [4] or nivolumab [5] in trials in the advanced setting. Although responses have only been present in a limited number of patients in these trials with monotherapy, these appear to be durable and in some cases can extend into years, highlighting the potential for clinical benefit in a select group [4]. However, it has become apparent that blocking a single checkpoint is not sufficient to produce significant tumour responses in the majority of patients with BTC due to primary or adaptive resistance [6].

3 Strategies for Overcoming Primary resistance

Given the limited activity seen with monotherapy, there is growing interest in developing combination strategies to enhance the efficacy of checkpoint inhibition in advanced BTC. Potential strategies for this include enhancing antigen release and presentation, as well as activation and infiltration of T cells into the tumour microenvironment. There are a large number of trials that are currently underway investigating combination therapies in BTC, aiming to enhance the immune response. The use of ICIs in combination with locoregional therapy, chemotherapy, targeted therapy, granulocyte-macrophage-colony-stimulating factor (GM-CSF) and other immunotherapy agents will now be discussed further (Fig. 1).

4 Combined PD-1 and CTLA-4 Inhibition

Programmed cell death-1 (PD-1) and cytotoxic T lymphocyte-associated protein 4 (CTLA-4) are co-inhibitory receptors that are expressed on the surface of T cells and work by suppressing their activation [7]. It is thought that CTLA-4 and PD-1 inhibit T-cell activation at separate time points in T-cell evolution and via distinct pathways; therefore, blocking of CTLA-4 can act synergistically with PD-1 blockade, to enhance the antitumor immune response [8]. This combination has been effective in several tumour types such as advanced melanoma, where OS at 5 years is 52% when treated with first-line nivolumab plus ipilimumab [9]. Dual-checkpoint inhibition may therefore also enhance the immune response in BTC.

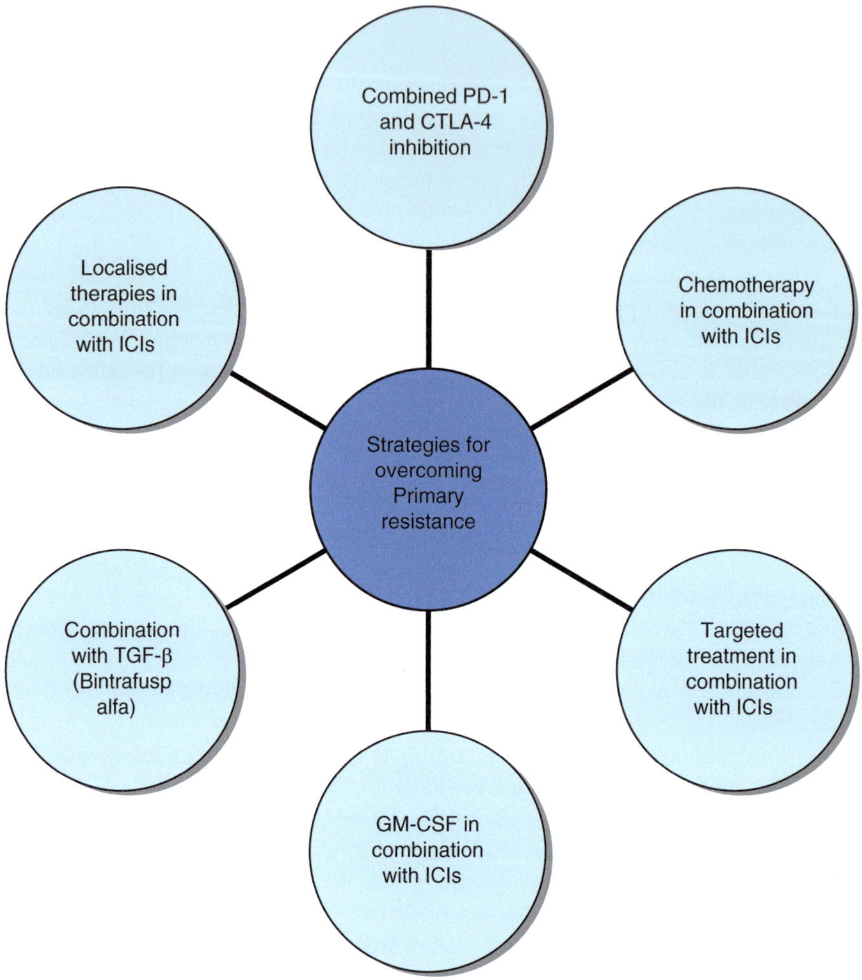

Fig. 1 Strategies to overcome primary resistance to immunotherapy in BTC
ICIs: immune checkpoint inhibitors, PD-1: Programmed cell death-1, CTLA-4: cytotoxic T lymphocyte-associated protein 4, GM-CSF: Granulocyte-macrophage-colony-stimulating factor; TGF-β: transforming growth factor-β

A phase I study of durvalumab (anti-PD-L1) and tremelimumab (anti-CTLA-4) in pre-treated (median 2 prior chemotherapy regimens) patients from Asia with advanced BTC demonstrated a median OS of 10.1 months with combination therapy compared to 8.1 months with monotherapy alone [10]. There is, however, an increased risk of immune-related adverse events associated with combination therapy that needs to be studied further.

There are several trials underway in the phase II setting, assessing the efficacy and safety of dual-checkpoint inhibition in BTC. NCT02834013 is a phase II study of nivolumab and ipilimumab in patients with rare tumours, including a subset of patients with advanced BTC who have progressed following systemic therapy. NCT03101566 is a phase II study of nivolumab in combination with cisplatin and gemcitabine or ipilimumab in patients with untreated, advanced BTC.

5 Chemotherapy in Combination with ICIs

Chemotherapy can enhance the effects of immunotherapy and the immune response by increasing the release and presentation of tumour antigens. The most promising data on IO in BTC have been from early-phase trials combining chemotherapy and checkpoint inhibitors in untreated, advanced BTC, with overall response rates between 36.7% and 73.4% [11–13]. The interaction between checkpoint inhibition and chemotherapy in BTC warrants further investigation. There are currently two global phase III trials underway: cisplatin and gemcitabine chemotherapy in combination with either durvalumab/placebo (TOPAZ-1; NCT03875235) or pembrolizumab/placebo (KEYNOTE-966; NCT04003636). Table 1 highlights the ongoing clinical trials assessing the combination of immunotherapy and chemotherapy in BTC in the adjuvant and advanced setting.

6 Targeted Treatment in Combination with ICIs

Angiogenesis is a hallmark of cancer and plays a key role in tumour growth and metastases. Vascular endothelial growth factor (VEGF) is involved in regulating angiogenesis and has been found to be overexpressed in BTC [14]. VEGF inhibitors can downregulate angiogenic signalling and increase T-cell trafficking and infiltration into tumour cells, and therefore may help enhance the efficacy of checkpoint inhibition [15, 16]. The effectiveness of this combination has been shown in several solid tumour types such as advanced hepatocellular carcinoma (HCC) with first-line bevacizumab (anti-VEGF) and atezolizumab (PD-L1 inhibitor) significantly improving OS compared to sorafenib (median OS 19.2 months vs. 13.4 months; hazard ratio for death: 0.66; 95% confidence interval [CI] 0.52–0.85, p-value = 0.0009), thus becoming the new standard of care in this disease group [17]. NCT04677504 is a randomised phase II study currently assessing the efficacy of this combination, atezolizumab with bevacizumab vs. atezolizumab alone, in conjunction with cisplatin and gemcitabine in patients with untreated, advanced BTC.

Ramucirumab is a monoclonal antibody that binds to the VEGF2 receptor (VEGFR), thus inhibiting VEGF and angiogenesis. Ramucirumab plus pembrolizumab was found to be a safe combination in the phase I setting; however, it demonstrated limited efficacy (ORR 4%) in patients with heavily pre-treated advanced BTC [18]. NCT02443324 is a phase I study currently evaluating the efficacy of this combination in a larger cohort of patients with advanced BTC, who have received up to 2 lines of prior systemic therapy.

Multi-tyrosine kinase inhibitors can target several pathways in addition to VEGFR, such as fibroblast growth factor receptor (FGFR), which may enhance ICI

Table 1 Summary of some ongoing clinical trials evaluating immunotherapy in combination with chemotherapy in patients with biliary tract cancer (BTC)

Study	Phase	Setting	Line of therapy	Drug combination	Target recruitment (n)	Primary endpoint	Location
NCT03260712	II	Advanced BTC	1st	CisGem + pembrolizumab	50	PFS at 6 months	Germany, Spain, UK
NCT03111732	II	Advanced BTC	At least one prior chemotherapy	Oxaliplatin, capecitabine + pembrolizumab	NOS	PFS at 5 months	USA
NCT03046862	II	Advanced BTC	1st	CisGem + durvalumab, tremelimumab	31	RR	Korea
NCT03704480	II	Advanced BTC	After failure of platinum-based chemotherapy	Durvalumab, tremelimumab ± paclitaxel	106	OS	France
NCT04308174	II	Neoadjuvant	N/a	CisGem ± durvalumab	45	R0 resection rate	Korea
NCT04413734	II	Advanced iCCA	NOS	CisGem ± triprilumab	120	PFS	China
NCT03101566	II	Advanced BTC	1st	Nivolumab + CisGem/ Ipilimumab	75	PFS at 6 months	USA
NCT03875235	III	Advanced BTC	1st	CisGem + durvalumab/placebo	757	OS	Global
NCT04003636	III	Advanced BTC	1st	CisGem + pembrolizumab/ placebo	1,048	OS	Global

CisGem: cisplatin and gemcitabine chemotherapy, PFS: progression-free survival, OS: overall survival, RR: response rate, iCCA: intrahepatic cholangiocarcinoma, NOS; not otherwise specified, N/a: not applicable activity. Lenvatinib plus pembrolizumab has shown promising antitumor activity in a phase Ib study of unresectable HCC, with an objective response rate of 46.0% per modified RECIST and median OS of 22 months [19]. NCT03797326 is a phase II study assessing the efficacy of lenvatinib in combination with pembrolizumab in patients with previously treated solid tumours, including advanced BTC. There are other phase II trials evaluating the use of anti-PD-1 toripalimab in conjunction with the multi-kinase inhibitors lenvatinib (NCT04211168) and axitinib (NCT04010071) as second-line treatment in advanced BTC.

7 GM-CSF in Combination with ICIs

Granulocyte-macrophage-colony-stimulating factor (GM-CSF) mediates proliferation and differentiation of dendritic cells, which are involved in tumour antigen presentation for priming of CD8+ T cells [20]. GM-CSF can therefore be used as an adjunct to immunotherapy to stimulate an antitumour immune response. This has been observed in previously treated advanced melanoma, where treatment with GM-CSF and ipilimumab resulted in longer median OS than ipilimumab alone (17.5 months vs. 12.7 months) [21]. The results of the NCT02703714 study, assessing the use of pembrolizumab in conjunction with GM-CSF in patients with advanced BTC in a phase II setting, are awaited.

8 Bintrafusp alfa

Another mechanism potentially involved in the progression of BTC is the transforming growth factor-β (TGF-β) pathway. TGF-β signalling can cause alterations in both the cancer and immune cells in the tumour microenvironment and enhances tumour growth [22]. Bintrafusp alfa is a bifunctional protein composed of TGF-β receptor II and human IgG1 antibody blocking PD-L1 [22]. This treatment can therefore help to overcome TGF-β-mediated immune evasion and resistance to checkpoint inhibition. A phase I study of bintrafusp alfa in 30 patients with advanced BTC, who had failed prior chemotherapy, demonstrated objective response rates of 20% with PFS of 2.5 months and OS 12.7 months [22].

There are currently two trials underway assessing the use of bintrafusp alpha as second-line therapy for patients with advanced BTC (NCT03833661) in the phase II setting, or in combination with standard-of-care chemotherapy (NCT04066491) in patients who are treatment-naïve (phase III).

9 Localised Therapies in Combination with ICIs

In a select group of patients with localised, unresectable BTC, there are several localised therapies which may provide an alternative management option to standard-of-care chemotherapy. These treatments can vary according to local expertise and availability and include external beam radiotherapy, transarterial chemoembolisation (TACE), radiofrequency ablation (RFA) and selective internal radiation therapy (SIRT) [23].

Radiotherapy has been shown to result in antigen release from tumour sites and has the potential to generate antitumour responses in both locally irradiated and non-irradiated metastatic lesions [24]. The combination of ICIs and radiotherapy can work synergistically to increase the susceptibility of tumour cells to an immune response. The KEYNOTE-001 study found that patients with pre-treated non-small-cell lung cancer (NSCLC), who had previously received any radiotherapy prior to pembrolizumab, had significantly longer OS (10.7 months vs. 5·3 months; HR 0·58, $p = 0{\cdot}026$) and PFS (4.4 months vs. 2·1 months; HR 0·56, $p = 0{\cdot}019$) than those that did not [25]. A pilot study of 15 patients with microsatellite-stable, advanced BTC, who had progressed on at least one line of previous therapy, demonstrated good response to durvalumab and tremelimumab in combination with radiotherapy. This showed a disease control rate of 33% with 17% of patients achieving a partial response and 8% a complete response [26]. The study demonstrates some activity with this combination and an expansion cohort is underway to assess this further (NCT03482102) [26].

Ablative procedures involve the use of chemicals or heat to destroy abnormal tissues and have been used in patients with BTC to manage biliary strictures to promote stent patency [27]. A pilot study assessed whether the combination of tremelimumab and microwave ablation could overcome resistance to CTLA-4 inhibition in patients with refractory, advanced BTC [28]. Although limited by a small sample size (n = 16), the study demonstrated increased circulating activated CD8+ T cells following treatment, and 12.5% of patients achieved a partial response and 31.3% achieved stable disease. The combination of ablative therapies with ICIs is being evaluated in a phase II trial (NCT02821754) in patients with advanced HCC and BTC, who have failed at least one line of chemotherapy.

Radioembolisation delivers high-dose radiotherapy to liver tumours using radiation-labelled microspheres [23]. The phase II NASIR-HCC Trial assessed the combination of nivolumab and SIRT (SIR-Spheres yttrium-90 microspheres) in 42 patients with unresectable HCC. Preliminary data presented shows a favourable safety profile and good responses, with 11.9% of patients achieving a complete response and an overall response rate of 38%, measured according to RECIST v1 [29]. This concept is currently being evaluated in NCT04238637: durvalumab and tremelimumab in combination with SIRT, following adjuvant or first-line chemotherapy in patients with locally advanced or limited metastasised intrahepatic BTC.

10 Microsatellite Instability-High Tumours

Patients with BTC who possess mismatch repair protein deficiency (MMR) have demonstrated improved outcomes with ICIs. The mismatch repair system is responsible for correcting DNA damage introduced into microsatellites during replication [30]. Defects in the MMR system can lead to accumulation of mutations in microsatellites and therefore microsatellite instability [30]. Tumours with high microsatellite instability (MSI-H) can express a high number of neoantigens and therefore are potentially more susceptible to immunotherapy [30]. Pembrolizumab was approved by the FDA in 2017 for patients with MMR-deficient or microsatellite instability-high (MSI-H) solid tumours.

MSI-high phenotypes in BTC are rare; approximately 2% of BTCs have a reported dMMR phenotype [23]. Despite this, there should be an increased drive in clinical trials to evaluate patients for MMR or MSI expression in BTC as a biomarker for response to immunotherapy [31].

11 Expert Opinion

The development of BTC has an established link to chronic inflammation (e.g. primary sclerosing cholangitis, ulcerative colitis, Crohn's and liver cirrhosis). Harnessing the immune response is therefore an attractive proposition, an approach that has shifted the paradigm of treatment for a number of malignancies. Given the modest efficacy of systemic therapy for patients with advanced BTC, novel therapies are needed.

To date, it is evident that ICI in monotherapy in an unselected patient population (either by anatomical site of origin or molecular signature) is of limited benefit. The observation that, in a small number of cases, there is prolonged progression-free survival benefit suggests that there may be factors (yet to be identified) that may predict the benefit for ICIs.

Many studies are underway, aiming to enhance the activity of ICIs through enhancement of antigen release and presentation, as well as activation and infiltration of T cells into the tumour microenvironment. As discussed above, these include physical/mechanical approaches (microwave ablation, TACE, SIRT); combined-modality approaches (ICI in combination with chemotherapy, radiotherapy [external beam or SIRT] or targeted therapies); or approaches aimed at maximising immune blockade/priming (combinations with CTLA-4 inhibitors, GM-CSF and bintrafusp alfa, for example). Most of these approaches are still in early-phase development, likely in highly selected patients, and initial signals of activity will need to undergo subsequent robust evaluation in randomised controlled studies.

Many unanswered questions remain; we are only at the start of this journey. Beyond the combination approach detailed above, future studies need to explore primary and acquired resistance to ICIs; the role of ICI beyond first disease progression; the impact of factors other than immediately tumour related (e.g. the microbiome); and the role in patients usually excluded from clinical trials (e.g. in the elderly, or in patients with poorer performance status, background autoimmune conditions, impaired end-organ function).

Most imminently, it is hoped that the results of the two global phase III studies evaluating the activity of durvalumab (TOPAZ-1) or pembrolizumab (KEYNOTE-966) in addition to cisplatin and gemcitabine in previously untreated patients with advanced BTC will provide a step-change in the understanding of the role of immunotherapy in these patients. Both studies have included patients from all anatomical subgroups and no molecular preselection criteria have been applied. Whilst the primary end point will be analysed by intention-to-treat analysis, the large size of the studies and associated translational analyses will enable exploratory subgroup analysis to gauge which patients are most likely to benefit from ICI. Until then, the role of ICI (with the exception of patients with MSI-H tumours) remains investigational.

Compliance with Ethical Standards

Funding This chapter did not receive a specific grant from funding agencies in the public, commercial or non-profit sectors.

Disclosure of Interests Dinakshi Shah: No conflicts of interest to declare.

Angela Lamarca: Travel and educational support from Ipsen, Pfizer, Bayer, AAA, Sirtex, Novartis, Mylan and Delcath. Speaker honoraria from Merck, Pfizer, Ipsen and Incyte. Advisory honoraria from EISAI, Nutricia Ipsen, QED and Roche. Member of the Knowledge Network and NETConnect Initiatives funded by Ipsen.

Mairéad G McNamara: Received research grant support from Servier, Ipsen and NuCana. She has received travel and accommodation support from Bayer and Ipsen and speaker honoraria from Pfizer, Ipsen, NuCana and Mylan. She has served on advisory boards for Celgene, Ipsen, Sirtex and Baxalta.

Juan W Valle: Consulting or Advisory role for Agios, AstraZeneca, Delcath Systems, Keocyt, Genoscience Pharma, Incyte, Ipsen, Merck, Mundipharma EDO, Novartis, PCI Biotech, Pfizer, Pieris Pharmaceuticals, QED and Wren Laboratories; Speakers' Bureau for Imaging Equipment Limited, Ipsen, Novartis and Nucana, and received Travel Grants from Celgene and Nucana.

Ethical approval This chapter does not contain any studies with human participants performed by any of the authors.

References

1. Malenica I, Donadon M, Lleo A (2020) Molecular and immunological characterization of biliary tract cancers: a paradigm shift towards a personalized medicine. Cancers (Basel) 12:1–19
2. Valle J, Wasan H, Palmer DH et al (2010) Cisplatin plus Gemcitabine versus Gemcitabine for biliary tract cancer. N Engl J Med. https://doi.org/10.1056/nejmoa0908721
3. Lamarca A, Palmer DH, Wasan HS et al (2021) Second-line FOLFOX chemotherapy versus active symptom control for advanced biliary tract cancer (ABC-06): a phase 3, open-label, randomised, controlled trial. Lancet Oncol. https://doi.org/10.1016/S1470-2045(21)00027-9
4. Bang Y-J, Ueno M, Malka D et al (2019) Pembrolizumab (pembro) for advanced biliary adenocarcinoma: results from the KEYNOTE-028 (KN028) and KEYNOTE-158 (KN158) basket studies. J Clin Oncol. https://doi.org/10.1200/jco.2019.37.15_suppl.4079
5. Kim RD, Chung V, Alese OB et al (2020) A Phase 2 multi-institutional study of Nivolumab for patients with advanced refractory biliary tract cancer. JAMA Oncol. https://doi.org/10.1001/jamaoncol.2020.0930
6. Sharma P, Hu-Lieskovan S, Wargo JA, Ribas A (2017) Primary, adaptive, and acquired resistance to cancer immunotherapy. Cell. https://doi.org/10.1016/j.cell.2017.01.017
7. Perkhofer L, Beutel AK, Ettrich TJ (2019) Immunotherapy: pancreatic cancer and extrahepatic biliary tract cancer. Visc Med. https://doi.org/10.1159/000497291

8. Willsmore ZN, Coumbe BGT, Crescioli S et al (2021) Combined anti-PD-1 and anti-CTLA-4 checkpoint blockade: treatment of melanoma and immune mechanisms of action. Eur J Immunol. https://doi.org/10.1002/eji.202048747
9. Larkin J, Chiarion-Sileni V, Gonzalez R et al (2019) Five-year survival with combined nivolumab and ipilimumab in advanced melanoma. N Engl J Med. https://doi.org/10.1056/nejmoa1910836
10. Ioka T, Ueno M, Oh D-Y et al (2019) Evaluation of safety and tolerability of durvalumab (D) with or without tremelimumab (T) in patients (pts) with biliary tract cancer (BTC). J Clin Oncol. https://doi.org/10.1200/jco.2019.37.4_suppl.387
11. Ueno M, Ikeda M, Morizane C et al (2019) Nivolumab alone or in combination with cisplatin plus gemcitabine in Japanese patients with unresectable or recurrent biliary tract cancer: a non-randomised, multicentre, open-label, phase 1 study. Lancet Gastroenterol Hepatol. https://doi.org/10.1016/S2468-1253(19)30086-X
12. Feng K, Liu Y, Zhao Y, Yang Q, Dong L, Liu J, Li X, Zhao Z, Mei Q, Han W (2020) Efficacy and biomarker analysis of nivolumab plus gemcitabine and cisplatin in patients with unresectable or metastatic biliary tract cancers: results from a phase II study. J Immunother Cancer. https://doi.org/10.1136/jitc-2019-000367
13. Do-Youn Oh, Kyung-Hun Lee, Dae-Won Lee, Tae Yong Kim, Ju-Hee Bang, Ah-Rong Nam, Young Lee, Qu Zhang, Marlon Rebelatto, Weimin Li and Kim JW (2020) Phase II study assessing tolerability, efficacy, and biomarkers for durvalumab (D) ± tremelimumab (T) and gemcitabine/cisplatin (GemCis) in chemo-naïve advanced biliary tract cancer (aBTC). J Clin Oncol 38:15: 4520–4520
14. Yoshikawa D, Ojima H, Iwasaki M, Hiraoka N, Kosuge T, Kasai S, Hirohashi S, Shibata T (2008) Clinicopathological and prognostic significance of EGFR, VEGF, and HER2 expression in cholangiocarcinoma. Br J Cancer. https://doi.org/10.1038/sj.bjc.6604129
15. Vogel A, Bathon M, Saborowski A (2021) Immunotherapies in clinical development for biliary tract cancer. Expert Opin Investig Drugs. https://doi.org/10.1080/13543784.2021.1868437
16. Song Y, Fu Y, Xie Q, Zhu B, Wang J, Zhang B (2020) Anti-angiogenic agents in combination with immune checkpoint inhibitors: a promising strategy for cancer treatment. Front Immunol. https://doi.org/10.3389/fimmu.2020.01956
17. Finn RS, Qin S, Ikeda M et al (2021) IMbrave150: updated overall survival (OS) data from a global, randomized, open-label phase III study of atezolizumab (atezo) + bevacizumab (bev) versus sorafenib (sor) in patients (pts) with unresectable hepatocellular carcinoma (HCC). J Clin Oncol. https://doi.org/10.1200/jco.2021.39.3_suppl.267
18. Arkenau H, Martin-Liberal J, Calvo E et al (2018) Ramucirumab Plus pembrolizumab in patients with previously treated advanced or metastatic biliary tract cancer: nonrandomized, open-label, phase I trial (JVDF). Oncologist. https://doi.org/10.1634/theoncologist.2018-0044
19. Finn RS, Ikeda M, Zhu AX et al (2020) Phase ib study of lenvatinib plus pembrolizumab in patients with unresectable hepatocellular carcinoma. J Clin Oncol. https://doi.org/10.1200/JCO.20.00808
20. Hong IS (2016) Stimulatory versus suppressive effects of GM-CSF on tumor progression in multiple cancer types. Exp Mol Med. https://doi.org/10.1038/emm.2016.64
21. Hodi FS, Lee S, McDermott DF, Rao UN, Butterfield LH, Tarhini AA, Leming P, Puzanov I, Shin D, Kirkwood JM (2014) Ipilimumab plus sargramostim vs. ipilimumab alone for treatment of metastatic melanoma: a randomized clinical trial. J Am Med Assoc. https://doi.org/10.1001/jama.2014.13943
22. Yoo C, Oh DY, Choi HJ et al (2020) Phase i study of bintrafusp alfa, a bifunctional fusion protein targeting TGF-β and PD-L1, in patients with pretreated biliary tract cancer. J Immunother Cancer. https://doi.org/10.1136/jitc-2020-000564
23. Valle JW, Kelley RK, Nervi B, Oh DY, Zhu AX (2021) Biliary tract cancer. Lancet. https://doi.org/10.1016/S0140-6736(21)00153-7
24. Jagodinsky JC, Harari PM, Morris ZS (2020) The promise of combining radiation therapy with immunotherapy. Int J Radiat Oncol Biol Phys. https://doi.org/10.1016/j.ijrobp.2020.04.023

25. Shaverdian N, Lisberg AE, Bornazyan K, Veruttipong D, Goldman JW, Formenti SC, Garon EB, Lee P (2017) Previous radiotherapy and the clinical activity and toxicity of pembrolizumab in the treatment of non-small-cell lung cancer: a secondary analysis of the KEYNOTE-001 phase 1 trial. Lancet Oncol. https://doi.org/10.1016/S1470-2045(17)30380-7
26. Hong TS, Goyal L, Parikh AR et al (2020) A pilot study of durvalumab/tremelimumab (durva/treme) and radiation (XRT) for metastatic biliary tract cancer (mBTC): preliminary safety and efficacy. J Clin Oncol. https://doi.org/10.1200/jco.2020.38.4_suppl.547
27. Satiya J, Schwartz I, Tabibian JH, Kumar V, Girotra M (2020) Ablative therapies for hepatic and biliary tumors: endohepatology coming of age. Transl Gastroenterol Hepatol. https://doi.org/10.21037/TGH.2019.10.17
28. Xie C, Duffy AG, Mabry-Hrones D et al (2019) Tremelimumab in combination with microwave ablation in patients with refractory biliary tract cancer. Hepatology. https://doi.org/10.1002/hep.30482
29. De La Torre M, Matilla A, Varela M et al. Nivolumab after selective internal radiation therapy using sir spheres resin microspheres in patients with hepatocellular carcinoma: the NASIR HCC trial. In: Proceedings of the 14th Annual Conference of the International Liver Cancer Association (ILCA); 2020
30. Marcus L, Lemery SJ, Keegan P, Pazdur R (2019) FDA approval summary: Pembrolizumab for the treatment of microsatellite instability-high solid tumors. Clin Cancer Res. https://doi.org/10.1158/1078-0432.CCR-18-4070
31. Le DT, Uram JN, Wang H et al (2015) PD-1 Blockade in tumors with mismatch-repair deficiency. N Engl J Med. https://doi.org/10.1056/nejmoa1500596

Part VII

Pancreas

Immune Landscape of Pancreas Ductal Adenocarcinoma: Current Therapeutic Strategies and Future Perspective

Binbin Zheng-Lin and Eileen M. O'Reilly

Contents

B. Zheng-Lin
Department of Medicine, Icahn School of Medicine at Mount Sinai Morningside and Mount Sinai West, New York, NY, USA

Department of Medicine, Memorial Sloan Kettering Cancer Center, New York, NY, USA

E. M. O'Reilly (✉)
Department of Medicine, Memorial Sloan Kettering Cancer Center, New York, NY, USA

Weill Cornell Department of Medicine, Weill Cornell Medicine, New York, NY, USA

David M. Rubenstein Center for Pancreatic Research, Memorial Sloan Kettering Cancer Center, New York, NY, USA
e-mail: oreillye@mskcc.org

Cancer Immunotherapy (2021)
https://doi.org/10.1007/13905_2021_8,
Published Online: 25 August 2021

Abstract

Regardless of success of immunotherapy in other tumor types, pancreatic ductal adenocarcinoma (PDAC) has remained largely resistant to the benefit of immunotherapy. The unique immune resistance of PDAC arises from multiple non-redundant pathways which lead to tumor immune escape and T effector cell anergy. Cellular and acellular components of the PDAC tumor microenvironment further exacerbate its immunosuppressant phenotype. Despite yielding negative results, trials with single modality immunotherapy have deepened our understanding of the PDAC immune landscape. Current research efforts have shifted to combined immunomodulatory strategies seeking to amplify the activity of chemotherapy and immune checkpoint inhibition. In this article, we will review the relevant developments of IO applied to PDAC treatment.

Keywords

Cancer vaccine · CAR T cell therapy · Immune checkpoint inhibitor · Immunotherapy · *KRAS* · Pancreatic cancer

1 Background

Pancreatic ductal adenocarcinoma (PDAC) affects over 60,000 adults/year in the USA while retaining one of the lowest 5-year survival rate of 10% amongst all solid tumors [1]. PDAC is forecast to be the second leading cause of cancer death within this decade due to its late clinical presentation, complex pathobiology, resistance to conventional chemotherapy, and limited breakthroughs in new therapy development [2]. In spite of the successes of immunotherapy in other types of malignancies, PDAC exhibits an inherent immune resistance phenotype that arises from its complex genetic landscape. While most pancreatic tumors share common oncogenic pathways affecting Kirsten rat sarcoma viral oncogene homolog (*KRAS*), tumor protein P53 (TP53), mothers against decapentaplegic homolog 4 (*SMAD4*), and cyclin dependent kinase inhibitor 2A (*CDKN2A*), less recurring alterations in DNA damage response (DDR) genes, chromatin modifications, and copy number variations lead to a diversity of genotypes and clinical phenotypes [3, 4]. Beyond intrinsic effects on tumor growth and survival, mutated *KRAS* signaling contributes directly to PDAC immune evasion via autophagosome-mediated degradation of histocompatibility complex class I (MHC-I) and upregulation of inhibitory immune checkpoint molecules including programmed death (PD) ligand 1 (PD-L1) [5, 6]. Another distinctive feature of PDAC is a dense stroma comprised of non-immune cells, immune cells, and the extracellular matrix which account for more than 70% of tumor volume. The presence of immunosuppressive cells in the tumor microenvironment (TME) is acquired in a premalignant stage of pancreatic intraepithelial neoplasia (PanIN) and develops in parallel with tumor progression [7]. Under normal circumstances, dendritic cells (DCs) present tumor antigens to naïve CD8 T cells in secondary lymphoid organs which then undergo antigen-specific activation and acquire cytotoxic activity and effector differentiation. In the PDAC TME, tumor-infiltrating T regulatory (Treg) cells attenuate the response of T effector cells and promote their quiescence via IL-10 and TGF-β signaling [8]. Concomitantly, tumor-associated macrophages (TAMs) and myeloid-derived suppressor cells (MDSCs) induce T cell apoptosis and anergy via PD-1 and cytotoxic T-lymphocyte-associated protein 4 (CTLA-4) inhibitory signaling and reactive oxygen and nitrogen species generation [9]. Mutated *KRAS* promotes macrophage colony-stimulating factor (GM-CSF) and chemokine C-X-C motif ligand (CXCL) 1 contributing recruitment of these pro-tumorigenic cells while excluding antitumor T effector cells and DCs [10, 11]. Non-immune cells in the TME also participate in downregulation of immune response and enhancement of tumor growth. *KRAS*-mediated deregulation of Hedgehog signaling induces activation of cancer-associated fibroblasts (CAFs) and pancreatic stellate cells (PSCs) with subsequent stromal deposition of hyaluronic acid (HA), collagen, laminin, and fibronectin. Resultant dense desmoplasia impairs the activity of therapeutic agents by altering their pharmacokinetics and pharmacodynamics [12]. PSCs also secrete growth factors and cytokines favoring recruitment of inhibitory immune cells hence exacerbating the immunosuppressant phenotype of the TME [13, 14].

Due to limited clinical activity of single-agent immunotherapy agents in PDAC (Table 1) [15, 16], current research focus is shifting towards immunomodulatory combination strategies aimed at enhancing endogenous T cell function, providing exogenously tumor-specific T cell activity via adoptive transfer, and neutralizing immunosuppressive properties of the TME. Herein, we review the relevant immunotherapy strategies applied to PDAC treatment (Fig. 1).

2 Immune Checkpoint Blockade (ICB)

Pembrolizumab is currently approved by the Food and Drug Administration (FDA) as treatment for patients with metastatic PDAC (mPDAC) patients with mismatch repair-deficient (dMMR) and microsatellite instability-high (MSI-H) status [17]. dMMR/MSI-H tumors are characterized by high tumor mutational burden (TMB), greater intra-tumoral immune cell infiltration, and improved response to ICB regardless of primary tumor type [18, 19]. Notwithstanding, the clinical use of ICB in PDAC is greatly limited as less than 1% of tumors harbor dMMR/MSI-H status [20]. Additionally, the benefit of ICB in dMMR/MSI-H PDAC is comparatively blunted as opposed to other solid malignancies. KEYNOTE-158 trial is a non-randomized multi-cohort phase 2 study that enrolled patients with 27 tumor types treated with pembrolizumab. Amongst all cancer types, endometrial and gastric showed the highest objective response rates (ORRs) which were, respectively, 57.1% (95% CI 42.2–71.2) and 45.8% (95% CI 25.6–67.2). In the PDAC cohort with 22 patients with advanced disease, pembrolizumab achieved modest activity: ORR was 18.2% (95% CI 5.2–40.3) which included one case of one

Table 1 Characteristics of selective completed clinical trials evaluating immunotherapeutic agents in pancreas cancer. Completed studies without results on clinical activity were not included; trials with unknown, suspended, or terminated status were also excluded

Study	Phase	Experimental arm (N of PDAC)	Control arm (*N*)	Patient population	Results in the PDAC cohort
Immune Checkpoint Blockade					
Brahmer et al. [15]	1	BMS-936559 (*N* = 14)	NA	Advanced solid tumors including PDAC	No responder reported
Royal et al. [16]	2	Ipilimumab (*N* = 27)	NA	PDAC, locally advanced or metastatic	No responder reported
O'Reilly et al. [22]	2	• Durvalumab plus tremelimumab (*N* = 32) • Durvalumab alone (*N* = 33)	NA	PDAC, metastatic	• Durvalumab plus tremelimumab: ORR 3.1% (95% CI 0.08–16.22) • Durvalumab alone: ORR 0% (95% CI 0.00–10.58)
Le et al. [18]	NA	Pembrolizumab (*N* = 8)	NA	Advanced dMMR solid tumors including PDAC	Two CR and three PR in the PDAC cohort
Marabelle et al. [21]	2	Pembrolizumab (*N* = 22)	NA	Advanced solid tumors including PDAC	ORR 18.2% (95% CI 5.2–40.3%); median OS (95% CI 2.1–9.8)
ICB and Chemotherapy					
Weiss et al. [29]	1b/2	GnP plus pembrolizumab (*N* = 17)	NA	PDAC, metastatic	PFS 9.1 months (95% CI 4.9–15.3); median OS 15 months (95% CI 6.8–22.6)
Wainberg et al. [30]	1	GnP plus nivolumab (*N* = 50)	NA	PDAC, locally advanced or metastatic	ORR 18% (95% CI 8.6–31.4); median OS 9.9 months (95% CI 6.74–12.16)

Renouf et al. [31]	2	Durvalumab/tremelimumab plus GnP ($N = 119$)	GnP ($N = 61$)	PDAC, metastatic	Overlapping median OS (9.8 months in experimental arm vs. 8.8 month in control arm, HR = 0.94, 90% 0.71–1.25, $P = 0.72$). Respective ORR were 30.3% vs. 23.0% (OR 1.49, 90% CI 0.81–2.72, $P = 0.28$)
ICB and Other Agents					
O'Hara et al. [34]	1b	• Cohort B1 ($N = 6$): GnP + sotigalimab at 0.1 mg/kg • Cohort B2 ($N = 6$): GnP + sotigalimab at 0.3 mg/kg • Cohort C1 ($N = 6$): GnP + nivolumab + sotigalimab at 0.1 mg/kg • Cohort C2 ($N = 6$): GnP + nivolumab + sotigalimab at 0.3 mg/kg	NA	PDAC, metastatic	• B1: median OS 12.7 months (95% CI 1.1–NR) • B2: median OS 20.1 months (95% CI 7.2–NR) • C1: median OS 15.9 months (95% CI 0.5–NR) • C2: median OS not evaluable
Manji et al. [44]	1	AB680 + zimberelimab + GnP ($N = 16$)	NA	PDAC, metastatic	In nine response-evaluable patients, three with a PR and five with SD were observed
Ko et al. [47]	1/2	Atezolizumab + PEGPH20 ($N = 66$)	GnP or mFOLFOX-6 ($N = 42$)	PDAC, metastatic	Experimental arm: ORR 6.1% (95% CI 1.7–14.8) Control arm: 2.4% (95% CI 0.06–12.6)
Cho et al. [48]	1/2	Atezolizumab + cobimetinib ($N = 14$)	GnP ($N = 15$)	PDAC, metastatic	No responder in either study arm
Oh et al. [49]	1/2	Atezolizumab + BL-8040 ($N = 15$)	mFOLFOX-6 or GnP ($N = 15$)	PDAC, metastatic	No responder in either study arm

(continued)

Table 1 (continued)

Study	Phase	Experimental arm (N of PDAC)	Control arm (*N*)	Patient population	Results in the PDAC cohort
Chung et al. [50]	1/2	Atezolizumab + RO6874281 ($N = 29$)	mFOLFOX-6 ($N = 23$) or GnP ($N = 23$)	PDAC, metastatic	Experimental arm: one participant with a PR was reported
Bockorny et al. [115]	2	Pembrolizumab + BL-8040 + liposomal irinotecan/5-fluorouracil/leucovorin	NA	PDAC, metastatic	Seven patients had a PR, ten experienced SD
Wainberg et al. [92]	1	Cabiralizumab + nivolumab ($N = 33$)	NA	Advanced solid tumors including PDAC	Durable response reported in three patients with a PR and one with SD; all four patients had MSS disease
Cassier et al. [94]	1	Pexidartinib + durvalumab (*N* unspecified)	NA	Advanced solid tumors including PDAC	Four patients with SD amongst all enrolled patients, PDAC-specific survival data not reported
O'Hara et al. [114]	1	LY2510924 + durvalumab ($N = 8$)	NA	Advanced solid tumors including PDAC	Three PDAC patients achieved SD
Adoptive Cell Therapy					
Thistlethwaite et al. [54]	1	Anti-CEACAM5 CAR T cell + preconditioning fludarabine + IL2 ($N = 1$)	NA	Advanced solid tumors including PDAC	No objective response was reported. Autoimmune pneumonitis observed in four patients including the one PDAC patient
Beatty et al. [59]	1	Anti-MSLN CAR T cell ($N = 6$)	NA	PDAC, metastatic	Two cases with SD, durations of response were 3.8–5.4 months
Haas et al. [60]	1	Anti-MSLN CAR T cell ($N = 5$)	NA	Advanced solid tumors including PDAC	Two cases with SD, durations of response were 2 and 3 months
Wang et al. [63]	1	Anti-MSLN CAR T cells with PD-1 disruption ($N = 6$)	NA	Advanced solid tumors including PDAC	Overall response included four cases with SD and two with a PR

Ferrandina et al. [64]	1	Anti-CD133 CAR T cell ($N = 7$)	NA	Advanced solid tumors including PDAC	Two reported a PR and three had SD
Shaw et al. [68]	1	BPX-601 ($N = 18$)	NA	PDAC, metastatic	Amongst 13 response-evaluable patients, eight experienced a SD
Lum et al. [71]	1/2	EGFR BATs ($N = 7$)	NA	PDAC, locally advanced or metastatic	Median OS was 31 months (CI not reported)
Cancer Vaccines					
Hardacre et al. [73]	2	Adjuvant Algenpantucel-L + gemcitabine- or 5-fluorouracil-based chemoradiotherapy ($N = 70$)	NA	Resected PDAC	Median DFS 14.1 months (CI not reported) 12-month survival was 86% (CI not reported)
Le et al. [119]	1	• Ipilimumab alone ($N = 15$) • Ipilimumab plus GVAX vaccine ($N = 15$)	NA	PDAC, locally advanced or metastatic	One SD in ipilimumab, three cases with SD in ipilimumab plus GVAX arm. Median OS were, respectively, 3.6 vs. 5.7 months (HR 0.51, 95% CI 0.23–1.08, $P = 0.072$)
Le et al. [77]	2	• Cy + GVAX + CRS-207 ($N = 61$) • Cy + GVAX ($N = 29$)	NA	PDAC, metastatic	Median OS was 6.1 months in triplet arm vs. 3.9 months in doublet group (HR 0.59, 95% CI 0.36–0.97, $P = 0.02$).
Tsujikawa et al. [79]	2	• Cy + GVAX + CRS-207 ($N = 42$) • Cy + GVAX + CRS-207 + nivolumab ($N = 51$)	NA	PDAC, metastatic	• Cy + GVAX + CRS-207: median OS 6.1 months (95% CI 3.5–7) • Cy + GVAX + CRS-207 + nivolumab: median OS 5.9 months (95% CI 4.75–8.6)

(continued)

Table 1 (continued)

Study	Phase	Experimental arm (N of PDAC)	Control arm (*N*)	Patient population	Results in the PDAC cohort
Wu et al. [80]	2	Maintenance GVAX + Cy + ipilimumab ($N = 40$)	Maintenance FOLFIRINOX ($N = 42$)	Metastatic PDAC treated with FOLFIRINOX	Median OS was 9.38 (95% CI 5.0–12.2) in experimental arm vs. 14.7 months (95% CI 11.6–20) in control arm (HR 1.75, 95% CI 1.09–2.79, $P = 0.019$)
Rong et al. [82]	1	MUC-1-peptide-pulsed DC cell vaccine ($N = 7$)	NA	PDAC, locally advanced or metastatic	No responders reported
Mehrotra et al. [83]	1	Poly-ICLC plus autologous DCs pulsed with hTERT, CEA, and survivin	NA	PDAC, locally advanced or metastatic	Four patients with SD reported in eight response-evaluable patients. Median OS was 7.7 months (CI not reported)
Middleton et al. [74]	3	• Concurrent GV1001 + gemcitabine + capecitabine ($N = 354$) • Gemcitabine + capecitabine followed by sequential GV1001 ($N = 350$)	Gemcitabine + capecitabine ($N = 358$)	PDAC, locally advanced or metastatic	Compared to chemotherapy alone (median OS 7.9 months, 95% CI 7.1–8.8), median OS did not improve with concurrent vaccination (median OS 6.9 months; HR 1.19, 98.25% CI 0.97–1.48, $P = 0.05$) or with sequential vaccination (median OS 8.4 months; HR 1.05, 98.25% CI 0.85–1.29, $P = 0.64$)
Shima et al. [75]	2	• SVN-2B + IFNβ ($N = 30$) • SVN-2B ($N = 34$)	Placebo ($N = 19$)	HLA-A24-positive advanced PDAC	No difference in PFS reported across SVN-2B + IFNβ groups, SVN-2B, or placebo group, respective PFS were 102 days (95% CI 77–144), 96.5 days (95% CI 66–131), and 111 days (95% CI 63–150), $P = 0.4565$

Yamaue et al. [76]	2/3	Elpamotide + gemcitabine (*N* = 100)	Placebo + gemcitabine (*N* = 53)	PDAC, locally advanced or metastatic	Median OS in experimental arm was 8.36 months, and 8.54 months in control arm (HR 0.87, 95% CI 0.486–1.557)
Feng et al. [120]	1	Anti-HER2 CAR T cells with preconditioning nab-paclitaxel and Cy (*N* = 2)	NA	Advanced solid tumors including PDAC	Two PDAC patients experienced SD ranging 5.3–8.3 months

CEA carcinoembryonic agent; *Cy* cyclophosphamide; *DC* dendritic cell; *DFS* disease-free survival; *dMMR* mismatch repair-deficient; *FOLFIRINO* folinic acid, fluorouracil, irinotecan, oxaliplatin; *GnP* gemcitabine and nab-paclitaxel; *hTERT* human telomerase reverse transcriptase; *ICI* immune checkpoint inhibitor; *IL* interleukin; *mFOLFOX6* folinic acid, fluorouracil, oxaliplatin; *MSS* microsatellite stable; *NR* not reached; *ORR* objective response; *OS* overall survival; *PARPi* poly-ADP ribose polymerase inhibitor; *PBL* peripheral blood lymphocytes; *PDAC* pancreatic ductal adenocarcinoma; *PFS* progression-free survival

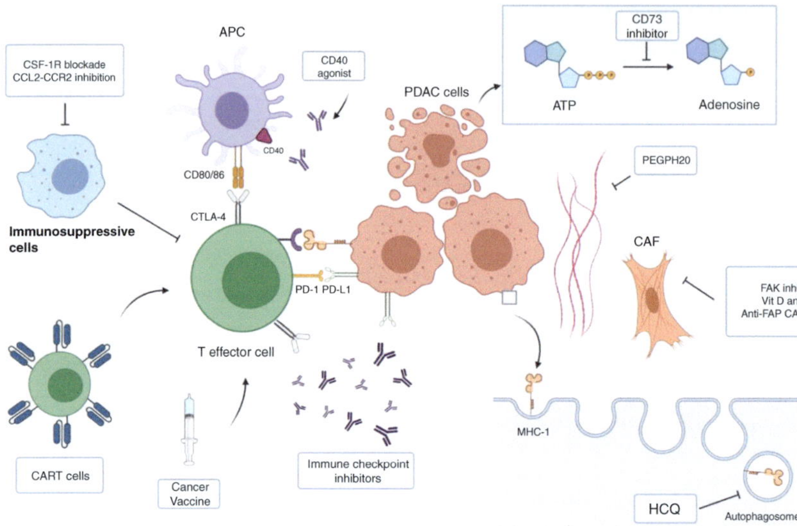

Fig. 1 Current therapeutic approaches to PDAC immune resistance. Multiple non-redundant mechanisms mediate PDAC immune escape. Combined regimens (e.g., ICB with chemotherapy and CD40 agonist) seek to overcome PDAC resistance to ICB. Cancer vaccines and CAR T cells aim to enhance T effector cell activity. HCQ inhibits autophagosome-mediated MHC-1 degradation hence preventing T cell anergy. Multiple experimental agents have been developed to modulate the immunosuppressant phenotype of TME via inhibition of immunosuppressive cells (e.g., tumor-associated macrophages and myeloid-derived suppressor cells) and stromal components. Ectonucleotidase CD73 blockade limits accumulation of immunosuppressant adenosine in the extracellular space. *APC* antigen-presenting cell; *CAF* cancer-associated fibroblast; *CAR* chimeric antigen receptor; *CCL2* CC chemokine ligand 2; *CCR2* CC chemokine receptor 2; *CTLA-4* cytotoxic T-lymphocyte-associated protein 4; *CSF-1R* colony-stimulating factor 1 receptor; *FAK* focal adhesion kinase; *FAP* fibroblast, activation protein; *HCQ* hydroxychloroquine; ICB immune checkpoint inhibitor; *MHC-1* major histocompatibility complex class I; *PEGPH20* pegvorhyaluronidase alfa; *PD-1* programmed cell death protein 1; *PD-L1* programmed death-ligand 1; *PDAC* pancreatic ductal adenocarcinoma; *TME* tumor microenvironment

complete response (CR) and three with a partial response (PR). Median progression-free survival (PFS) and median overall survival (OS) in PDAC patients were, respectively, 2.1 months (95% CI 1.9–3.4) and 4 months (95% CI 2.1–9.8) [21].

As for the remaining majority of microsatellite stable (MSS) PDAC, single or combination immune checkpoint inhibitors showed minimal response. In a phase 2 trial with 27 advanced or mPDAC patients, no responder was observed with ipilimumab [16]. In mPDAC patients whose disease progressed after first-line chemotherapy, tremelimumab plus durvalumab showed an ORR of 3.1% (95% CI 0.08–16.22), while durvalumab alone had an ORR of 0% (95% CI 0.0–10.6) [22]. Indeed, MSS PDAC is an immunologically "cold" tumor characterized by a low median TMB of 2.7 mutations/megabase, limited neoantigenic targets, low MHC-I expression, as well as a TME-mediated suppression of T cell priming [5, 13, 23, 24]. To overcome the inherent limitations of ICI therapy in PDAC, multiple combination approaches are being developed.

2.1 Combined Chemo-Immunotherapy Approaches

In addition to direct cytotoxic effect on tumor cells, chemotherapy synergizes with immunotherapy by increasing tumor expression of MHC-I [25]. Furthermore, tumor cell death releases pathogen-associated molecular patterns and damage-associated molecular patterns (DAMPs), which are then detected by innate immune cells via toll-like receptors (TLRs) and cyclic GMP-AMP synthase–stimulator of interferon genes (cGAS–STING) DNA sensing pathway. Pattern recognition triggers release of inflammatory cytokines and type I interferons (IFN) leading to subsequent adaptive immune cell activation [26, 27]. The result is an immunopotentiation effect with T cell priming, enhanced intra-tumoral T cell infiltration, and T cell receptor (TCR) repertoire expansion [28]. In a phase 1b/2 study with treatment-naïve mPDAC patients, pembrolizumab plus gemcitabine/nab-paclitaxel (GnP) resulted in a median PFS of 9.1 months (95% CI 4.9–15.3) and median OS of 15 months (95% CI 6.8–22.6), respectively [29]. Whereas in another phase 1 study with advanced PDAC treated with nivolumab plus GnP, grade 3/4 adverse events were observed in 48 out of 50 patients, which led to treatment discontinuation in 18 patients. The ORR was 18% (95% CI 8.6–31.4), and the median OS was 9.9 months (95% CI 6.74–12.16) [30]. In a large randomized phase 2 trial conducted in Canada with 180 mPDAC patients, durvalumab/tremelimumab plus GnP as compared to GnP did not improve survival (respective median OS were 9.8 months and 8.8 months; HR 0.94, 90% CI 0.71–1.25, $P = 0.72$) or ORR (30.3% vs. 23.0% respectively; OR 1.49, 90% CI 0.81–2.72, $P = 0.28$) [31]. Additional clinical trials on combined chemo-immunotherapy in PDAC are underway (Table 2).

2.2 CD40 Agonism

Activation of CD40, a tumor necrosis factor receptor on DC surface, promotes adaptive immune activity via upregulation of MHC molecules and stimulatory cytokines including interleukin (IL) 12 [32]. In murine models, the agonistic CD40 monoclonal antibody sotigalimab (APX005M) co-administered with GnP sensitized pancreatic tumor cells to ICB via antigen-presenting cell (APC) and T cell priming [33]. The PRINCE trial is an open-label, multicenter study evaluating sotigalimab plus GnP with/without nivolumab in mPDAC patients. The non-randomized phase 1b experience with four cohorts has recently been reported. Patients in cohorts B received GnP plus sotigalimab at a lower dose of 0.1 mg/kg (cohort B1) and higher dose of 0.3 mg/kg (cohort B2), while cohorts C received GnP, nivolumab plus lower (cohort C1) and higher dosing (cohort C2) of sotigalimab [34]. The combination regimen demonstrated a favorable safety profile with dose-limiting toxicity (DLTs) observed in 2 of 24 evaluable patients (both febrile neutropenia). At a median follow-up of 17.8 months, a total of 14 patients experienced a PR while 7 had stable disease (SD). Median OS in cohorts B1 and B2 were 12.7 months (95% CI 1.1–not reached [NR]) and 20.1 months (95% CI 7.2–NR), respectively. Cohort C1 reported a median OS of 15.9 months (95% CI 0.5–NR). Median OS in C2 was not evaluable due to limited number of mortality events at data cut-off. The

Table 2 Ongoing registered clinical trials evaluating experimental immunotherapeutic agents in pancreas cancer

NCT Identifier	Phase	Experimental arm	Control arm	Target population	Primary endpoints	Status	Estimated completion
ICB and Chemotherapy							
NCT03264404	2	Azacitidine + pembrolizumab	None	PDAC, locally advanced or metastatic	PFS	Recruiting	December 31, 2021
NCT02879318	2	GnP + durvalumab + tremelimumab	GnP	PDAC, stage IV	OS	Active, not recruiting	June 30, 2021
ICI plus PARPi							
NCT03404960	1/2	Niraparib + nivolumab or ipilimumab	None	PDAC, locally advanced or metastatic	PFS	Recruiting	June 2021
NCT03851614	2	Durvalumab + cediranib or olaparib	None	Locally advanced or metastatic mismatch repair proficient solid tumors including PDAC	Changes in genomic and immune biomarkers	Recruiting	March 1, 2022
NCT03637491	1/2	Binimetinib ± avelumab ± talazoparib	None	Locally advanced or metastatic *RAS*-mutant solid tumor including PDAC	DLT, ORR	Recruiting	November 28, 2024
NCT04666740	2	Pembrolizumab + olaparib	None	Metastatic PDAC with homologous recombination gene alterations or platinum sensitivity	PFS	Recruiting	January 2024
ICB and Purinergic Modulators							
NCT03454451	1	CPI-006 alone and combined with pembrolizumab or ciforadenant	None	Locally advanced or metastatic solid tumor including PDAC	DLT, AE, MTD	Recruiting	December 2023

NCT03207867	2	NIR178 + PDR001	None	Locally advanced or metastatic solid tumor including PDAC	ORR	Recruiting	December 1, 2021
NCT03884556	1	TTX-030 ± pembrolizumab ± docetaxel ± GnP	None	Locally advanced or metastatic solid tumor including PDAC	RP2D	Recruiting	March 2022
Additional ICB Combined Therapies							
NCT03214250	1/2	GnP ± nivolumab ± APX005M	None	PDAC, stage IV	AE, OS	Active, not recruiting	September 1, 2022
NCT02907099	2	Pembrolizumab + CXCR4 Antagonist BL-8040	None	PDAC, stage IV	ORR	Active, not recruiting	December 31, 2022
NCT04007744	1	Sonidegib + pembrolizumab	None	Locally advanced or metastatic solid tumor including PDAC	MTD, ORR	Recruiting	July 31, 2022
NCT04050085	1	Nivolumab + radiation + TLR9 Agonist SD-101	None	PDAC, stage IV	AE	Recruiting	November 5, 2021
NCT03723915	2	Pembrolizumab + Pelareorep	None	PDAC, locally advanced or metastatic	ORR	Active, not recruiting	June 15, 2021
NCT03193190	1/2	Atezolizumab with and without GnP ± third targeted agent[a]	GnP or mFOLFOX6	PDAC, stage IV	ORR, AE	Recruiting	November 3, 2021
NCT04327986	1/2	M7824 + M7824 ± SBRT	None	Unresectable or borderline resectable PDAC	ORR, RP2D	Not yet recruiting	December 31, 2025
NCT03841110	1	FT500 ± ICI (nivolumab, pembrolizumab, or atezolizumab)	None	Advanced solid tumor including PDAC	AE	Recruiting	June 2022

(continued)

Table 2 (continued)

NCT Identifier	Phase	Experimental arm	Control arm	Target population	Primary endpoints	Status	Estimated completion
Adoptive Cell Therapy							
NCT03638193	NA	Anti-MSLN CAR T cell	None	PDAC, locally advanced or metastatic	AE	Recruiting	February 1, 2022
NCT03323944	1	Anti-MSLN CAR T cell	None	PDAC, locally advanced or metastatic	AE	Recruiting	September 2021
NCT03638206	1/2	Anti-MSLN CAR T cell	None	MSLN-expressing PDAC	AE	Recruiting	March 1, 2023
NCT03682744	1	Anti-CEA CAR T cell	None	CEA-expressing adenocarcinoma peritoneal metastases or malignant ascites including PDAC	AE	Active, not recruiting	March 2021
NCT04037241	2/3	Anti-CEA CAR T cell ± irinotecan + 5FU ± GnP ± capecitabine	GnP, rirnotecan + 5FU, or capecitabine	CEA-expressing PDAC with unresectable liver metastases	OS	Not yet recruiting	January 1, 2022
NCT03818165	1	Anti-CEA CAR T cell	None	PDAC, stage IV	OS	Active, not recruiting	February 1, 2022
NCT02850536	1	Anti-CEA CAR T cell	None	CEA-expressing liver metastases or PDAC	AE	Active, not recruiting	February 2021
NCT02744287	1/2	Anti-PSCA CAR T cell (BPX-601) + Rimiducid	None	Metastatic solid tumor including PDAC	DLT, AE, MTD	Recruiting	February 2024

NCT03302403	NA	Anti-claudin 18 CAR T cell	None	Advanced tumor including PDAC	AE	Active, not recruiting	December 12, 2023
NCT03159819	NA	Anti-claudin 18 CAR T cell	None	Advanced tumor including PDAC	AE	Recruiting	December 31, 2021
NCT04404595	1	Anti-claudin 18 CAR T cell	None	CLDN18.2-positive tumor including PDAC	AE, MTD	Recruiting	September 1, 2035
NCT04581473	1/2	Anti-claudin 18 CAR T cell	None	CLDN18.2-positive advanced solid tumor including PDAC	AE, MTD, ORR	Recruiting	December 1, 2022
NCT01420874	1	EGFR BATs + FOLFOX6	None	Advanced tumor including PDAC	AE	Active, not recruiting	June 2021
NCT03269526	1/2	EGFR BATs	None	PDAC, locally advanced or metastatic	AE, OS	Recruiting	March 1, 2023
NCT04137536	1	EGFR BATs	None	PDAC, stage IV	AE	Recruiting	April 2022
NCT03093688	1/2	Anti-KRN7000 invariant Natural killer T cell + PD-1 + CD8 + T cell	None	Advanced tumor including PDAC	AE, ORR	Recruiting	June 30, 2022
Cancer Vaccines							
NCT03136406	1/2	GI-4000 + chemotherapy	None	PDAC progressed on or after chemotherapy	AE, ORR	Active, not recruiting	April 2021
NCT03329248	1/2	GI-4000 ± SRBT ± chemotherapy	None	PDAC progressed on or after chemotherapy	AE, ORR	Active, not recruiting	NA
NCT03387098	1/2	GI-4000 ± SRBT ± chemotherapy	None	PDAC progressed on or after chemotherapy	AE, ORR	Active, not recruiting	NA

(continued)

Table 2 (continued)

NCT Identifier	Phase	Experimental arm	Control arm	Target population	Primary endpoints	Status	Estimated completion
NCT00669734	1	PANVAC-F (falimarev) vaccine + PANVAC-V (inalimarev)	None	PDAC, locally advanced or metastatic	MTD	Active, not recruiting	March 1, 2021
NCT01595321	NA	PANC 10.05 pcDNA-1/GM-Neo and PANC 6.03 pcDNA-1/GM-Neo vaccine ± SBRT, FOLFIRINOX, and Cy	None	Chemotherapy-naïve resected PDAC	AE	Active, not recruiting	August 2021
NCT03153410	1	GVAX, Cy, pembrolizumab, and IMC-CS4 (LY3022855)	None	Borderline resectable PDAC	AE, tumor CD8 T cell density	Recruiting	September 2021
NCT02648282	2	GVAX, Cy, pembrolizumab, and SBRT	None	PDAC, locally advanced	DMFS	Active, not recruiting	July 2021
NCT03161379	2	GVAX, Cy, nivolumab, and SBRT	None	Borderline resectable PDAC	Tumor CD8 T cell density	Recruiting	January 2023
NCT03190265	2	Nivolumab + ipilimumab + CRS-207 ± GVAX/Cy	None	PDAC, stage IV	ORR	Recruiting	October 2023
NCT03006302	2	Epacadostat + pembrolizumab + GVAX/Cy or CRS-207	None	PDAC, stage IV	Recommended dose, 6-month survival	Recruiting	June 2023
NCT03552718	1	Personalized neoepitope yeast-based vaccine (YE-NEO-001)	None	Surgically resectable solid tumor including PDAC	AE, RP2D	Recruiting	NA
NCT01088789	2	PANC 10.05 pcDNA-1/GM-Neo and PANC 6.03 pcDNA-1 neo vaccine ± Cy	None	PDAC, stage I or II	DFS	Recruiting	April 2023
NCT02600949	1	Synthetic Tumor-Associated Peptide Vaccine Therapy + pembrolizumab + imiquimod	None	Metastatic solid tumor including PDAC	DLT, proportion of patients that receives personalized vaccine	Recruiting	May 31, 2021

KRAS-Targeted Therapy							
NCT03608631	1	Mesenchymal Stromal Cells-derived Exosomes with $KRAS^{G12D}$ siRNA	None	PDAC, stage IV	MTD, OS, PFS, minimal residual disease rate	Not yet recruiting	March 2022
NCT03948763	1	V941(mRNA-5671/V941) ± pembrolizumab	None	Locally advanced or metastatic solid tumor including PDAC	DLT, AE, discontinuation rate	Recruiting	November 19, 2026
Autophagy inhibitor							
NCT01506973	1/2	Hydroxychloroquine + GnP	None	PDAC, locally advanced or metastatic	OS	Active, not recruiting	March 2021
NCT03825289	1	Hydroxychloroquine + trametinib	None	PDAC, stage II to IV	DLT, RP2D	Recruiting	January 18, 2025
NCT04132505	1	Hydroxychloroquine + binimetinib	None	PDAC, stage IV	MTD	Recruiting	May 31, 2020
NCT04214418	1/2	Cobimetinib + Hydroxychloroquine + Atezolizumab	None	Locally advanced or metastatic solid tumor including PDAC	MTD	Recruiting	September 2023
Stroma-Modulating Agents							
NCT03941093	3	Pamrevlumab + GnP	GnP	PDAC, locally advanced	OS, resection rate	Recruiting	December 2023
NCT03415854	2	Paricalcitol, cisplatin, GnP	None	PDAC, stage IV	Pathologic complete response rate	Active, not recruiting	December 31, 2020
NCT03520790	1/2	Paricalcitol + GnP	GnP	PDAC, stage IV	AE, OS	Active, not recruiting	November 30, 2025

(continued)

Table 2 (continued)

NCT Identifier	Phase	Experimental arm	Control arm	Target population	Primary endpoints	Status	Estimated completion
NCT02546531	1	Defactinib plus pembrolizumab, with or without gemcitabine	None	Locally advanced or metastatic solid tumor including PDAC	RP2D, MTD	Active, not recruiting	July 31, 2021
NCT02758587	1/2	Defactinib plus pembrolizumab	None	Locally advanced or metastatic solid tumor including PDAC	AE	Recruiting	December 2021

5-FU fluorouracil; *AE* adverse events; *Cy* cyclophosphamide; *DC* dendritic cell; *DLT* dose-limiting toxicity; *DMFS* distant metastasis free survival; *EGFR BATs* anti-CD3 and anti-EGFR bispecific antibody armed activated T cells; *GnP* gemcitabine and nab-paclitaxel; *ICI* immune checkpoint inhibitor; *MTD* maximum tolerated dose; *mTCR* murine T-cell receptor; *NK* natural killer; *ORR* objective response; *OS* overall survival; *PARPi* poly-ADP ribose polymerase inhibitor; *PBL* peripheral blood lymphocytes; *PDAC* pancreatic ductal adenocarcinoma; *PFS* progression-free survival; *RP2D* recommended phase 2 dose; *siRNA* small interference RNA; *SBRT* stereotactic radiation therapy

[a]Targeted agents include Cobimetinib, PEGPH20, BL-8040, Selicrelumab, Bevacizumab, RO6874281, AB928, Tiragolumab, and Tocilizumab

randomized phase 2 component of this trial has completed recruitment and is pending results (NCT03214250).

2.3 Immune Checkpoint Blockade and DNA Damage Response

Altered DNA damage response (DDR) genes lead to abundant tumor somatic mutations and neoantigen production which in turn favors T cell activation [35]. In particular, mutated *BRCA1/2* results in homologous recombination deficiency (HRD) leading to impaired DNA double-strand break repair [36]. In a tumor sample set from Caris Life Sciences of 2824 patients, 124 (4.4%) PDAC patients harbored *BRCA1/2* mutations which were significantly associated with higher PD-L1 expression (22% vs. 11%, $P < 0.001$), elevated TMB (mean 8.7 mutations/megabase vs. 6.5, $P < 0.001$), as well as higher MSI-H frequency (4.8% vs. 1.2%, $P = 0.002$) [37]. Poly-ADP-ribose polymerase (PARP) inhibition prevents DNA single-strand breaks repair causing synthetic lethality in HRD tumor cells [38]. The phase 3 POLO (Pancreas OLaparib Ongoing) trial enrolled germline *BRCA1/2*-mutated mPDAC patients who had stable or responding disease to first-line platinum-based therapy. In this randomized study, maintenance dose of PARP inhibitor (PARPi) olaparib was associated with a significantly longer median PFS as compared to placebo (7.4 vs. 3.8 months, respectively; HR 0.53, 95% CI 0.35–0.82, $P = 0.004$), albeit median OS were overlapping (18.9 months with olaparib vs. 18.1 months with placebo; HR 0.91, 95% CI 0.56–1.46, $P = 0.68$) [39].

The clinical activity of combined ICB plus PARPi is being evaluated by multiple ongoing trials. The PARPVAX trial is a phase 1/2, randomized, open-label study examining the efficacy of niraparib plus nivolumab or ipilimumab in patients with advanced or mPDAC who have received ≥16 weeks of therapy without evidence of disease progression (NCT03404960). Similarly, mPDAC patients with a germline *BRCA1/2* mutation with stable/responding disease to platinum-based therapy are randomized to olaparib with/without pembrolizumab in a phase 2 trial from the South West Oncology Group (NCT04548752). The phase 2 POLAR trial is currently examining the efficacy of pembrolizumab plus olaparib in mPDAC patients (NCT04666740). Enrolled individuals will be assigned to three cohorts based on their status of HRD status (mutations in core HDR genes [*BRCA1/2* or *PALB2*] vs. in non-core HRD genes) and a third cohort who have had an exceptional response to prior platinum therapy. Additional ongoing trials are displayed in Table 2.

2.4 Purinergic Signaling and Immunotherapy

Tumor cell lysis and subsequent leakage of adenosine triphosphate (ATP) to the extracellular space constitute an immunostimulant purinergic signal that promotes DC activation, chemotaxis, and T cell effector priming. Conversely, extracellular catalysis of ATP by ectonucleotidases generates adenosine nucleosides which suppress immune responses and limit T cell response to ICB [40]. Overexpression of ectonucleotidase CD73 in PDAC TME is correlated with an increased tumor burden, treatment resistance, metastasis, and poor prognosis [41, 42]. Preclinical studies have demonstrated inhibition of CD73 synergized antitumor activity of anti-PD-1 and anti-CTLA-4 therapies [43]. Clinical evidence of CD73 blockade in PDAC is emerging. ARC-8 is an ongoing phase 1, open-label study with therapy-naïve mPDAC patients treated with escalating dose of CD73 inhibitor AB680 in addition to PD-1 inhibitor zimberelimab and GnP (NCT04104672). Preliminary analyses of 16 patients showed favorable safety and tolerability profile with one case of DLT (grade 2 autoimmune hepatitis). Amongst nine response-evaluable patients, three PRs and five patients with SD were observed [44]. In another phase 1 open-label study with advanced PDAC and colorectal cancer, no DLT was reported in 42 patients treated with the anti-CD73 monoclonal antibody (mAb) oleclumab or in 24 treated with oleclumab plus durvalumab [45]. Out of 20 PDAC patients, 2 PRs and 3 SD were reported.

The MORPHEUS platform is a phase 1b/2, open-label, multicenter, randomized umbrella study that aims to compare safety and efficacy of multiple ICB-based combined regimens across different cancer types [46]. The MORPHEUS-Pancreatic Cancer trial is enrolling untreated and chemotherapy-pre-treated patients with advanced mPDAC (NCT03193190). The control arm patients receive GnP, while participants in multiple experimental arms will receive atezolizumab with/without GnP plus a third targeted agent with immunomodulatory activity. In the previously treated disease setting, interim analyses from an atezolizumab-based regimen without chemotherapy demonstrated limited benefit when combined with the HA-degrading enzyme pegvorhyaluronidase alfa (PEGPH20) (ORR 0%, 95% CI 0–24.7) [47], cobimetinib (MEK inhibitor) (ORR 0%, CI not reported) [48], BL-8040 (C-X-C chemokine receptor [CXCR] 4 antagonist) (ORR 0%, 95% CI 0–23) [49], or with RO6874281 (anti-FAP/IL-2 fusion protein) (ORR 7.1% in the every other week arm, 95% CI not reported) [50]. The efficacy and safety of ICB-based regimen combined with front-line chemotherapy are being explored in junction with tocilizumab (anti-IL6), selicrelumab (CD40), tiragolumab (anti-T cell immunoglobulin and ITIM domain [TIGIT]), and AB928 (adenosine modulator) amongst other novel agents.

3 Adoptive Cell Therapy

Adoptive T cell therapy is designed to induce specific antitumor activity against genetically pre-selected tumor surface proteins, carbohydrates, or glycolipids [51]. Chimeric antigen receptor (CAR) T cells have led to therapeutic breakthroughs in many hematological malignancies, albeit their application in solid tumor remains limited. This is partly due to poor engraftment and expansion of infused CAR T cells exacerbated by an immunosuppressive TME [52]. Preconditioning with chemotherapy (e.g., cyclophosphamide with/without fludarabine) has been shown to increase the release of proinflammatory cytokine and efficacy in CAR T cell-treated leukemia [52, 53]. Furthermore, CAR T cell therapy in solid tumors is hindered by lack of identification of an ideal antigen target, as expression of tumor-associated antigens in normal tissues leads to dose-limiting on-target/off-tumor toxicity [54, 55]. In the treatment of PDAC, CAR T cell therapy is in the preclinical and early-clinical phase of development (Tables 1 and 2).

Carcinoembryonic antigen (CEA) is a cell surface glycoprotein that plays an essential role in cell adhesion in the gastrointestinal tract during early fetal development [56]. CEA as tumor marker is overexpressed in 75% of PDAC as well as in colorectal, liver, and gastric tumors [56]. Despite low expression in the normal respiratory and gastrointestinal epithelia, first generation anti-CEA CAR T cells led to severe autoimmune colitis and pneumonitis in treated individuals [54, 55]. Raj et al. developed CAR T cells targeted against CEA-related cell adhesion molecule 7 (CEACAM7), which is found on the surface of PDAC cells and restrictively expressed in normal colon and pancreatic tissues. Anti-CEACAM7 CAR T cells induced complete regression of primary tumors and hepatic metastases in three of five treated murine models, and improved median OS as compared to control mice treated with non-modified CAR T cells (61 vs. 29 days, respectively, range not reported, $P < 0.05$) [57]. On a cautionary note, all surviving mice in the experimental arm developed graft versus host syndrome and were euthanized. The role of CEACAM7 as target for CAR T cell in PDAC warrants further exploration.

Mesothelin (MSLN) is a glycoprotein present in more than 80% of PDAC, as well as in normal pleura, pericardium, and peritoneum at low levels. MSLN is postulated to promote tumor cell adhesion, invasion, and survival [58]. To limit duration of toxicity, mRNA-based method has been applied to develop T cells that transiently express CAR, albeit it required frequent infusions to sustain immunologic activity. In a phase 1 trial with mPDAC patients whose disease has progressed on chemotherapy, six patients received anti-MSLN CAR T cell therapy with scheduled infusions of three times weekly for up to 3 weeks [59]. The study demonstrated a favorable safety and tolerability without any DLT. Two patients experienced SD with respective PFS of 3.8 and 5.4 months. In another study with 19 patients with solid tumors, 5 PDAC patients treated with anti-MSLN CAR T cells were included. Of these, 2 SD with limited response duration of 2 and 3 months were observed. In the same study, pre-treatment cyclophosphamide (Cy) enhanced initial CAR T cell expansion, albeit did not improve graft survival beyond 28 days [60]. Anti-MSLN CAR T cells co-delivered with Cy and B cell-depleting anti-CD19 CAR T cells were tested in three patients with chemo-refractory mPDAC [61]. Despite overall safety profile without DLT and successful B cell depletion in all patients, anti-MSLN CAR T cell levels became undetectable by post-infusion day 7–10. Concurrent PD-1 blockade showed potentiation of CAR T cell therapy and TME remodeling in murine models [62]. In a pilot study, patients harboring MSLN-positive advanced tumors received anti-MSLN CAR T cells with PD-1 disruption by CRISPR-Cas9 system (NCT03747965). Interim analysis with nine patients including six cases of PDAC showed no significant on-target/off-tumor toxicity or autoimmune toxicity. Overall, seven patients were response-evaluable, four achieved SD and two a PR. PDAC-specific survival or response data was not reported [63].

Overexpression of CD133, a biomarker for cancer stem cell linked to tumor survival and metastasis, is detected in 50% of PDAC [64]. A single-arm phase 1 trial enrolled 23 patients with metastatic solid tumors treated with anti-CD133 CAR T cells [65]. In the mPDAC cohort with seven participants, two experienced a PR lasting 2 and 4 months; three had SD lasting 3 to 10 months at study cut-off. No DLT was observed. All treated mPDAC patients exhibited leukopenia, which included one case of grade 3 and one of grade 4 of severity.

Prostate stem cell antigen (PSCA) is normally detected at low levels in prostate, kidney, bladder, stomach, and esophagus [66]. It is overexpressed in 60–80% of PDAC and also detected in PanIN [66, 67]. BPX-601 is an autologous anti-PSCA CAR T cell that harbors a MyD88/CD40 co-activation domain inducible by administration of rimiducid and its safety and efficacy are being examined by an ongoing phase 1/2 open-label, non-randomized trial with metastatic solid tumors (NCT02744287). In a preliminary analysis with 18 PSCA-positive mPDAC patients, 13 individuals had evaluable response which included 8 with a SD and 5 with progression of disease (PD) (duration of response not reported) [68].

Despite epidermal growth factor receptor (EGFR) blockade demonstrating only modest clinical activity in advanced PDAC patients [69], preclinical evidence suggests that dual inhibition of EGFR and CD3-positive T cells enhances T-cell mediated cytotoxicity in *EGFR*-positive tumor cells [70]. In a phase 1/2 study, anti-CD3 and anti-EGFR bispecific antibody armed activated T cells (EGFR BATs) were infused in advanced PDAC patients [71]. There were no associated DLTs or persistent grade 3/4 adverse events. Post-apheresis peripheral blood mononuclear cells showed specific cytotoxicity and increased natural killer (NK) cell activity. Median OS and median time to progression in seven evaluable patients were, respectively, 31 months and 7 months (CI not reported). The safety and early efficacy profile of EGFR BATs is being examined in an ongoing phase 1 study with mPDAC patients whose disease progressed on first-line chemotherapy (NCT04137536).

Adoptive cell therapy is a rapidly growing field and its efficacy, safety, optimal dosing schedules, and preconditioning regimens in PDAC treatment are currently under evaluation in multiple early-phase clinical trials. Additional antigen targets evaluated with CAR T cell therapy are described in Tables 1 and 2.

4 Therapeutic Vaccines

Cancer vaccines trigger or expand patients' own tumoricidal T cell response by delivering tumor antigen in the forms of peptide, DNA plasmid, mRNA, DCs, or whole tumor cell [72]. Despite induction of T cell immunity in patients, confirmatory trials yielded negative results with vaccine therapies targeting murine alpha-1,3-galactosyltransferase (Algenpantucel-L) [73], human telomerase reverse transcriptase (hTERT) peptide [74], survivin [75], and vascular endothelial growth factor receptor 2 peptide (elpamotide) [76]. Additional antigen targets for vaccine approach are under investigation.

GVAX is an irradiated allogeneic whole pancreatic cancer cell-based vaccine. In addition to antigen presentation, these cells are designed to stimulate antigen-presenting cell (APC) uptake and T cell priming by expressing GM-CSF. Despite initial promising results in previously treated mPDAC patients [77], combination regimens of GVAX with Cy plus CRS-207, a live attenuated mesothelin-expression *Listeria monocytogenes*, failed to meet the primary efficacy endpoint when compared to physician's choice of single-agent chemotherapy. Median OS in comparator arms were overlapping: 3.7 months (95% CI 2.9–5.3) in GVAX/Cy/CRS-207 arm, 5.4 months (95% CI 4.2–6.4) in CRS alone arm, and 4.6 months (95% CI 4.2–5.7) in control arm [78]. In another phase 2 open-label study with 93 mPDAC patients, GVAX/Cy/CRS-207 demonstrated similar median OS of 6.1 months (95% CI 3.5–7), whereas concomitant nivolumab did not provide an additive survival benefit (median OS 5.9 months, 95% CI 4.75–8.6) [79]. In a maintenance setting for mPDAC patients treated with front-line folinic acid, fluorouracil, irinotecan, and oxaliplatin (FOLFIRINOX), a randomized phase 2 trial of GVAX/Cy/ipilimumab versus continuation of FOLFIRINOX did not improve outcomes with respective median OS 9.38 (95% CI 5.0–12.2) and 14.7 months (95% CI 11.6–20) (HR 1.75, 95% CI 1.09–2.79, $P = 0.019$) [80]. Notably, in GVAX-treated patients who experienced longer survival, TME acquired an immunostimulant phenotype with a higher intra-tumoral density of T helper cells, T effector cells, and NK cells, as well as depleted immunosuppressant myeloid cell lineages [78–80].

Upon vaccine delivery, antigen is captured by peripheral APCs which undergo activation and then migration to lymph nodes for antigen presentation to T cells. In vitro generated DC-based vaccine displays direct homing from peripheral injection site to lymphoid organs, bypassing these first steps. DNA, mRNA, whole-cell antigens, or peptides may be used to generate antigen-pulsed DCs [81]. In a phase 1 pilot trial with seven PDAC patients whose disease progressed following surgery and chemotherapy, MUC-1-peptide-pulsed DC cells administration was safe with no reported grade 3/4 toxicities, albeit no disease control was attained [82]. In another study, DCs were pulsed with three tumor peptides (hTERT, CEA, and survivin). TLR-3 agonist poly-ICLC was co-delivered to trigger direct DC activation and to augment T cell responses [83]. Twelve patients with locally advanced or mPDAC received treatment without DLT. In eight response-evaluable patients, four experienced SD with three showing antigen-specific T cell generation. Overall median OS was 7.7 months (CI not reported), with one patient surviving 28 months post-apheresis.

4.1 Cancer Vaccines and a Renewed Approach to Target *KRAS*

Abou-Alfa et al. administered a *KRAS* peptide vaccine specific to patient tumor's *KRAS* mutation boosted with recombinant human GM-CSF [84]. Twenty-four PDAC patients received *KRAS* vaccine as an adjuvant therapy. No grade 3 or 4 adverse effect was reported. Amongst nine evaluable patients, only one exhibited a specific immune response to *KRAS* on delayed-type hypersensitivity test. Overall median OS was 20.3 months (95% CI 11.6–45.3), which was similar to median OS observed in patients who received only adjuvant *KRAS* vaccine (19 months, 95% CI 3.6–45.9). In another cohort of PDAC patients treated with adjuvant anti-*KRAS* peptide vaccines, long-term follow-up demonstrated 10-year survival rates of 16% in all vaccinated patients (3 in 19 patients, CI not reported) and of 19% amongst the immune responders (3 out of 16 patients, CI not reported) [85]. No survivors from non-vaccinated cohort were reported at 10-year follow-up. An ongoing open-label phase 1 trial is exploring the safety of adjuvant *KRAS* long peptide vaccine combined with poly-ICLC adjuvant, nivolumab, and ipilimumab (NCT04117087). Similarly, an open-label phase 1 with mature DCs-based vaccine pulsed with HLA-specific *KRAS* short peptide (mDC3/8-*KRAS* vaccine) is currently in the recruitment phase (NCT03592888). mRNA-derived cancer vaccine V941 harbors immunostimulatory activity against $KRAS^{G12D}$, $KRAS^{G12V}$, $KRAS^{G13D}$, and $KRAS^{G12C}$, and its safety with/without pembrolizumab is being examined in an ongoing phase 1 trial (NCT03948763).

Despite modest activity, these studies highlight the safety and feasibility of administering vaccine-based therapies to PDAC patients. More importantly, vaccine-induced tumor-specific T cell priming and TME remodeling suggest potential therapeutic synergy with immunomodulatory agents [86]. Preclinical models have shown vaccine-induced tumor regression may be amplified with concomitant inhibition of ICB, and CD40 [87–89], albeit clinical efficacy remains to be verified.

5 Targeting the Tumor Microenvironment

PDAC TME provides a therapeutic obstacle hindering the delivery and efficacy of chemotherapy, immunotherapy, and adoptive cell therapy. The cellular component of TME comprised of TAMs, T regulatory (Treg) cells, and myeloid-derived suppressor cells (MDSCs) promotes an immunosuppressive phenotype constraining cytotoxic T cell responses. These cells also release proinflammatory cytokines that upregulate PSCs and CAFs, which in turn promotes a highly fibrotic stroma limiting drug delivery and cytotoxic T cell infiltration [13]. Diverse therapeutic strategies to target PDAC TME are being investigated preclinically and clinically.

5.1 Targeting Tumor-Adjacent Immunosuppressive Cells

TAMs promote tumor angiogenesis, metastasis, chemoresistance, and immune evasion via secretion of immunosuppressive cytokines [9, 90]. In murine models, colony-stimulating factor-1 receptor (CSF-1R) inhibition led to TAMs depletion, intratumor T cell infiltration, and enhancement of ICB activity [91]. Despite encouraging early-phase results [92], a phase 2 open-label study with the anti-CSF-1R monoclonal antibody, cabiralizumab, plus nivolumab with/without chemotherapy (GnP or folinic acid/fluorouracil/oxaliplatin [FOLFOX]), did not meet the primary endpoint of PFS benefit when compared to chemotherapy alone (GnP or fluorouracil/leucovorin/liposomal irinotecan [FOLFIRI]) [93]. Specific details are pending. In another phase 1 study, the CSF-1R inhibitor, pexidartinib, plus durvalumab achieved SD in 4 (21%, range not reported) of 19 patients with advanced PDAC and colon cancer, PDAC-specific survival data has not been reported [94]. Enrollment of the expansion cohort of the same study was completed, updated results are pending (NCT02777710).

The activation of CC chemokine ligand 2 (CCL2) and receptor 2 (CCR2) axis promotes mobilization and conversion of bone marrow monocytes to TAMs. In an open-label, non-randomized phase 1b study, patients with borderline resectable or locally advanced PDAC received either FOLFIRINOX alone ($N = 8$) or combined with oral CCR2 inhibitor PF-04136309 ($N = 39$) [95]. After median follow-up of 77 days (IQR 70–90), over 10% of the patients in the experimental arm developed grade 3 or higher adverse events, and DLTs were observed in two (5%) participants. Within the response-evaluable cohort of the PF-04136309 arm ($N = 33$), a PR was reported in 16 patients (48.5%, 95% CI 30.8–66.5), 10 (30%, CI not reported) of which underwent successful excisional surgery. In another study with treatment-naïve mPDAC patients, PF-04136309 plus GnP showed ORR in five patients (23.8%, 95% CI 8.2–47.2) which were all PRs [96]. Four DLTs were seen in three patients. Phase 2 of the study appeared to be terminated due to business-related decisions (NCT02732938).

MDSC recruitment due to compensatory granulocytic chemokine release by fibroblasts may mediate resistance to CSF-1R blockade therapy [97, 98]. MDSCs exert immunosuppressive activity and their levels have been correlated with disease progression in PDAC [9], albeit clinical data on MDSCs suppression is limited. In murine models, dual blockade of MDSCs and TAMs via respective inhibition of CXCR2 and CCR2 augmented antitumor response to FOLFORINOX [99]. In PDAC patients, preconditioning gemcitabine/fluorouracil decreased peripheral blood MDSCs, and improved median OS when combined with cytokine-induced killer (CIK) cells vs. CIK alone (14.9 months vs. 5.6 months, respectively, CI not reported, $P = 0.001$) [100]. In another study, peripheral MDSCs depletion was achieved with an agonistic TRAIL-R2 antibody, DS-8273a, in patients with advanced cancer including one case of PDAC [101]. Despite no difference in clinical response was observed (data not reported), lower post-treatment levels of MDSC were significantly correlated with longer time to progression (at post-treatment at day 42, Spearman $R = -0.98$, $P < 0.0001$).

5.2 Targeting Stromal Elements

The dense stroma produced by tumor-adjacent PSCs and CAFs is composed of abundant HA, collagen, and fibronectin [13]. HA-degrading therapy with PEGPH20 demonstrated promising results from early trials in advanced PDAC patients [102, 103]. Notwithstanding, a phase 2 trial with modified FOLFIRINOX with/without

PEGPH20 was prematurely closed due to increased mortality and toxicity in enrolled mPDAC patients with an unselected HA status. The interim analyses favored modified FOLFIRINOX over combined regimen with PEGPH20, respective median OS were 14.4 months (95% CI 10.1–15.7) vs. 7.7 months (95% CI 4.6–9.3) (HR = 2.07, 95% CI 1.28–3.34, $P < 0.01$) [104]. In parallel, the phase 3 HALO 109-301 trial with mPDAC patients with high HA-expressing tumors, the addition of PEGPH20 to GnP did not improve survival as compared to GnP alone, respective median OS were 11.2 (95% CI 10.3–12.3) and 11.5 months (95% CI 9.0–12.5) (HR 1.00, 95% CI 0.80–1.27, $P = 0.97$) [105].

Overexpressed connective tissue growth factor (CTGF) correlates with high degrees of tumor desmoplasia [106]. In a randomized phase 1/2 trial in locally advanced PDAC patients, adding anti-CTGF mAb pamrevlumab to neoadjuvant GnP improved patient eligibility for surgical exploration (17 patients in the combination arm vs. 2 in GnP arm, $P = 0.0019$), albeit tumor resection rates were not significantly different (8 of 17 patients vs. 1 in 3 patients, respectively, $P = 0.119$) [107]. Median OS were similar and were 19.3 months (95% CI 13.3–27.7) and 19 months (95% CI 13.2–NR), respectively. A phase 3 of the trial is currently assessing the safety and efficacy of neoadjuvant pamrevlumab plus GnP in locally advanced PDAC (NCT03941093).

Fibroblast activation protein (FAP) expressed in CAFs has been implicated in tumorigenesis, metastasis, and poor prognosis in PDAC [108]. Under physiological circumstances, FAP is undetectable in intact healthy tissue and only expressed during tissue remodeling, wound healing, and embryogenesis [109]. Anti-FAP CAR T cells decreased tumor growth, stromagenesis, and angiogenesis in syngeneic murine PDAC models [110], albeit lethal bone toxicity and cachexia were observed in other tumor models [111]. FAP-expressing fibroblasts also secrete CXCL12 which ligates CXCR4 on PDAC cells resulting in tumor survival and growth [112]. An inhibited CXCR4-CXCL12 axis facilitated T cell infiltration in the TME and enhanced anti-PD-1 activity in PDAC cell models [113]. In an open-label phase 1a study, LY2510924, a selective CXCR4 antagonist, combined with durvalumab, was administered to eight patients with PDAC and one with rectal cancer [114]. The combined regimen had a favorable safety profile without DLT. Of four patients who experienced SD, three were PDAC patients. Preliminary analyses from MORPHEUS-Pancreatic Cancer trial in patients with previously treated mPDAC (second line setting), atezolizumab plus motixafortide (BL-8040) showed limited clinical efficacy with reported SD in 1 (7.1%, 95% CI 0.18–33.87) of 14 patients, as opposed to 6 (40%, 95% CI 16.34–67.71) out of 15 patients treated with chemotherapy (modified FOLFOX-6 or GnP) [49]. In the phase 2 COMBAT trial with 22 mPDAC patients, motixafortide plus pembrolizumab plus chemotherapy (liposomal irinotecan/5-fluorouracil/leucovorin) showed disease control in 17 (77%, 95% CI not reported) patients, including 7 with a PR and 10 with SD [115], which was modestly higher than the historically reported disease control rate (DCR) with chemotherapy alone in the NAPOLI-1 study (DCR 52%, 95% CI 43–61) [116].

Vitamin D receptor (VDR) acts as a transcriptional regulator implicated in PSCs quiescence, and VDR agonism in murine models leads to stromal remodeling and putatively enhanced response to chemotherapy [117]. The efficacy of the vitamin D analog paricalcitol is being evaluated in mPDAC patients in combination with GnP (NCT03520790), GnP and cisplatin (NCT03415854) as well as a maintenance therapy with pembrolizumab (NCT03331562).

6 Autophagy Inhibition

KRAS-upregulated autophagy enables cancer cells to recycle their own intracellular compounds as an energy source hence ensuring growth and survival. Furthermore, autophagy contributes to immune escape by selectively targeting MHC-I molecules for lysosomal degradation. Inhibition of autophagy leads to enhanced antitumor immune response to dual PD-1 and CTLA-4 blockade in preclinical studies [5]. In a phase 2 trial with locally advanced and mPDAC patients, the autophagy inhibitor hydroxychloroquine (HCQ) plus GnP demonstrated a higher ORR compared to GnP alone (38% vs. 21% respectively, range not reported, $P = 0.047$), albeit 1-year survival rates were similar (41% vs. 49%, $P = 0.44$) [118]. HCQ combined with atezolizumab and cobimetinib is being examined by phase 1/2 MEKiAUTO trial (NCT04214418). This study is in the recruitment phase and will include a cohort of patients with *KRAS*-mutant advanced PDAC.

7 Future Perspectives

The complex oncogenic landscape of PDAC contributes to tumor growth while also fueling its immune resistance. Limited single-agent ICB activity points to the necessity of overcoming T cell anergy intrinsic to MSS pancreatic tumors. Whereas crosstalk between cancer cells and cellular and non-cellular elements in the stroma further exacerbates immunologic "coldness" of PDAC. The activity of chemo-immunotherapy in settings of a depleted or re-educated TME warrants further clinical exploration. Finally, quasi-universal *KRAS* mutations contribute to various non-redundant immune escape mechanisms in PDAC. Developing cancer vaccines and adoptive cell therapies enabled new pathways to abate the "undruggability" of *KRAS*, albeit their activities are yet to be translated into clinical responses. Trials such as MORPHEUS-Pancreatic cancer platform (NCT03193190) and PRINCE trial (NCT03214250) seek to combine tumoricidal effect of chemotherapy and ICB, while also promoting T cell priming or TME modulation via a third agent. Indeed, immunotherapy applied to PDAC is rapidly evolving towards a combined immune modulatory strategy. While novel multi-agent regimens may promise exciting theoretical antitumor synergy, the tolerability and toxicity associated with polypharmacy will assuredly remain as prospective challenges.

Compliance with Ethical Standards

Conflict of Interest/Disclosure Statement EOR: Research funding to MSK: Genentech-Roche, Celgene-BMS, BioNTech, BioAtla, AstraZeneca, Arcus.

Consulting/Advisory/DSMB: Cytomx Therapeutics, Rafael Therapeutics, Noxxon, Sobi, Silenseed, Molecular Templates, Boehringer Ingelheim, BioNTech, Ipsen, Polaris, Merck, AstraZeneca, Bayer, Genentech-Roche, Celgene-BMS, Eisai. MSK Institutional COI: BioNTech.

Funding NCI Cancer Center Support Grant: P30 CA008478.

David M. Rubenstein Center for Pancreas Cancer Research.

References

1. Siegel RL, Miller KD, Fuchs HE, Jemal A (2021) Cancer statistics, 2021. CA Cancer J Clin 71(1):7–33. https://doi.org/10.3322/caac.21654
2. Rahib L, Smith BD, Aizenberg R, Rosenzweig AB, Fleshman JM, Matrisian LM (2014) Projecting cancer incidence and deaths to 2030: the unexpected burden of thyroid, liver, and pancreas cancers in the United States. Cancer Res 74(11):2913–2921. https://doi.org/10.1158/0008-5472.CAN-14-0155
3. Torres C, Grippo PJ (2018) Pancreatic cancer subtypes: a roadmap for precision medicine. Ann Med 50(4):277–287. https://doi.org/10.1080/07853890.2018.1453168
4. Biankin AV, Waddell N, Kassahn KS, Gingras MC, Muthuswamy LB, Johns AL et al (2012) Pancreatic cancer genomes reveal aberrations in axon guidance pathway genes. Nature 491(7424):399–405. https://doi.org/10.1038/nature11547
5. Yamamoto K, Venida A, Yano J, Biancur DE, Kakiuchi M, Gupta S et al (2020) Autophagy promotes immune evasion of pancreatic cancer by degrading MHC-I. Nature 581(7806):100–105. https://doi.org/10.1038/s41586-020-2229-5
6. Coelho MA, de Carne Trecesson S, Rana S, Zecchin D, Moore C, Molina-Arcas M et al (2017) Oncogenic RAS signaling promotes tumor immunoresistance by stabilizing PD-L1 mRNA. Immunity 47(6):1083–99.e6. https://doi.org/10.1016/j.immuni.2017.11.016
7. Clark CE, Hingorani SR, Mick R, Combs C, Tuveson DA, Vonderheide RH (2007) Dynamics of the immune reaction to pancreatic cancer from inception to invasion. Cancer Res 67(19):9518–9527. https://doi.org/10.1158/0008-5472.CAN-07-0175
8. Cardenas MA, Prokhnevska N, Kissick HT (2021) Organized immune cell interactions within tumors sustain a productive T-cell response. Int Immunol 33(1):27–37. https://doi.org/10.1093/intimm/dxaa057
9. Davidov V, Jensen G, Mai S, Chen SH, Pan PY (2020) Analyzing one cell at a TIME: analysis of myeloid cell contributions in the tumor immune microenvironment. Front Immunol 11:1842. https://doi.org/10.3389/fimmu.2020.01842
10. Li J, Byrne KT, Yan F, Yamazoe T, Chen Z, Baslan T et al (2018) Tumor cell-intrinsic factors underlie heterogeneity of immune cell infiltration and response to immunotherapy. Immunity 49(1):178–93.e7. https://doi.org/10.1016/j.immuni.2018.06.006
11. Bayne LJ, Beatty GL, Jhala N, Clark CE, Rhim AD, Stanger BZ et al (2012) Tumor-derived granulocyte-macrophage colony-stimulating factor regulates myeloid inflammation and T cell immunity in pancreatic cancer. Cancer Cell 21(6):822–835. https://doi.org/10.1016/j.ccr.2012.04.025
12. Dias Carvalho P, Guimaraes CF, Cardoso AP, Mendonca S, Costa AM, Oliveira MJ et al (2018) KRAS oncogenic signaling extends beyond cancer cells to orchestrate the microenvironment. Cancer Res 78(1):7–14. https://doi.org/10.1158/0008-5472.CAN-17-2084

13. Oliver AJ, Lau PKH, Unsworth AS, Loi S, Darcy PK, Kershaw MH et al (2018) Tissue-dependent tumor microenvironments and their impact on immunotherapy responses. Front Immunol 9:70. https://doi.org/10.3389/fimmu.2018.00070
14. Gu D, Schlotman KE, Xie J (2016) Deciphering the role of hedgehog signaling in pancreatic cancer. J Biomed Res 30(5):353–360. https://doi.org/10.7555/JBR.30.20150107
15. Brahmer JR, Tykodi SS, Chow LQ, Hwu WJ, Topalian SL, Hwu P et al (2012) Safety and activity of anti-PD-L1 antibody in patients with advanced cancer. N Engl J Med 366(26):2455–2465. https://doi.org/10.1056/NEJMoa1200694
16. Royal RE, Levy C, Turner K, Mathur A, Hughes M, Kammula US et al (2010) Phase 2 trial of single agent Ipilimumab (anti-CTLA-4) for locally advanced or metastatic pancreatic adenocarcinoma. J Immunother 33(8):828–833. https://doi.org/10.1097/CJI.0b013e3181eec14c
17. Sohal DPS, Kennedy EB, Cinar P, Conroy T, Copur MS, Crane CH et al (2020) Metastatic pancreatic cancer: ASCO guideline update. J Clin Oncol 2010:JCO2001364. https://doi.org/10.1200/JCO.20.01364
18. Le DT, Durham JN, Smith KN, Wang H, Bartlett BR, Aulakh LK et al (2017) Mismatch repair deficiency predicts response of solid tumors to PD-1 blockade. Science 357(6349):409–413. https://doi.org/10.1126/science.aan6733
19. Le DT, Uram JN, Wang H, Bartlett BR, Kemberling H, Eyring AD et al (2015) PD-1 blockade in tumors with mismatch-repair deficiency. N Engl J Med 372(26):2509–2520. https://doi.org/10.1056/NEJMoa1500596
20. Hu ZI, Shia J, Stadler ZK, Varghese AM, Capanu M, Salo-Mullen E et al (2018) Evaluating mismatch repair deficiency in pancreatic adenocarcinoma: challenges and recommendations. Clin Cancer Res 24(6):1326–1336. https://doi.org/10.1158/1078-0432.CCR-17-3099
21. Marabelle A, Le DT, Ascierto PA, Di Giacomo AM, De Jesus-Acosta A, Delord JP et al (2020) Efficacy of pembrolizumab in patients with noncolorectal high microsatellite instability/mismatch repair-deficient cancer: results from the phase II KEYNOTE-158 Study. J Clin Oncol 38(1):1–10. https://doi.org/10.1200/JCO.19.02105
22. O'Reilly EM, Oh DY, Dhani N, Renouf DJ, Lee MA, Sun W et al (2019) Durvalumab with or without tremelimumab for patients with metastatic pancreatic ductal adenocarcinoma: a phase 2 randomized clinical trial. JAMA Oncol. https://doi.org/10.1001/jamaoncol.2019.1588
23. Alexandrov LB, Nik-Zainal S, Wedge DC, Aparicio SA, Behjati S, Biankin AV et al (2013) Signatures of mutational processes in human cancer. Nature 500(7463):415–421. https://doi.org/10.1038/nature12477
24. Chalmers ZR, Connelly CF, Fabrizio D, Gay L, Ali SM, Ennis R et al (2017) Analysis of 100,000 human cancer genomes reveals the landscape of tumor mutational burden. Genome Med 9(1):34. https://doi.org/10.1186/s13073-017-0424-2
25. Liu WM, Fowler DW, Smith P, Dalgleish AG (2010) Pre-treatment with chemotherapy can enhance the antigenicity and immunogenicity of tumours by promoting adaptive immune responses. Br J Cancer 102(1):115–123. https://doi.org/10.1038/sj.bjc.6605465
26. Pfirschke C, Engblom C, Rickelt S, Cortez-Retamozo V, Garris C, Pucci F et al (2016) Immunogenic chemotherapy sensitizes tumors to checkpoint blockade therapy. Immunity 44(2):343–354. https://doi.org/10.1016/j.immuni.2015.11.024
27. Woo SR, Fuertes MB, Corrales L, Spranger S, Furdyna MJ, Leung MY et al (2014) STING-dependent cytosolic DNA sensing mediates innate immune recognition of immunogenic tumors. Immunity 41(5):830–842. https://doi.org/10.1016/j.immuni.2014.10.017
28. Bear AS, Vonderheide RH, O'Hara MH (2020) Challenges and opportunities for pancreatic cancer immunotherapy. Cancer Cell 38(6):788–802. https://doi.org/10.1016/j.ccell.2020.08.004
29. Weiss GJ, Blaydorn L, Beck J, Bornemann-Kolatzki K, Urnovitz H, Schutz E et al (2018) Phase Ib/II study of gemcitabine, nab-paclitaxel, and pembrolizumab in metastatic pancreatic adenocarcinoma. Investig New Drugs 36(1):96–102. https://doi.org/10.1007/s10637-017-0525-1
30. Wainberg ZA, Hochster HS, Kim EJ, George B, Kaylan A, Chiorean EG et al (2020) Open-label, phase I study of nivolumab combined with nab-paclitaxel plus gemcitabine in advanced

pancreatic cancer. Clin Cancer Res 26(18):4814–4822. https://doi.org/10.1158/1078-0432.CCR-20-0099
31. Renouf DJ, Knox JJ, Kavan P, Jonker DJ, Welch S, Couture F et al (2020) The Canadian Cancer Trials Group PA.7 trial: Results of a randomized phase II study of gemcitabine (GEM) and nab-paclitaxel (Nab-P) vs. GEM, nab-P, durvalumab (D) and tremelimumab (T) as first line therapy in metastatic pancreatic ductal adenocarcinoma (mPDAC). ESMO Virtual Congress 2020. Ann Oncol 31:S1142–SS215. https://doi.org/10.1016/annonc/annonc325
32. Vonderheide RH (2020) CD40 agonist antibodies in cancer immunotherapy. Annu Rev Med 71:47–58. https://doi.org/10.1146/annurev-med-062518-045435
33. Winograd R, Byrne KT, Evans RA, Odorizzi PM, Meyer AR, Bajor DL et al (2015) Induction of T-cell immunity overcomes complete resistance to PD-1 and CTLA-4 blockade and improves survival in pancreatic carcinoma. Cancer Immunol Res 3(4):399–411. https://doi.org/10.1158/2326-6066.CIR-14-0215
34. O'Hara MH, O'Reilly EM, Varadhachary G, Wolff RA, Wainberg ZA, Ko AH et al (2021) CD40 agonistic monoclonal antibody APX005M (sotigalimab) and chemotherapy, with or without nivolumab, for the treatment of metastatic pancreatic adenocarcinoma: an open-label, multicentre, phase 1b study. Lancet Oncol 22(1):118–131. https://doi.org/10.1016/S1470-2045(20)30532-5
35. Connor AA, Denroche RE, Jang GH, Timms L, Kalimuthu SN, Selander I et al (2017) Association of distinct mutational signatures with correlates of increased immune activity in pancreatic ductal adenocarcinoma. JAMA Oncol 3(6):774–783. https://doi.org/10.1001/jamaoncol.2016.3916
36. Holter S, Borgida A, Dodd A, Grant R, Semotiuk K, Hedley D et al (2015) Germline BRCA mutations in a large clinic-based cohort of patients with pancreatic adenocarcinoma. J Clin Oncol 33(28):3124–3129. https://doi.org/10.1200/JCO.2014.59.7401
37. Seeber A, Puccini A, Xiu J, Goldberg RM, Grothey A, Shields AF et al (2019) Association of BRCA-mutant pancreatic cancer with high tumor mutational burden (TMB) and higher PD-L1 expression. J Clin Oncol 37(15_Suppl):4133. https://doi.org/10.1200/JCO.2019.37.15_suppl.4133
38. Francica P, Rottenberg S (2018) Mechanisms of PARP inhibitor resistance in cancer and insights into the DNA damage response. Genome Med 10(1):101. https://doi.org/10.1186/s13073-018-0612-8
39. Golan T, Hammel P, Reni M, Van Cutsem E, Macarulla T, Hall MJ et al (2019) Maintenance olaparib for germline BRCA-mutated metastatic pancreatic cancer. N Engl J Med 381(4):317–327. https://doi.org/10.1056/NEJMoa1903387
40. Allard B, Longhi MS, Robson SC, Stagg J (2017) The ectonucleotidases CD39 and CD73: novel checkpoint inhibitor targets. Immunol Rev 276(1):121–144. https://doi.org/10.1111/imr.12528
41. Zhou L, Jia S, Chen Y, Wang W, Wu Z, Yu W et al (2019) The distinct role of CD73 in the progression of pancreatic cancer. J Mol Med (Berl) 97(6):803–815. https://doi.org/10.1007/s00109-018-01742-0
42. Allard D, Allard B, Gaudreau PO, Chrobak P, Stagg J (2016) CD73-adenosine: a next-generation target in immuno-oncology. Immunotherapy 8(2):145–163. https://doi.org/10.2217/imt.15.106
43. Allard B, Pommey S, Smyth MJ, Stagg J (2013) Targeting CD73 enhances the antitumor activity of anti-PD-1 and anti-CTLA-4 mAbs. Clin Cancer Res 19(20):5626–5635. https://doi.org/10.1158/1078-0432.CCR-13-0545
44. Manji GA, Wainberg ZA, Krishnan K, Giafis N, Udyavar A, Quah CS et al (2021) ARC-8: phase I/Ib study to evaluate safety and tolerability of AB680 + chemotherapy + zimberelimab (AB122) in patients with treatment-naive metastatic pancreatic adenocarcinoma (mPDAC). J Clin Oncol 39(3_Suppl):404. https://doi.org/10.1200/JCO.2021.39.3_suppl.404
45. Overman MJ, LoRusso P, Strickler JH, Patel SP, Clarke SJ, Noonan AM et al (2018) Safety, efficacy and pharmacodynamics (PD) of MEDI9447 (oleclumab) alone or in combination with durvalumab in advanced colorectal cancer (CRC) or pancreatic cancer (panc). J Clin Oncol 36(15_Suppl):4123. https://doi.org/10.1200/JCO.2018.36.15_suppl.4123

46. Desai J, Kortmansky JS, Segal NH, Fakih M, Oh D-Y, Kim K-P et al (2019) MORPHEUS: a phase Ib/II study platform evaluating the safety and clinical efficacy of cancer immunotherapy (CIT)–based combinations in gastrointestinal (GI) cancers. J Clin Oncol 37(4_Suppl):TPS467. https://doi.org/10.1200/JCO.2019.37.4_suppl.TPS467
47. Ko AH, Lee J, Alsina M, Ajani JA, Bang Y-J, Chung HC et al (2020) Phase Ib/II open-label, randomized evaluation of 2L atezolizumab (atezo) + PEGPH20 versus control in MORPHEUS-pancreatic ductal adenocarcinoma (M-PDAC) and MORPHEUS-gastric cancer (M-GC). J Clin Oncol 38(15_Suppl):4540. https://doi.org/10.1200/JCO.2020.38.15_suppl.4540
48. Cho BC, Bahary N, Bendell J, Felip E, Johnson M, Kang Y-K et al (2020) Abstract CT201: Phase Ib/II open-label, randomized evaluation of atezolizumab + cobimetinib vs. control in MORPHEUS-NSCLC (non-small cell lung cancer), MORPHEUS-PDAC (pancreatic ductal adenocarcinoma) and MORPHEUS-GC (gastric cancer). Cancer Res 80(16 Suppl):CT201. https://doi.org/10.1158/1538-7445.AM2020-CT201
49. Oh D-Y, Ajani JA, Bang Y-J, Chung HC, Lacy J, Lee J et al (2020) Phase Ib/II open-label, randomized evaluation of 2L atezolizumab (atezo) + BL-8040 versus control in MORPHEUS-pancreatic ductal adenocarcinoma (M-PDAC) and MORPHEUS-gastric cancer (M-GC). J Clin Oncol 38(4_Suppl):712. https://doi.org/10.1200/JCO.2020.38.4_suppl.712
50. Chung V, Alistar A, George B, Kim K, Kindler H, Oh D et al (2020) SO-4 phase Ib/II, open-label, randomised evaluation of atezolizumab plus RO6874281 vs. control in MORPHEUS–pancreatic ductal adenocarcinoma. Ann Oncol 31:S218. https://doi.org/10.1016/j.annonc.2020.04.019
51. Sadelain M, Brentjens R, Riviere I (2013) The basic principles of chimeric antigen receptor design. Cancer Discov 3(4):388–398. https://doi.org/10.1158/2159-8290.CD-12-0548
52. Geyer MB, Brentjens RJ (2016) Review: Current clinical applications of chimeric antigen receptor (CAR) modified T cells. Cytotherapy 18(11):1393–1409. https://doi.org/10.1016/j.jcyt.2016.07.003
53. DeSelm CJ, Tano ZE, Varghese AM, Adusumilli PS (2017) CAR T-cell therapy for pancreatic cancer. J Surg Oncol 116(1):63–74. https://doi.org/10.1002/jso.24627
54. Thistlethwaite FC, Gilham DE, Guest RD, Rothwell DG, Pillai M, Burt DJ et al (2017) The clinical efficacy of first-generation carcinoembryonic antigen (CEACAM5)-specific CAR T cells is limited by poor persistence and transient pre-conditioning-dependent respiratory toxicity. Cancer Immunol Immunother 66(11):1425–1436. https://doi.org/10.1007/s00262-017-2034-7
55. Parkhurst MR, Yang JC, Langan RC, Dudley ME, Nathan DA, Feldman SA et al (2011) T cells targeting carcinoembryonic antigen can mediate regression of metastatic colorectal cancer but induce severe transient colitis. Mol Ther 19(3):620–626. https://doi.org/10.1038/mt.2010.272
56. Hammarstrom S (1999) The carcinoembryonic antigen (CEA) family: structures, suggested functions and expression in normal and malignant tissues. Semin Cancer Biol 9(2):67–81. https://doi.org/10.1006/scbi.1998.0119
57. Raj D, Nikolaidi M, Garces I, Lorizio D, Castro NM, Caiafa SG et al (2021) CEACAM7 is an effective target for CAR T-cell therapy of pancreatic ductal adenocarcinoma. Clin Cancer Res. https://doi.org/10.1158/1078-0432.CCR-19-2163
58. Hassan R, Thomas A, Alewine C, Le DT, Jaffee EM, Pastan I (2016) Mesothelin immunotherapy for cancer: ready for prime time? J Clin Oncol 34(34):4171–4179. https://doi.org/10.1200/JCO.2016.68.3672
59. Beatty GL, O'Hara MH, Lacey SF, Torigian DA, Nazimuddin F, Chen F et al (2018) Activity of mesothelin-specific chimeric antigen receptor T cells against pancreatic carcinoma metastases in a phase 1 trial. Gastroenterology 155(1):29–32. https://doi.org/10.1053/j.gastro.2018.03.029
60. Haas AR, Tanyi JL, O'Hara MH, Gladney WL, Lacey SF, Torigian DA et al (2019) Phase I study of lentiviral-transduced chimeric antigen receptor-modified T cells recognizing mesothelin in advanced solid cancers. Mol Ther 27(11):1919–1929. https://doi.org/10.1016/j.ymthe.2019.07.015

61. Ko AH, Jordan AC, Tooker E, Lacey SF, Chang RB, Li Y et al (2020) Dual targeting of mesothelin and CD19 with chimeric antigen receptor-modified T cells in patients with metastatic pancreatic cancer. Mol Ther 28(11):2367–2378. https://doi.org/10.1016/j.ymthe.2020.07.017
62. John LB, Devaud C, Duong CP, Yong CS, Beavis PA, Haynes NM et al (2013) Anti-PD-1 antibody therapy potently enhances the eradication of established tumors by gene-modified T cells. Clin Cancer Res 19(20):5636–5646. https://doi.org/10.1158/1078-0432.CCR-13-0458
63. Wang Z, Chen M, Zhang Y, Liu Y, Yang Q, Nie J et al (2020) Phase I study of CRISPR-engineered CAR-T cells with PD-1 inactivation in treating mesothelin-positive solid tumors. J Clin Oncol 38(15_Suppl):3038. https://doi.org/10.1200/JCO.2020.38.15_suppl.3038
64. Ferrandina G, Petrillo M, Bonanno G, Scambia G (2009) Targeting CD133 antigen in cancer. Expert Opin Ther Targets 13(7):823–837. https://doi.org/10.1517/14728220903005616
65. Wang Y, Chen M, Wu Z, Tong C, Dai H, Guo Y et al (2018) CD133-directed CAR T cells for advanced metastasis malignancies: A phase I trial. Oncoimmunology 7(7):e1440169. https://doi.org/10.1080/2162402X.2018.1440169
66. Argani P, Rosty C, Reiter RE, Wilentz RE, Murugesan SR, Leach SD et al (2001) Discovery of new markers of cancer through serial analysis of gene expression: prostate stem cell antigen is overexpressed in pancreatic adenocarcinoma. Cancer Res 61(11):4320–4324
67. Feldmann G, Beaty R, Hruban RH, Maitra A (2007) Molecular genetics of pancreatic intraepithelial neoplasia. J Hepato-Biliary-Pancreat Surg 14(3):224–232. https://doi.org/10.1007/s00534-006-1166-5
68. Shaw J, Ballard B, Yi X, Malankar A, Collinson-Pautz MR, Becerra CR et al (2020) Tumor infiltration and cytokine biomarkers of prostate stem cell antigen (PSCA)-directed GOCAR-T cells in patients with advanced pancreatic tumors. J Clin Oncol 38(4_Suppl):734. https://doi.org/10.1200/JCO.2020.38.4_suppl.734
69. Moore MJ, Goldstein D, Hamm J, Figer A, Hecht JR, Gallinger S et al (2007) Erlotinib plus gemcitabine compared with gemcitabine alone in patients with advanced pancreatic cancer: a phase III trial of the National Cancer Institute of Canada Clinical Trials Group. J Clin Oncol 25(15):1960–1966. https://doi.org/10.1200/JCO.2006.07.9525
70. Reusch U, Sundaram M, Davol PA, Olson SD, Davis JB, Demel K et al (2006) Anti-CD3 x anti-epidermal growth factor receptor (EGFR) bispecific antibody redirects T-cell cytolytic activity to EGFR-positive cancers in vitro and in an animal model. Clin Cancer Res 12(1):183–190. https://doi.org/10.1158/1078-0432.CCR-05-1855
71. Lum LG, Thakur A, Choi M, Deol A, Kondadasula V, Schalk D et al (2020) Clinical and immune responses to anti-CD3 × anti-EGFR bispecific antibody armed activated T cells (EGFR BATs) in pancreatic cancer patients. Oncoimmunology 9(1):1773201. https://doi.org/10.1080/2162402X.2020.1773201
72. Zhang Y, Ma JA, Zhang HX, Jiang YN, Luo WH (2020) Cancer vaccines: targeting KRAS-driven cancers. Expert Rev Vaccines 19(2):163–173. https://doi.org/10.1080/14760584.2020.1733420
73. Hardacre JM, Mulcahy M, Small W, Talamonti M, Obel J, Krishnamurthi S et al (2013) Addition of algenpantucel-L immunotherapy to standard adjuvant therapy for pancreatic cancer: a phase 2 study. J Gastrointest Surg 17(1):94–100; discussion 101. https://doi.org/10.1007/s11605-012-2064-6
74. Middleton G, Silcocks P, Cox T, Valle J, Wadsley J, Propper D et al (2014) Gemcitabine and capecitabine with or without telomerase peptide vaccine GV1001 in patients with locally advanced or metastatic pancreatic cancer (TeloVac): an open-label, randomised, phase 3 trial. Lancet Oncol 15(8):829–840. https://doi.org/10.1016/S1470-2045(14)70236-0
75. Shima H, Tsurita G, Wada S, Hirohashi Y, Yasui H, Hayashi H et al (2019) Randomized phase II trial of survivin 2B peptide vaccination for patients with HLA-A24-positive pancreatic adenocarcinoma. Cancer Sci 110(8):2378–2385. https://doi.org/10.1111/cas.14106
76. Yamaue H, Tsunoda T, Tani M, Miyazawa M, Yamao K, Mizuno N et al (2015) Randomized phase II/III clinical trial of elpamotide for patients with advanced pancreatic cancer: PEGASUS-PC Study. Cancer Sci 106(7):883–890. https://doi.org/10.1111/cas.12674

77. Le DT, Wang-Gillam A, Picozzi V, Greten TF, Crocenzi T, Springett G et al (2015) Safety and survival with GVAX pancreas prime and Listeria monocytogenes-expressing mesothelin (CRS-207) boost vaccines for metastatic pancreatic cancer. J Clin Oncol 33(12):1325–1333. https://doi.org/10.1200/JCO.2014.57.4244
78. Le DT, Picozzi VJ, Ko AH, Wainberg ZA, Kindler H, Wang-Gillam A et al (2019) Results from a phase IIb, randomized, multicenter study of GVAX pancreas and CRS-207 compared with chemotherapy in adults with previously treated metastatic pancreatic adenocarcinoma (ECLIPSE Study). Clin Cancer Res 25(18):5493–5502. https://doi.org/10.1158/1078-0432.CCR-18-2992
79. Tsujikawa T, Crocenzi T, Durham JN, Sugar EA, Wu AA, Onners B et al (2020) Evaluation of cyclophosphamide/GVAX pancreas followed by Listeria-Mesothelin (CRS-207) with or without nivolumab in patients with pancreatic cancer. Clin Cancer Res 26(14):3578–3588. https://doi.org/10.1158/1078-0432.CCR-19-3978
80. Wu AA, Bever KM, Ho WJ, Fertig EJ, Niu N, Zheng L et al (2020) A phase II study of allogeneic GM-CSF-transfected pancreatic tumor vaccine (GVAX) with ipilimumab as maintenance treatment for metastatic pancreatic cancer. Clin Cancer Res 26(19):5129–5139. https://doi.org/10.1158/1078-0432.CCR-20-1025
81. Baldin AV, Savvateeva LV, Bazhin AV, Zamyatnin AA Jr (2020) Dendritic cells in anticancer vaccination: rationale for ex vivo loading or in vivo targeting. Cancers (Basel) 12(3). https://doi.org/10.3390/cancers12030590
82. Rong Y, Qin X, Jin D, Lou W, Wu L, Wang D et al (2012) A phase I pilot trial of MUC1-peptide-pulsed dendritic cells in the treatment of advanced pancreatic cancer. Clin Exp Med 12(3):173–180. https://doi.org/10.1007/s10238-011-0159-0
83. Mehrotra S, Britten CD, Chin S, Garrett-Mayer E, Cloud CA, Li M et al (2017) Vaccination with poly(IC:LC) and peptide-pulsed autologous dendritic cells in patients with pancreatic cancer. J Hematol Oncol 10(1):82. https://doi.org/10.1186/s13045-017-0459-2
84. Abou-Alfa GK, Chapman PB, Feilchenfeldt J, Brennan MF, Capanu M, Gansukh B et al (2011) Targeting mutated K-ras in pancreatic adenocarcinoma using an adjuvant vaccine. Am J Clin Oncol 34(3):321–325. https://doi.org/10.1097/COC.0b013e3181e84b1f
85. Weden S, Klemp M, Gladhaug IP, Moller M, Eriksen JA, Gaudernack G et al (2011) Long-term follow-up of patients with resected pancreatic cancer following vaccination against mutant K-ras. Int J Cancer 128(5):1120–1128. https://doi.org/10.1002/ijc.25449
86. Wang QJ, Yu Z, Griffith K, Hanada K, Restifo NP, Yang JC (2016) Identification of T-cell receptors targeting KRAS-mutated human tumors. Cancer Immunol Res 4(3):204–214. https://doi.org/10.1158/2326-6066.CIR-15-0188
87. Zaidi N, Quezada SA, Kuroiwa JMY, Zhang L, Jaffee EM, Steinman RM et al (2019) Anti-CTLA-4 synergizes with dendritic cell-targeted vaccine to promote IL-3-dependent CD4(+) effector T cell infiltration into murine pancreatic tumors. Ann N Y Acad Sci 1445(1):62–73. https://doi.org/10.1111/nyas.14049
88. Fu J, Malm IJ, Kadayakkara DK, Levitsky H, Pardoll D, Kim YJ (2014) Preclinical evidence that PD1 blockade cooperates with cancer vaccine TEGVAX to elicit regression of established tumors. Cancer Res 74(15):4042–4052. https://doi.org/10.1158/0008-5472.CAN-13-2685
89. Vonderheide RH, Glennie MJ (2013) Agonistic CD40 antibodies and cancer therapy. Clin Cancer Res 19(5):1035–1043. https://doi.org/10.1158/1078-0432.CCR-12-2064
90. Lankadasari MB, Mukhopadhyay P, Mohammed S, Harikumar KB (2019) TAMing pancreatic cancer: combat with a double edged sword. Mol Cancer 18(1):48. https://doi.org/10.1186/s12943-019-0966-6
91. Zhu Y, Knolhoff BL, Meyer MA, Nywening TM, West BL, Luo J et al (2014) CSF1/CSF1R blockade reprograms tumor-infiltrating macrophages and improves response to T-cell checkpoint immunotherapy in pancreatic cancer models. Cancer Res 74(18):5057–5069. https://doi.org/10.1158/0008-5472.CAN-13-3723
92. Wainberg ZA, Piha-Paul SA, Luke JJ, Kim EJ, Thompson J, Britten C et al (2017) First-in-human phase 1 dose escalation and expansion of a novel combination, anti-CSF-1 receptor

(cabiralizumab) plus anti-PD-1 (nivolumab), in patients with advanced solid tumors. 32nd SITC Annual Meeting. National Harbor, MD

93. Five prime therapeutics provides update on phase 2 trial of cabiralizumab combined with Opdivo® in pancreatic cancer (2020). https://www.businesswire.com/news/home/20200218005144/en/. Accessed 8 Feb 2021
94. Cassier PA, Garin G, Eberst L, Delord J-P, Chabaud S, Terret C et al (2019) MEDIPLEX: a phase 1 study of durvalumab (D) combined with pexidartinib (P) in patients (pts) with advanced pancreatic ductal adenocarcinoma (PDAC) and colorectal cancer (CRC). J Clin Oncol 37(15_Suppl):2579. https://doi.org/10.1200/JCO.2019.37.15_suppl.2579
95. Nywening TM, Wang-Gillam A, Sanford DE, Belt BA, Panni RZ, Cusworth BM et al (2016) Targeting tumour-associated macrophages with CCR2 inhibition in combination with FOLFIRINOX in patients with borderline resectable and locally advanced pancreatic cancer: a single-centre, open-label, dose-finding, non-randomised, phase 1b trial. Lancet Oncol 17(5):651–662. https://doi.org/10.1016/S1470-2045(16)00078-4
96. Noel M, O'Reilly EM, Wolpin BM, Ryan DP, Bullock AJ, Britten CD et al (2020) Phase 1b study of a small molecule antagonist of human chemokine (C-C motif) receptor 2 (PF-04136309) in combination with nab-paclitaxel/gemcitabine in first-line treatment of metastatic pancreatic ductal adenocarcinoma. Investig New Drugs 38(3):800–811. https://doi.org/10.1007/s10637-019-00830-3
97. Thyagarajan A, Alshehri MSA, Miller KLR, Sherwin CM, Travers JB, Sahu RP (2019) Myeloid-derived suppressor cells and pancreatic cancer: implications in novel therapeutic approaches. Cancers (Basel) 11(11). https://doi.org/10.3390/cancers11111627
98. Kumar V, Donthireddy L, Marvel D, Condamine T, Wang F, Lavilla-Alonso S et al (2017) Cancer-associated fibroblasts neutralize the anti-tumor effect of CSF1 receptor blockade by inducing PMN-MDSC infiltration of tumors. Cancer Cell 32(5):654–68.e5. https://doi.org/10.1016/j.ccell.2017.10.005
99. Nywening TM, Belt BA, Cullinan DR, Panni RZ, Han BJ, Sanford DE et al (2018) Targeting both tumour-associated CXCR2(+) neutrophils and CCR2(+) macrophages disrupts myeloid recruitment and improves chemotherapeutic responses in pancreatic ductal adenocarcinoma. Gut 67(6):1112–1123. https://doi.org/10.1136/gutjnl-2017-313738
100. Wang Z, Liu Y, Zhang Y, Shang Y, Gao Q (2016) MDSC-decreasing chemotherapy increases the efficacy of cytokine-induced killer cell immunotherapy in metastatic renal cell carcinoma and pancreatic cancer. Oncotarget 7(4):4760–4769. https://doi.org/10.18632/oncotarget.6734
101. Dominguez GA, Condamine T, Mony S, Hashimoto A, Wang F, Liu Q et al (2017) Selective targeting of myeloid-derived suppressor cells in cancer patients using DS-8273a, an agonistic TRAIL-R2 antibody. Clin Cancer Res 23(12):2942–2950. https://doi.org/10.1158/1078-0432.CCR-16-1784
102. Hingorani SR, Zheng L, Bullock AJ, Seery TE, Harris WP, Sigal DS et al (2018) HALO 202: randomized phase II study of PEGPH20 plus nab-paclitaxel/gemcitabine versus nab-paclitaxel/gemcitabine in patients with untreated, metastatic pancreatic ductal adenocarcinoma. J Clin Oncol 36(4):359–366. https://doi.org/10.1200/JCO.2017.74.9564
103. Hingorani SR, Harris WP, Beck JT, Berdov BA, Wagner SA, Pshevlotsky EM et al (2016) Phase Ib study of PEGylated recombinant human hyaluronidase and gemcitabine in patients with advanced pancreatic cancer. Clin Cancer Res 22(12):2848–2854. https://doi.org/10.1158/1078-0432.CCR-15-2010
104. Ramanathan RK, McDonough SL, Philip PA, Hingorani SR, Lacy J, Kortmansky JS et al (2019) Phase IB/II randomized study of FOLFIRINOX plus Pegylated recombinant human hyaluronidase versus FOLFIRINOX alone in patients with metastatic pancreatic adenocarcinoma: SWOG S1313. J Clin Oncol 37(13):1062–1069. https://doi.org/10.1200/JCO.18.01295
105. Van Cutsem E, Tempero MA, Sigal D, Oh DY, Fazio N, Macarulla T et al (2020) Randomized phase III trial of Pegvorhyaluronidase alfa with nab-paclitaxel plus gemcitabine for patients with hyaluronan-high metastatic pancreatic adenocarcinoma. J Clin Oncol 38(27):3185–3194. https://doi.org/10.1200/JCO.20.00590

106. Armstrong T, Packham G, Murphy LB, Bateman AC, Conti JA, Fine DR et al (2004) Type I collagen promotes the malignant phenotype of pancreatic ductal adenocarcinoma. Clin Cancer Res 10(21):7427–7437. https://doi.org/10.1158/1078-0432.CCR-03-0825
107. Picozzi V, Alseidi A, Winter J, Pishvaian M, Mody K, Glaspy J et al (2020) Gemcitabine/nab-paclitaxel with pamrevlumab: a novel drug combination and trial design for the treatment of locally advanced pancreatic cancer. ESMO Open 5(4). https://doi.org/10.1136/esmoopen-2019-000668
108. Cohen SJ, Alpaugh RK, Palazzo I, Meropol NJ, Rogatko A, Xu Z et al (2008) Fibroblast activation protein and its relationship to clinical outcome in pancreatic adenocarcinoma. Pancreas 37(2):154–158. https://doi.org/10.1097/MPA.0b013e31816618ce
109. Ali AI, Oliver AJ, Samiei T, Chan JD, Kershaw MH, Slaney CY (2019) Genetic redirection of T cells for the treatment of pancreatic cancer. Front Oncol 9:56. https://doi.org/10.3389/fonc.2019.00056
110. Lo A, Wang LS, Scholler J, Monslow J, Avery D, Newick K et al (2015) Tumor-promoting desmoplasia is disrupted by depleting FAP-expressing stromal cells. Cancer Res 75(14):2800–2810. https://doi.org/10.1158/0008-5472.CAN-14-3041
111. Tran E, Chinnasamy D, Yu Z, Morgan RA, Lee CC, Restifo NP et al (2013) Immune targeting of fibroblast activation protein triggers recognition of multipotent bone marrow stromal cells and cachexia. J Exp Med 210(6):1125–1135. https://doi.org/10.1084/jem.20130110
112. Furusato B, Mohamed A, Uhlen M, Rhim JS (2010) CXCR4 and cancer. Pathol Int 60(7):497–505. https://doi.org/10.1111/j.1440-1827.2010.02548.x
113. Seo YD, Jiang X, Sullivan KM, Jalikis FG, Smythe KS, Abbasi A et al (2019) Mobilization of CD8(+) T cells via CXCR4 blockade facilitates PD-1 checkpoint therapy in human pancreatic cancer. Clin Cancer Res 25(13):3934–3945. https://doi.org/10.1158/1078-0432.CCR-19-0081
114. O'Hara MH, Messersmith W, Kindler H, Zhang W, Pitou C, Szpurka AM et al (2020) Safety and pharmacokinetics of CXCR4 peptide antagonist, LY2510924, in combination with durvalumab in advanced refractory solid tumors. J Pancreat Cancer 6(1):21–31. https://doi.org/10.1089/pancan.2019.0018
115. Bockorny B, Semenisty V, Macarulla T, Borazanci E, Wolpin BM, Stemmer SM et al (2020) BL-8040, a CXCR4 antagonist, in combination with pembrolizumab and chemotherapy for pancreatic cancer: the COMBAT trial. Nat Med 26(6):878–885. https://doi.org/10.1038/s41591-020-0880-x
116. Wang-Gillam A, Hubner RA, Siveke JT, Von Hoff DD, Belanger B, de Jong FA et al (2019) NAPOLI-1 phase 3 study of liposomal irinotecan in metastatic pancreatic cancer: final overall survival analysis and characteristics of long-term survivors. Eur J Cancer 108:78–87. https://doi.org/10.1016/j.ejca.2018.12.007
117. Sherman MH, Yu RT, Engle DD, Ding N, Atkins AR, Tiriac H et al (2014) Vitamin D receptor-mediated stromal reprogramming suppresses pancreatitis and enhances pancreatic cancer therapy. Cell 159(1):80–93. https://doi.org/10.1016/j.cell.2014.08.007
118. Karasic TB, O'Hara MH, Loaiza-Bonilla A, Reiss KA, Teitelbaum UR, Borazanci E et al (2019) Effect of gemcitabine and nab-paclitaxel with or without hydroxychloroquine on patients with advanced pancreatic cancer: a phase 2 randomized clinical trial. JAMA Oncol 5(7):993–998. https://doi.org/10.1001/jamaoncol.2019.0684
119. Le DT, Lutz E, Uram JN, Sugar EA, Onners B, Solt S et al (2013) Evaluation of ipilimumab in combination with allogeneic pancreatic tumor cells transfected with a GM-CSF gene in previously treated pancreatic cancer. J Immunother 36(7):382–389. https://doi.org/10.1097/CJI.0b013e31829fb7a2
120. Feng K, Liu Y, Guo Y, Qiu J, Wu Z, Dai H et al (2018) Phase I study of chimeric antigen receptor modified T cells in treating HER2-positive advanced biliary tract cancers and pancreatic cancers. Protein Cell 9(10):838–847. https://doi.org/10.1007/s13238-017-0440-4

Perspective on the Immunotherapy of Pancreatic Cancer

Bridget Keenan and Margaret Tempero

Contents

Abstract

Pancreatic cancer has demonstrated low response rates to immunotherapy, due in part to late diagnosis, inherent immune resistance, and desmoplastic stroma. Signals in the tumor microenvironment that suppress effector immune cells include the physical barrier of the stroma and suppressive pro-oncogenic molecules secreted by immune myeloid cells and non-immune cells such as fibroblasts. Different strategies to overcome these barriers including vaccines, targeting suppressive myeloid cells, depleting stroma, and T cell therapy have been used thus far with mixed success. The outlook for pancreatic cancer includes rationale combinations of different treatment modalities and identification of biomarkers of response.

B. Keenan · M. Tempero (✉)
Division of Hematology/Oncology, Department of Medicine, University of California San Francisco, San Francisco, CA, USA
e-mail: bridget.keenan@ucsf.edu; margaret.tempero@ucsf.edu

Cancer Immunotherapy (2021)
https://doi.org/10.1007/13905_2021_9,

Published Online: 25 August 2021

Keywords

Cancer vaccines · CAR T cells · Immunotherapy · Pancreatic cancer · Tumor microenvironment

1 Introduction

Due to lack of symptoms until late stage disease, many cases of pancreatic cancer are diagnosed in advanced stages [1]. Among other factors, the clinical presentation in later stages when mechanisms of immunosuppression are well-established may make pancreatic cancer resistant to both standard therapies and immunotherapy. In addition, pancreatic cancer is thought to be "immunologically cold," lacking infiltrates of tumor-infiltrating anti-tumor T cells [2], which are seen in other tumor types such as melanoma [3]. T cells that do persist may be "exhausted" and dysfunctional due to epigenetic programs induced by chronic antigen stimulation [4, 5]. Tumor mutational burden (TMB) has been correlated with response to immunotherapy; pancreatic cancer has generally low TMB and accordingly, low rates of immunotherapy response [6]. Patients with pancreatic tumors that have microsatellite instability (MSI-high) have been shown to respond to immunotherapy (overall response rate of 18.2% in the KEYNOTE-158 study), in line with other MSI-high tumors [7]; however less than 2% of PDA are MSI-high [8]. However, beyond the quantity of tumor antigens, the character or "quality," such as structural similarity to infectious antigens, may be more predictive of response [9].

KRAS is mutated in the majority of human pancreatic adenocarcinomas [10] and the $KRAS^{G12D}$ mutation itself can contribute to immunosuppression by downstream signaling contributing to an inflammatory milieu and stromal activation [11]. In addition to tumor-intrinsic properties such as the type and quantity of mutations, the dense stroma and suppressive immune cells further contribute to resistance to immunotherapy. Suppressive myeloid cells inhibit $CD8^+$ T cells from entering tumor microenvironment [12] and can induce tumor cells to upregulate PD-L1 to suppress T cells [13]. In mouse models of Kras-driven pancreatic cancer that closely recapitulate the development of human cancer, it has been shown that suppressive myeloid and T regulatory cells accumulate in even pre-malignant stages (termed PanINs—pancreatic intra-epithelial neoplasia [14]) [2, 15] and myeloid cells can be recruited by tumor-secreted factors such as GM-CSF and IL-8 [16, 17]. In patients, T regulatory cells also accumulate with advancing stage of disease and inversely correlate with survival [18]. In systemic circulation, pro-inflammatory cytokines such as IL-6 and IL-10 in untreated patients correlate with poor prognosis [19].

Stroma refers to the non-tumor cells including the extracellular matrix, stromal cells such as fibroblasts, and the tumor vasculature; in pancreatic cancer, the dense stroma is a hallmark of the tumor microenvironment [20]. Malignant cells signal to cancer-associated fibroblasts (CAFs) which then produce ECM proteins; the outcome is desmoplasia, the stromal reaction to the presence of cancer. High interstitial pressures generated by the stroma can impede the delivery of chemotherapy;

hyaluronic acid (HA) has been identified as a major component of ECM that increases pressure and prevents extravasation of therapeutic agents [21]. Furthermore, dense ECM can impede the tumor-infiltrating T cells from accessing tumor cells [22]. In addition to producing ECM, CAFs are involved in bi-directional cross-talk with malignant and immune cells in the stroma, promoting tumor progression and immune evasion in pancreatic cancer and other cancer types [23, 24]. However, recent studies have revealed that there is a complex range of CAF phenotypes, including myofibroblasts that secrete stroma and inflammatory fibroblasts characterized by IL-6 production, a potentially immunosuppressive cytokine [25]. While CAFs are not immune-derived cells, single cell RNA sequencing revealed a fibroblast sub-type in human and mouse tumors capable of antigen presentation and thus of shaping the immune response to cancer [26].

While there are many challenges specific to pancreatic cancer that inhibit the efficacy of tumor immunotherapy, there has been significant progress made in the understanding of underlying suppressive mechanisms and into therapeutic avenues to surmount these challenges (Table 1). Targeting tumor stromal cells and matrix, re-invigorating exhausted T cells, and depleting suppressive myeloid cells are all

Table 1 Immunotherapy challenges and strategies in pancreatic cancer

Barrier to immunotherapy in pancreatic cancer	Immunotherapeutic strategy	Examples of clinical agents in past or current clinical trials for pancreatic cancer
Lack of T cell infiltration in tumors	Increase tumor infiltration by igniting T cell responses and converting immune "cold" to "hot" tumors	Vaccines, toll-like receptor agonists, oncolytic viruses
Exhausted T cell phenotype	Immune checkpoint inhibition (CPI)	CPI alone, CPI in combination with chemotherapy or radiation, bispecific T cell engagers
Low tumor mutational burden (TMB)	Identification of T cell receptors (TCR) with ability to bind tumor-associated antigens (TAA), identification of "high quality" TAA for targeting with vaccines	T cell therapy (CAR T or endogenous TCR T cells), vaccines
Kras pathway-mediated suppression	Inhibition of Kras	Vaccines targeting Kras, direct Kras inhibitors
Stromal desmoplasia	Targeting of dense extracellular matrix (ECM), increase penetration of immune cells, inhibit suppressive stromal elements	Hyaluronidase (PEGPH20), FAP-targeted CAR T cells, Sonic hedgehog pathway inhibitors, ECM/matrix metalloproteinase inhibitors
Myeloid cell-mediated suppression	Inhibit suppressive myeloid cells, re-polarize myeloid cells to immunogenic phenotype	CCR2 inhibitors, CSF1R inhibitors, CD40 agonists
Fibroblasts	Deplete or inhibit fibroblasts and fibroblast activation protein (FAP)	FAP inhibitors, FAP-targeted CAR T cell therapy
Immunosuppressive B cells	Depletion of B cells	CD19-directed CAR T cell therapy, ibrutinib

potential strategies that have been tested both pre-clinically and clinically thus far. Cellular therapies using transgenic T cell receptor (TCR) or chimeric antigen receptor (CAR) T cells represent the most recent efforts to harness the potential of the immune response to treat pancreatic cancer.

2 Cancer Vaccines

Vaccines, one strategy to treat cancers with immunotherapy, rely on rational selection of both vector and target antigen, by necessity these must be designed to overcome immunosuppression and/or tolerance to tumor antigens. In pancreatic cancer, numerous delivery approaches have been used such as whole tumor cells [27, 28], dendritic cells [29], attenuated bacteria [30] or viruses [31], and peptides [32, 33]. Whole tumor cells circumvent the challenge of tumor-antigen selection by allowing the immune system to process and present antigens present in the vaccine in a manner unique to each patient [34], while dendritic cell vaccines take advantage of the immune system's most potent antigen presenting cell to initiate a response to selected antigens [35]. In addition, vaccine vectors have been modified to express co-stimulatory molecules [31] and secrete cytokines such as GM-CSF [27], and vaccines have been co-administered with immunostimulatory adjuvants [32, 36] or cytokines such as IL-2 [37]. Ideal vaccine targets are proteins over-expressed or mutated within the tumor and are common to many patients' tumors. Tumor-associated antigens targeted with vaccines in pancreatic cancer thus far include survivin [38], vascular endothelial growth factor receptor 2 (VEGFR2) [39], mesothelin [30], Wilms' tumor gene 1 (WT1) [40], telomerase [33, 41], MUC1 [29], CEA [31], and KRAS [37, 42]. There have been modest clinical benefits observed across different platforms and targeted antigens, but there has yet to be major progress leading to the incorporation of vaccines into standard practice. A recent development, capitalizing on these early efforts as well as advances in sequencing technology, is the creation of personalized vaccines based on neoantigens specific to each patient [43]. Thus far, this strategy has proven feasible in melanoma, with early clinical efficacy [44], and a trial is ongoing to study a personalized neoantigen vaccine in pancreatic cancer (NCT03956056).

Many of these vaccines have been shown to have the ability to induce antigen-specific T cell responses [27, 29, 36, 37]; however, the induction of tumor-antigen specific T cells alone in mouse models with cancer vaccines does not translate into increased survival due to additional barriers that prevent T cell trafficking to tumors [15]. Despite the immunosuppressive tumor microenvironment, neoadjuvant cancer vaccines given prior to surgery can convert "immunologically cold" tumors into "hot" tumors with T cell infiltration and tertiary lymphoid structure formation, giving some hope that immunotherapy can be used successfully in pancreatic cancer when additional immunosuppressive factors are overcome [45]. This result also suggests that vaccines may be useful in earlier stages of pre-malignancy [46]. Vaccines may not be sufficient for anti-tumor efficacy in pancreatic cancer; however, they may be useful in igniting an antigen-specific T cell response that could then be augmented with other therapies that increase T cell trafficking or efficacy.

3 Checkpoint Inhibitors

Monoclonal antibodies targeting the immune "checkpoints" CTLA-4, PD-1, or PD-L1 can overcome T cell exhaustion and show efficacy in many tumor types [47, 48]. However, in unselected pancreatic cancer patients (without microsatellite instability in the tumor, for example), attempts to use checkpoint inhibitors as monotherapy have been met with failure, despite demonstration of markers such as CTLA-4 expressed in pancreatic cancer patients [19]. In a Phase II trial of ipilimumab (anti-CTLA-4) alone, 27 patients with metastatic or locally advanced previously treated disease, there were no responders by criteria specified although one patient had a delayed response after initial progressive disease; the authors concluded that anti-CTLA-4 was not effective for pancreatic cancer [49]. Compared to ipilimumab alone, ipilimumab combined with GVAX resulted in several patients with a period of disease stabilization, although there were no patients with tumor regression, despite the induction of mesothelin-specific T cell responses in patients with longer overall survival [50]. In a study of an anti-PD-L1 therapeutic antibody for advanced solid tumors, there were no objective responses in 14 patients enrolled with pancreatic cancer [51]. Similarly, in a trial of patients with different advanced tumor types treated with pembrolizumab, pancreatic cancer patients ($n = 24$) had an overall response rate of 0% [52].

Pre-clinical studies suggest that combinatorial therapy, for example, chemotherapy, and CD40 agonism, may be needed to overcome resistance to checkpoint inhibition [53]. A CD40 agonist antibody combined with gemcitabine chemotherapy resulted in tumor regressions in several patients [54, 55]. In mice, the mechanism of CD40 agonism relied on macrophages capable of infiltrating and depleting tumor stroma [54]; thus, there is rationale to combine CD40 agonists (macrophage activation) with checkpoint inhibition (T cell invigoration) in further studies, and trials are ongoing to investigate this approach (NCT02482168). Chemotherapy (nab-paclitaxel and gemcitabine) in combination with nivolumab or pembrolizumab for chemotherapy-naïve patients has alternately proven to be comparable or slightly improved (respectively) in terms of survival rates for chemotherapy alone [56, 57].

4 Inhibition of Suppressive Myeloid Cells

Depleting or re-polarizing myeloid cells to less suppressive phenotypes through the use of inhibitors targeting myeloid cell receptors CSF1R and CCR2 in pre-clinical models can augment anti-tumor T cell responses and improve chemotherapy effectiveness [58]. Clinically, decreased inflammatory monocytes in the peripheral blood have been demonstrated with myeloid inhibitors but efficacy has been variable [59]. In a Phase 1b study of an oral inhibitor of CCR2 (PF-04136309) in combination with gemcitabine and nab-paclitaxel, the overall response rate measured 23.8%, close to historical response rates for this chemotherapy regimen alone in the first line setting for metastatic pancreatic cancer [59, 60]. Furthermore, the combination of a CCR2 inhibitor and chemotherapy resulted in a 24% rate of pulmonary toxicity, raising concerns about the safety of this novel agent. The combination of a different

CCR2 antagonist, CCX872, and FOLFIRINOX in locally advanced or metastatic PDA resulted in an overall survival at 18 months of 29%, comparing favorably with previous response rates to FOLFIRINOX alone [61, 62]. Using a CCR2 antagonist in combination with FOLFIRINOX earlier in treatment in a Phase IB trial for neoadjuvant treatment of borderline resectable or locally advanced pancreatic cancer resulted in an improved response rate (49%) compared to FOLFIRINOX alone in other studies, with similar findings of monocyte depletion and without concerns of excessive toxicity [63–65]. Tumors harbor heterogeneous populations of suppressive myeloid cells derived from monocytic and granulocytic precursors and therefore combined targeting of multiple populations is one strategy to improve on the efficacy of myeloid-targeted agents [66]. Additionally, combining myeloid cell inhibitors with checkpoint inhibitors or other immunotherapies may prove an effective strategy [67].

5 Overcoming the Suppressive Tumor Microenvironment

Given the interactions of the immune cells in the pancreatic tumor microenvironment with stromal components, therapeutics aimed at ECM or fibroblasts in pancreatic cancer can be considered immunomodulatory. Unfortunately, thus far, these attempts have largely been unsuccessful in patients, despite anti-tumor efficacy and augmentation of the immune response in mice. In pre-clinical models, attempts to target the stroma using enzymatic degradation of HA have improved on the efficacy of chemotherapy alone [21]. A Phase IB/II trial combining pegylated recombinant human hyaluronidase (PEGPH20) with modified fluorouracil, leucovorin, irinotecan, and oxaliplatin (mFOLFIRINOX) for patients with metastatic pancreatic cancer was closed to accrual following the planned interim futility analysis, with an overall survival that favored mFOLFIRINOX alone (14.4 months) versus the combination (7.7 months) [68]. Of note, there was no selection for HA expression in this trial. In the HALO 202 trial comparing PEGPH20 combined with nab-paclitaxel/gemcitabine (AG) vs. AG alone, HA was measured retrospectively [69]. The HALO 202 trial demonstrated a PFS benefit for patients treated with the combination and patients with HA-expressing tumors (HA-high) had increased PFS compared to those with negative tumors in the PEGPH20-treated group. In both trials patients developed thromboembolic events with PEGPH20 that required prophylaxis with enoxaparin [68, 69]. Unfortunately, in a phase III trial of PEGPH20+AG compared to AG alone in patients with HA-high pancreatic tumors, PEGPH20+AG failed to show an overall survival or PFS benefit compared to AG alone [70], and so this strategy has been largely abandoned.

A variety of other stromal-targeted agents have been studied in trials to a lesser degree, including other extracellular matrix or fibroblast-targeted therapies. Fibroblast activation protein (FAP), a stromal protein that can promote tumor metastasis, is expressed by fibroblasts and malignant cells and expression of FAP in pancreatic tumors correlates with poor prognosis [71]. A small molecule inhibitor of FAP combined with gemcitabine resulted in some responses in pancreatic cancer patients [72]. The sonic hedgehog (SHH) pathway is pivotal in pancreatic cancer tumorigenesis, and inhibition of this pathway in pre-clinical models can improve survival and reduce desmoplasia [73, 74]. However, clinical trials of SHH inhibitors in combination with chemotherapy failed to demonstrate a benefit beyond rates of response to chemotherapy alone [75, 76]. Matrix metalloproteinases (MMP), capable of disintegrating stroma, and MMP inhibitors may work primarily by inhibiting tumor metastasis rather than having direct cytotoxic effects [77]. Marimastat, one such MMP inhibitor, showed a comparable one-year survival compared to gemcitabine chemotherapy in the first line for unresectable pancreatic cancer [78]. Despite pancreatic cancer being thought of as hypovascular, angiogenesis is involved in tumorigenesis and could therefore be targeted with existing inhibitors to vascular endothelial growth factor (VEGF) [79]. Bevacizumab, a VEGF-targeted monoclonal antibody used in multiple cancer types, has not been shown to be effective in combination with chemotherapy regimens compared to chemotherapy and placebo, and carries bleeding and thromboembolic risks which may be magnified in pancreatic cancer patients [80, 81].

6 T Cell Cellular Therapy

One of the most promising approaches currently is the use of ex vivo modified tumor antigen-specific T cells adoptively transferred into patients, based on the success of using chimeric antigen receptor (CAR) T cells in hematologic malignancies [82, 83]. The expansion of this type of immunotherapy to solid organ tumors is in the early stages, but several trials have been conducted thus far. Several small studies using mesothelin-directed CAR T cells have demonstrated the safety and feasibility of this approach [84–86]. A phase one trial of mesothelin-directed CARs was conducted with six patients with advanced chemo-refractory pancreatic cancer and demonstrated safety and tolerability. One patient whose tumor expressed mesothelin had reduction in FDG uptake in liver lesions by PET imaging; however, efficacy was limited overall with two patients experiencing a period of stable disease [85]. Another approach in addition to designing a CAR is to use autologous T cells with an endogenous and engineered T cell receptor to recognize antigens. In a phase I study of administration of autologous T cell lines targeting several tumor-associated antigens, 8 out of 13 patients had disease control following first line chemotherapy for longer than expected time per historical controls, with 4 patients demonstrating partial or complete responses [87].

Along with the challenge common to all solid tumors of antigen selection, pancreatic cancer presents the challenge of dense stroma impeding T cells. Targeting the stroma as well as tumor antigens, for example, with FAP-targeted CAR T cells that can act alone or in combination with tumor-antigen-targeted CAR T cells [88] or CAR T cells could be designed to withstand elements that make the tumor microenvironment inhospitable such as hypoxia [89]. In a trial of dual CAR T cells, targeting CD19 and targeting mesothelin, the CD19-targeted CAR T cells could effectively deplete potentially immunosuppressive B cells, but did not improve the persistence of the mesothelin-targeted CAR T cells [90]. One additional concern for the use of personalized T cell therapy in patients with advanced pancreatic cancer is the timeframe for personalized therapy development, which can take months to implement. Many novel technologic advances in the cellular therapy development pipeline are ongoing to enhance efficacy and safety.

7 Conclusions and Future Directions

Along with developing novel immunotherapies with improved efficacy, biomarkers are desperately needed for stratifying patients who may respond to immunotherapy. Biomarkers of response can shed light on mechanisms of response to immunotherapy and are of particular importance in pancreatic cancer when tissue-based sampling can be technically challenging. T cell receptor sequencing is one approach to understand how immunotherapy shapes the immune repertoire. For example, changes in T cell receptor diversity are correlated with ipilimumab therapy in pancreatic cancer patients, with an increasing number of clonal T cells following treatment associated with survival [91]. On the other hand, PD-L1 status, a biomarker of response for checkpoint inhibitors in other cancer types, did not correlate with response to checkpoint inhibitors [56]. Thus far, biomarkers have been challenging to identify due to low number of pancreatic cancer responders [52].

New therapeutic strategies are on the horizon and may include vaccines, cellular therapy, oncolytic viruses [92], and bispecific T cell engagers [93]. Combinations of immunotherapy with radiation and chemotherapy may be needed to overcome the immune suppression that characterizes pancreatic cancer. Finally, immunotherapy may be most effective when used in earlier stages of pancreatic cancer, and for that, we will also rely upon on technology to increase early detection.

Compliance with Ethical Standards

Funding Not applicable.

Disclosure of Interests B. Keenan has received research grants from Partner Therapeutics. M. Tempero has received grants from Celgene and Halozyme and is an advisory board member for AbbVie, AstraZeneca, Biotech Research Group, Boehriner Ingelheim, Bristol-Myers Squibb, Corcept Therapeutics, Geistlich Pharma, Merck & Co., Seagen, Inc., Swedish Orphan Biovitrum and an consultant for ISPEN, Incyte, and Karyopharm Therapeutics.

Studies involving humans
Ethical approval This article does not contain any studies with human participants performed by any of the authors.

Studies involving animals
Ethical approval This article does not contain any studies with animals performed by any of the authors.

Informed Consent Not applicable.

References

1. Vincent A, Herman J, Schulick R, Hruban RH, Goggins M (2011) Pancreatic cancer. Lancet 378(9791):607–620
2. Clark CE, Hingorani SR, Mick R, Combs C, Tuveson DA, Vonderheide RH (2007) Dynamics of the immune reaction to pancreatic cancer from inception to invasion. Cancer Res 67(19):9518–9527
3. Blando J, Sharma A, Higa MG, Zhao H, Vence L, Yadav SS et al (2019) Comparison of immune infiltrates in melanoma and pancreatic cancer highlights VISTA as a potential target in pancreatic cancer. Proc Natl Acad Sci U S A 116(5):1692–1697
4. Sen DR, Kaminski J, Barnitz RA, Kurachi M, Gerdemann U, Yates KB et al (2016) The epigenetic landscape of T cell exhaustion. Science 354(6316):1165–1169
5. Stromnes IM, Schmitt TM, Hulbert A, Brockenbrough JS, Nguyen H, Cuevas C et al (2015) T cells engineered against a native antigen can surmount immunologic and physical barriers to treat pancreatic ductal adenocarcinoma. Cancer Cell 28(5):638–652
6. Yarchoan M, Hopkins A, Jaffee EM (2017) Tumor mutational burden and response rate to PD-1 inhibition. N Engl J Med 377(25):2500–2501
7. Marabelle A, Fakih MG, Lopez J, Shah M, Shapira-Frommer R, Nakagawa K, Chung HC, Kindler HL, Lopez-Martin JA, Miller W, Italiano A, Kao S, Piha-Paul SA, Delord J-P, McWilliams RR, Aurora-Garg D, Chen M, Jin F, Norwood K, Bang Y-J (2019) Association of tumour mutational burden with outcomes in patients with select advanced solid tumours treated with pembrolizumab in KEYNOTE-158. Ann Oncol 30(Suppl. 5):v477–v4v8
8. Dudley JC, Lin MT, Le DT, Eshleman JR (2016) Microsatellite instability as a biomarker for PD-1 blockade. Clin Cancer Res 22(4):813–820
9. Balachandran VP, Luksza M, Zhao JN, Makarov V, Moral JA, Remark R et al (2017) Identification of unique neoantigen qualities in long-term survivors of pancreatic cancer. Nature 551(7681):512–516
10. Jones S, Zhang X, Parsons DW, Lin JC, Leary RJ, Angenendt P et al (2008) Core signaling pathways in human pancreatic cancers revealed by global genomic analyses. Science 321(5897):1801–1806
11. Collins MA, Bednar F, Zhang Y, Brisset JC, Galban S, Galban CJ et al (2012) Oncogenic Kras is required for both the initiation and maintenance of pancreatic cancer in mice. J Clin Invest 122(2):639–653
12. Lesokhin AM, Hohl TM, Kitano S, Cortez C, Hirschhorn-Cymerman D, Avogadri F et al (2012) Monocytic CCR2(+) myeloid-derived suppressor cells promote immune escape by limiting activated CD8 T-cell infiltration into the tumor microenvironment. Cancer Res 72(4):876–886
13. Zhang Y, Velez-Delgado A, Mathew E, Li D, Mendez FM, Flannagan K et al (2017) Myeloid cells are required for PD-1/PD-L1 checkpoint activation and the establishment of an immunosuppressive environment in pancreatic cancer. Gut 66(1):124–136
14. Hruban RH, Adsay NV, Albores-Saavedra J, Compton C, Garrett ES, Goodman SN et al (2001) Pancreatic intraepithelial neoplasia: a new nomenclature and classification system for pancreatic duct lesions. Am J Surg Pathol 25(5):579–586
15. Keenan BP, Saenger Y, Kafrouni MI, Leubner A, Lauer P, Maitra A et al (2014) A Listeria vaccine and depletion of T-regulatory cells activate immunity against early stage pancreatic intraepithelial neoplasms and prolong survival of mice. Gastroenterology 146(7):1784–94.e6
16. Bayne LJ, Beatty GL, Jhala N, Clark CE, Rhim AD, Stanger BZ et al (2012) Tumor-derived granulocyte-macrophage colony-stimulating factor regulates myeloid inflammation and T cell immunity in pancreatic cancer. Cancer Cell 21(6):822–835
17. Sparmann A, Bar-Sagi D (2004) Ras-induced interleukin-8 expression plays a critical role in tumor growth and angiogenesis. Cancer Cell 6(5):447–458
18. Hiraoka N, Onozato K, Kosuge T, Hirohashi S (2006) Prevalence of FOXP3+ regulatory T cells increases during the progression of pancreatic ductal adenocarcinoma and its premalignant lesions. Clin Cancer Res 12(18):5423–5434

19. Farren MR, Mace TA, Geyer S, Mikhail S, Wu C, Ciombor K et al (2016) Systemic immune activity predicts overall survival in treatment-naive patients with metastatic pancreatic cancer. Clin Cancer Res 22(10):2565–2574
20. Hosein AN, Brekken RA, Maitra A (2020) Pancreatic cancer stroma: an update on therapeutic targeting strategies. Nat Rev Gastroenterol Hepatol 17(8):487–505
21. Provenzano PP, Cuevas C, Chang AE, Goel VK, Von Hoff DD, Hingorani SR (2012) Enzymatic targeting of the stroma ablates physical barriers to treatment of pancreatic ductal adenocarcinoma. Cancer Cell 21(3):418–429
22. Salmon H, Franciszkiewicz K, Damotte D, Dieu-Nosjean MC, Validire P, Trautmann A et al (2012) Matrix architecture defines the preferential localization and migration of T cells into the stroma of human lung tumors. J Clin Invest 122(3):899–910
23. Hwang RF, Moore T, Arumugam T, Ramachandran V, Amos KD, Rivera A et al (2008) Cancer-associated stromal fibroblasts promote pancreatic tumor progression. Cancer Res 68(3):918–926
24. Sahai E, Astsaturov I, Cukierman E, DeNardo DG, Egeblad M, Evans RM et al (2020) A framework for advancing our understanding of cancer-associated fibroblasts. Nat Rev Cancer 20(3):174–186
25. Ohlund D, Handly-Santana A, Biffi G, Elyada E, Almeida AS, Ponz-Sarvise M et al (2017) Distinct populations of inflammatory fibroblasts and myofibroblasts in pancreatic cancer. J Exp Med 214(3):579–596
26. Elyada E, Bolisetty M, Laise P, Flynn WF, Courtois ET, Burkhart RA et al (2019) Cross-species single-cell analysis of pancreatic ductal adenocarcinoma reveals antigen-presenting cancer-associated fibroblasts. Cancer Discov 9(8):1102–1123
27. Laheru D, Lutz E, Burke J, Biedrzycki B, Solt S, Onners B et al (2008) Allogeneic granulocyte macrophage colony-stimulating factor-secreting tumor immunotherapy alone or in sequence with cyclophosphamide for metastatic pancreatic cancer: a pilot study of safety, feasibility, and immune activation. Clin Cancer Res 14(5):1455–1463
28. Hardacre JM, Mulcahy M, Small W, Talamonti M, Obel J, Krishnamurthi S et al (2013) Addition of algenpantucel-L immunotherapy to standard adjuvant therapy for pancreatic cancer: a phase 2 study. J Gastrointest Surg 17(1):94–100; discussion 101
29. Pecher G, Haring A, Kaiser L, Thiel E (2002) Mucin gene (MUC1) transfected dendritic cells as vaccine: results of a phase I/II clinical trial. Cancer Immunol Immunother 51(11–12): 669–673
30. Le DT, Wang-Gillam A, Picozzi V, Greten TF, Crocenzi T, Springett G et al (2015) Safety and survival with GVAX pancreas prime and Listeria monocytogenes-expressing mesothelin (CRS-207) boost vaccines for metastatic pancreatic cancer. J Clin Oncol 33(12): 1325–1333
31. Kaufman HL, Kim-Schulze S, Manson K, DeRaffele G, Mitcham J, Seo KS et al (2007) Poxvirus-based vaccine therapy for patients with advanced pancreatic cancer. J Transl Med 5:60
32. Ramanathan RK, Lee KM, McKolanis J, Hitbold E, Schraut W, Moser AJ et al (2005) Phase I study of a MUC1 vaccine composed of different doses of MUC1 peptide with SB-AS2 adjuvant in resected and locally advanced pancreatic cancer. Cancer Immunol Immunother 54(3):254–264
33. Middleton G, Silcocks P, Cox T, Valle J, Wadsley J, Propper D et al (2014) Gemcitabine and capecitabine with or without telomerase peptide vaccine GV1001 in patients with locally advanced or metastatic pancreatic cancer (TeloVac): an open-label, randomised, phase 3 trial. Lancet Oncol 15(8):829–840
34. Keenan BP, Jaffee EM (2012) Whole cell vaccines—past progress and future strategies. Semin Oncol 39(3):276–286
35. Greten TF, Jaffee EM (1999) Cancer vaccines. J Clin Oncol 17(3):1047–1060
36. Mehrotra S, Britten CD, Chin S, Garrett-Mayer E, Cloud CA, Li M et al (2017) Vaccination with poly(IC:LC) and peptide-pulsed autologous dendritic cells in patients with pancreatic cancer. J Hematol Oncol 10(1):82

37. Rahma OE, Hamilton JM, Wojtowicz M, Dakheel O, Bernstein S, Liewehr DJ et al (2014) The immunological and clinical effects of mutated ras peptide vaccine in combination with IL-2, GM-CSF, or both in patients with solid tumors. J Transl Med 12:55
38. Wobser M, Keikavoussi P, Kunzmann V, Weininger M, Andersen MH, Becker JC (2006) Complete remission of liver metastasis of pancreatic cancer under vaccination with a HLA-A2 restricted peptide derived from the universal tumor antigen survivin. Cancer Immunol Immunother 55(10):1294–1298
39. Miyazawa M, Ohsawa R, Tsunoda T, Hirono S, Kawai M, Tani M et al (2010) Phase I clinical trial using peptide vaccine for human vascular endothelial growth factor receptor 2 in combination with gemcitabine for patients with advanced pancreatic cancer. Cancer Sci 101(2):433–439
40. Nishida S, Koido S, Takeda Y, Homma S, Komita H, Takahara A et al (2014) Wilms tumor gene (WT1) peptide-based cancer vaccine combined with gemcitabine for patients with advanced pancreatic cancer. J Immunother 37(2):105–114
41. Bernhardt SL, Gjertsen MK, Trachsel S, Moller M, Eriksen JA, Meo M et al (2006) Telomerase peptide vaccination of patients with non-resectable pancreatic cancer: a dose escalating phase I/II study. Br J Cancer 95(11):1474–1482
42. Toubaji A, Achtar M, Provenzano M, Herrin VE, Behrens R, Hamilton M et al (2008) Pilot study of mutant ras peptide-based vaccine as an adjuvant treatment in pancreatic and colorectal cancers. Cancer Immunol Immunother 57(9):1413–1420
43. Schumacher TN, Schreiber RD (2015) Neoantigens in cancer immunotherapy. Science 348(6230):69–74
44. Ott PA, Hu Z, Keskin DB, Shukla SA, Sun J, Bozym DJ et al (2017) An immunogenic personal neoantigen vaccine for patients with melanoma. Nature 547(7662):217–221
45. Lutz ER, Wu AA, Bigelow E, Sharma R, Mo G, Soares K et al (2014) Immunotherapy converts nonimmunogenic pancreatic tumors into immunogenic foci of immune regulation. Cancer Immunol Res 2(7):616–631
46. Keenan B, Jaffee EM (2013) Immunotherapy in preneoplastic disease: targeting early procarcinogenic inflammatory changes that lead to immune suppression and tumor tolerance. Ann N Y Acad Sci 1284:12–16
47. Topalian SL, Hodi FS, Brahmer JR, Gettinger SN, Smith DC, McDermott DF et al (2012) Safety, activity, and immune correlates of anti-PD-1 antibody in cancer. N Engl J Med 366(26):2443–2454
48. Postow MA, Callahan MK, Wolchok JD (2015) Immune checkpoint blockade in cancer therapy. J Clin Oncol 33(17):1974–1982
49. Royal RE, Levy C, Turner K, Mathur A, Hughes M, Kammula US et al (2010) Phase 2 trial of single agent Ipilimumab (anti-CTLA-4) for locally advanced or metastatic pancreatic adenocarcinoma. J Immunother 33(8):828–833
50. Le DT, Lutz E, Uram JN, Sugar EA, Onners B, Solt S et al (2013) Evaluation of ipilimumab in combination with allogeneic pancreatic tumor cells transfected with a GM-CSF gene in previously treated pancreatic cancer. J Immunother 36(7):382–389
51. Brahmer JR, Tykodi SS, Chow LQ, Hwu WJ, Topalian SL, Hwu P et al (2012) Safety and activity of anti-PD-L1 antibody in patients with advanced cancer. N Engl J Med 366(26): 2455–2465
52. Ott PA, Bang YJ, Piha-Paul SA, Razak ARA, Bennouna J, Soria JC et al (2019) T-cell-inflamed gene-expression profile, programmed death ligand 1 expression, and tumor mutational burden predict efficacy in patients treated with pembrolizumab across 20 cancers: KEYNOTE-028. J Clin Oncol 37(4):318–327
53. Winograd R, Byrne KT, Evans RA, Odorizzi PM, Meyer AR, Bajor DL et al (2015) Induction of T-cell immunity overcomes complete resistance to PD-1 and CTLA-4 blockade and improves survival in pancreatic carcinoma. Cancer Immunol Res 3(4):399–411
54. Beatty GL, Chiorean EG, Fishman MP, Saboury B, Teitelbaum UR, Sun W et al (2011) CD40 agonists alter tumor stroma and show efficacy against pancreatic carcinoma in mice and humans. Science 331(6024):1612–1616

55. Beatty GL, Torigian DA, Chiorean EG, Saboury B, Brothers A, Alavi A et al (2013) A phase I study of an agonist CD40 monoclonal antibody (CP-870,893) in combination with gemcitabine in patients with advanced pancreatic ductal adenocarcinoma. Clin Cancer Res 19(22):6286–6295
56. Wainberg ZA, Hochster HS, Kim EJ, George B, Kaylan A, Chiorean EG et al (2020) Open-label, phase I study of nivolumab combined with nab-paclitaxel plus gemcitabine in advanced pancreatic cancer. Clin Cancer Res 26(18):4814–4822
57. Weiss GJ, Blaydorn L, Beck J, Bornemann-Kolatzki K, Urnovitz H, Schutz E et al (2018) Phase Ib/II study of gemcitabine, nab-paclitaxel, and pembrolizumab in metastatic pancreatic adenocarcinoma. Investig New Drugs 36(1):96–102
58. Mitchem JB, Brennan DJ, Knolhoff BL, Belt BA, Zhu Y, Sanford DE et al (2013) Targeting tumor-infiltrating macrophages decreases tumor-initiating cells, relieves immunosuppression, and improves chemotherapeutic responses. Cancer Res 73(3):1128–1141
59. Noel M, O'Reilly EM, Wolpin BM, Ryan DP, Bullock AJ, Britten CD et al (2020) Phase 1b study of a small molecule antagonist of human chemokine (C-C motif) receptor 2 (PF-04136309) in combination with nab-paclitaxel/gemcitabine in first-line treatment of metastatic pancreatic ductal adenocarcinoma. Investig New Drugs 38(3):800–811
60. Von Hoff DD, Ervin T, Arena FP, Chiorean EG, Infante J, Moore M et al (2013) Increased survival in pancreatic cancer with nab-paclitaxel plus gemcitabine. N Engl J Med 369(18):1691–1703
61. Linehan D, Noel MS, Hezel AF, Wang-Gillam A, Eskens F, Sleijfer S et al (2018) Overall survival in a trial of orally administered CCR2 inhibitor CCX872 in locally advanced/metastatic pancreatic cancer: correlation with blood monocyte counts. J Clin Oncol 36(5_Suppl):92
62. Conroy T, Desseigne F, Ychou M, Bouche O, Guimbaud R, Becouarn Y et al (2011) FOLFIRINOX versus gemcitabine for metastatic pancreatic cancer. N Engl J Med 364(19):1817–1825
63. Yoo C, Lee SS, Song KB, Jeong JH, Hyung J, Park DH et al (2020) Neoadjuvant modified FOLFIRINOX followed by postoperative gemcitabine in borderline resectable pancreatic adenocarcinoma: a Phase 2 study for clinical and biomarker analysis. Br J Cancer 123(3): 362–368
64. Murphy JE, Wo JY, Ryan DP, Jiang W, Yeap BY, Drapek LC et al (2018) Total neoadjuvant therapy with FOLFIRINOX followed by individualized chemoradiotherapy for borderline resectable pancreatic adenocarcinoma: a phase 2 clinical trial. JAMA Oncol 4(7):963–969
65. Nywening TM, Wang-Gillam A, Sanford DE, Belt BA, Panni RZ, Cusworth BM et al (2016) Targeting tumour-associated macrophages with CCR2 inhibition in combination with FOLFIRINOX in patients with borderline resectable and locally advanced pancreatic cancer: a single-centre, open-label, dose-finding, non-randomised, phase 1b trial. Lancet Oncol 17(5):651–662
66. Nywening TM, Belt BA, Cullinan DR, Panni RZ, Han BJ, Sanford DE et al (2018) Targeting both tumour-associated CXCR2(+) neutrophils and CCR2(+) macrophages disrupts myeloid recruitment and improves chemotherapeutic responses in pancreatic ductal adenocarcinoma. Gut 67(6):1112–1123
67. Jung H, Ertl L, Janson C, Schall T, Charo I (2016) Abstract A107: Inhibition of CCR2 potentiates the checkpoint inhibitor immunotherapy in pancreatic cancer. Cancer Immunol Res 4(11 Supplement):A107
68. Ramanathan RK, McDonough SL, Philip PA, Hingorani SR, Lacy J, Kortmansky JS et al (2019) Phase IB/II randomized study of FOLFIRINOX plus Pegylated recombinant human hyaluronidase versus FOLFIRINOX alone in patients with metastatic pancreatic adenocarcinoma: SWOG S1313. J Clin Oncol 37(13):1062–1069
69. Hingorani SR, Zheng L, Bullock AJ, Seery TE, Harris WP, Sigal DS et al (2018) HALO 202: randomized phase II study of PEGPH20 plus nab-paclitaxel/gemcitabine versus nab-paclitaxel/ gemcitabine in patients with untreated, metastatic pancreatic ductal adenocarcinoma. J Clin Oncol 36(4):359–366

70. Tempero MA, Cutsem EV, Sigal D, Oh D-Y, Fazio N, Macarulla T et al (2020) HALO 109-301: a randomized, double-blind, placebo-controlled, phase 3 study of pegvorhyaluronidase alfa (PEGPH20) + nab-paclitaxel/gemcitabine (AG) in patients (pts) with previously untreated hyaluronan (HA)-high metastatic pancreatic ductal adenocarcinoma (mPDA). J Clin Oncol 38(4_Suppl):638
71. Lo A, Li CP, Buza EL, Blomberg R, Govindaraju P, Avery D et al (2017) Fibroblast activation protein augments progression and metastasis of pancreatic ductal adenocarcinoma. JCI Insight 2(19)
72. Nugent FW, Cunningham C, Barve MA, Fisher W, Patel H, Meiri E et al (2007) Phase 2 study of talabostat/gemcitabine in Stage IV pancreatic cancer. J Clin Oncol 25(18_Suppl):4616
73. Bailey JM, Swanson BJ, Hamada T, Eggers JP, Singh PK, Caffery T et al (2008) Sonic hedgehog promotes desmoplasia in pancreatic cancer. Clin Cancer Res 14(19):5995–6004
74. Hidalgo M, Maitra A (2009) The hedgehog pathway and pancreatic cancer. N Engl J Med 361(21):2094–2096
75. De Jesus-Acosta A, Sugar EA, O'Dwyer PJ, Ramanathan RK, Von Hoff DD, Rasheed Z et al (2020) Phase 2 study of vismodegib, a hedgehog inhibitor, combined with gemcitabine and nab-paclitaxel in patients with untreated metastatic pancreatic adenocarcinoma. Br J Cancer 122(4):498–505
76. Catenacci DV, Junttila MR, Karrison T, Bahary N, Horiba MN, Nattam SR et al (2015) Randomized phase Ib/II study of gemcitabine plus placebo or vismodegib, a hedgehog pathway inhibitor, in patients with metastatic pancreatic cancer. J Clin Oncol 33(36):4284–4292
77. Watson SA, Morris TM, Robinson G, Crimmin MJ, Brown PD, Hardcastle JD (1995) Inhibition of organ invasion by the matrix metalloproteinase inhibitor batimastat (BB-94) in two human colon carcinoma metastasis models. Cancer Res 55(16):3629–3633
78. Bramhall SR, Rosemurgy A, Brown PD, Bowry C, Buckels JA, Marimastat Pancreatic Cancer Study Group (2001) Marimastat as first-line therapy for patients with unresectable pancreatic cancer: a randomized trial. J Clin Oncol 19(15):3447–3455
79. Vennin C, Murphy KJ, Morton JP, Cox TR, Pajic M, Timpson P (2018) Reshaping the tumor stroma for treatment of pancreatic cancer. Gastroenterology 154(4):820–838
80. Ko AH, Dito E, Schillinger B, Venook AP, Xu Z, Bergsland EK et al (2008) A phase II study evaluating bevacizumab in combination with fixed-dose rate gemcitabine and low-dose cisplatin for metastatic pancreatic cancer: is an anti-VEGF strategy still applicable? Investig New Drugs 26(5):463–471
81. Kindler HL, Niedzwiecki D, Hollis D, Sutherland S, Schrag D, Hurwitz H et al (2010) Gemcitabine plus bevacizumab compared with gemcitabine plus placebo in patients with advanced pancreatic cancer: phase III trial of the Cancer and Leukemia Group B (CALGB 80303). J Clin Oncol 28(22):3617–3622
82. Park JH, Riviere I, Gonen M, Wang X, Senechal B, Curran KJ et al (2018) Long-term follow-up of CD19 CAR therapy in acute lymphoblastic leukemia. N Engl J Med 378(5):449–459
83. Neelapu SS, Locke FL, Bartlett NL, Lekakis LJ, Miklos DB, Jacobson CA et al (2017) Axicabtagene ciloleucel CAR T-cell therapy in refractory large B-cell lymphoma. N Engl J Med 377(26):2531–2544
84. Beatty GL, Haas AR, Maus MV, Torigian DA, Soulen MC, Plesa G et al (2014) Mesothelin-specific chimeric antigen receptor mRNA-engineered T cells induce anti-tumor activity in solid malignancies. Cancer Immunol Res 2(2):112–120
85. Beatty GL, O'Hara MH, Lacey SF, Torigian DA, Nazimuddin F, Chen F et al (2018) Activity of mesothelin-specific chimeric antigen receptor T cells against pancreatic carcinoma metastases in a phase 1 trial. Gastroenterology 155(1):29–32
86. Haas AR, Tanyi JL, O'Hara MH, Gladney WL, Lacey SF, Torigian DA et al (2019) Phase I study of lentiviral-transduced chimeric antigen receptor-modified T cells recognizing mesothelin in advanced solid cancers. Mol Ther 27(11):1919–1929
87. Smaglo BG, Musher BL, Vasileiou S, Kuvalekar M, Watanabe A, Robertson C et al (2020) A phase I trial targeting advanced or metastatic pancreatic cancer using a combination of stan-

dard chemotherapy and adoptively transferred nonengineered, multiantigen specific T cells in the first-line setting (TACTOPS). J Clin Oncol 38(15_Suppl):4622
88. Kakarla S, Chow KK, Mata M, Shaffer DR, Song XT, Wu MF et al (2013) Antitumor effects of chimeric receptor engineered human T cells directed to tumor stroma. Mol Ther 21(8):1611–1620
89. Rodriguez-Garcia A, Palazon A, Noguera-Ortega E, Powell DJ Jr, Guedan S (2020) CAR-T cells hit the tumor microenvironment: strategies to overcome tumor escape. Front Immunol 11:1109
90. Ko AH, Jordan AC, Tooker E, Lacey SF, Chang RB, Li Y et al (2020) Dual targeting of mesothelin and CD19 with chimeric antigen receptor-modified T cells in patients with metastatic pancreatic cancer. Mol Ther 28(11):2367–2378
91. Hopkins AC, Yarchoan M, Durham JN, Yusko EC, Rytlewski JA, Robins HS et al (2018) T cell receptor repertoire features associated with survival in immunotherapy-treated pancreatic ductal adenocarcinoma. JCI Insight 3(13)
92. Watanabe K, Luo Y, Da T, Guedan S, Ruella M, Scholler J et al (2018) Pancreatic cancer therapy with combined mesothelin-redirected chimeric antigen receptor T cells and cytokine-armed oncolytic adenoviruses. JCI Insight 3(7)
93. Slaney CY, Wang P, Darcy PK, Kershaw MH (2018) CARs versus BiTEs: a comparison between T cell-redirection strategies for cancer treatment. Cancer Discov 8(8):924–934

Part VIII

Biomarkers for Immunotherapy in Gastrointestinal Cancers

Biomarkers for Immunotherapy in Gastrointestinal Cancers

Juliette Palle, Julien Taïeb, and Aziz Zaanan

Contents

J. Palle · J. Taïeb · A. Zaanan (✉)
Gastroenterology and Digestive Oncology Department, Georges Pompidou European Hospital, APHP, Université de Paris, Paris, France
e-mail: aziz.zaanan@aphp.fr

Cancer Immunotherapy (2021)
https://doi.org/10.1007/13905_2021_10,

Published Online: 25 August 2021

Abstract

Immunotherapy represents one of the most promising emerging therapies for the treatment of gastrointestinal (GI) cancers. As for targeted therapies, the results of the first trials have underlined the need for biomarkers to select patients who benefit from these molecules. After the first studies conducted in colorectal cancer, mismatch repair (MMR) deficiency, resulting in microsatellite instability (MSI), has been identified to predict response and survival to immunotherapy regardless of tumor origin. More recently, an elevated tumor mutational burden (TMB) was also validated as a tumor-origin independent predictive biomarker for response to pembrolizumab. Following the emerging concept of molecular diagnosis, the Food and Drug Administration (FDA) approved MSI/MMR deficiency and high-TMB as criteria for the indication of immunotherapy regardless of tumor origin. As in non-GI tumor locations, such as broncho-pulmonary cancer, PD-L1 overexpression in tumor cells and/or in immune cells of the tumor microenvironment has been identified and validated by the FDA as a biomarker for response to immunotherapy in gastric and esophageal cancers. However, optimal assessment method and definition of PD-L1 overexpression are still under investigation. Other immune-related biomarkers such as tumor-infiltrating lymphocyte assessment, inflamed-gene expression, or circulating neutrophil-to-lymphocyte ratio might correlate to response and/or survival in several tumor locations, but need to be further investigated. Lastly, several tumor location specific parameters appear to be promising biomarkers in selected indications, such as POLE mutations in colorectal cancer, EBV status in gastric cancer, and HPV status in anal cancer.

Keywords

Biomarkers · Microsatellite instability · Mismatch repair system · PD-L1 expression · Tumor mutational burden

1 Introduction

Since the apparition of immunotherapy in the therapeutic landscape of gastrointestinal (GI) cancers, the identification of predictive biomarkers has been a key objective to select patients who may benefit from these new treatments. As demonstrated by the large studies leading to authorization for immunotherapy in GI cancers, the assessment of biomarkers such as PD-L1 expression is necessary to predict response and survival in several tumor locations such as gastric and esophageal cancer. Moreover, other biomarkers such as mismatch repair (MMR) system status or tumor mutational burden (TMB) were shown to predict the efficacy of immunotherapy regardless of tumor origin, creating a true paradigm shift in cancer treatment.

In this chapter, we will first discuss the main biomarkers currently validated in immunotherapy for GI cancers (MMR status, TMB, and PD-L1 expression). Then, we will review the particularities of current knowledge and perspectives for each tumor location (Table 1).

Table 1 Main biomarkers of response to immunotherapy in gastrointestinal cancers

Biomarker	Assessment method	Routine use	Relevance in GI cancers	Approval	Remarks	Main references
PD-L1 expression	IHC	Yes	GC, EC: strong CRC, AC, HCC: unclear	FDA-approved for GC and EC	Different cutoffs and scores	Fuchs [59], Kato [87], Kojima [88]
dMMR and/or MSI	IHC/PCR	Yes	CRC: confirmed Tumor agnostic	FDA-approved for all solid advanced tumors		Le [5], Overman [3, 25]
Tumor mutational burden	NGS	Upcoming	Tumor agnostic	FDA-approved for all solid advanced tumors	Cutoff for FDA approval (>10 mutations/megabase)	Marabelle [9]
POLE mutations	PCR	Not yet	CRC: suggested	No		Forgo [55], Gong [56]
EBV status	IHC, ISH, PCR	Not yet	GC: suggested	No		Kim [70]
Gene expression profiling	NGS	No	GC, HCC: suggested	No		Fuchs [59], Jianjigian [61], Melero [103]
PD-L1 amplification	ISH	No	CRC: unclear	No		Sorscher [40]
Tumor-infiltrating lymphocytes	IHC	No	CRC, HCC: suggested	No		Loupakis [47], Melero [103]

dMMR mismatch repair deficiency, *MSI* microsatellite instability, *IHC* immunohistochemistry, *PCR* polymerase chain reaction, *NGS* next generation sequencing, *ISH* in situ hybridization, *GC* gastric cancer, *EC* esophageal cancer, *CRC* colorectal cancer, *AC* anal cancer, *HCC* hepatocellular carcinoma, *FDA* Food and Drug Administration

2 Main Biomarkers for Immunotherapy in GI Cancers

2.1 Microsatellite Instability/Mismatch Repair Deficiency

Microsatellite instability (MSI) is observed when the DNA MMR system is impaired. This deficiency can be caused by germline mutations of the *MLH1*, *MSH2*, *MSH6*, or *PMS2* genes, leading to the autosomal dominant Lynch syndrome that predisposes to gastrointestinal, gynecologic, and urothelial cancers. Sporadic deficiency in MMR system (dMMR) can also occur through the hypermethylation of the *MLH1* promoter resulting in the silencing of this gene [1]. There is a strong rationale to support that immunotherapy could be particularly effective in dMMR/MSI tumors. Indeed, dMMR is associated with an increased number of mutation-associated neoantigens, which may lead to a high immune infiltration within the tumor microenvironment. However these immune populations express high levels of inhibitory checkpoints (such as PD-1, CTLA-4, LAG-3) counteracting an effective immune response [2]. The demonstration that MMR status can predict response to immunotherapy was firstly brought by colorectal cancer (CRC) studies that will be described further [3, 4]. In 2017, a pivotal study by Le et al. included 86 patients with advanced dMMR/MSI tumors (including patients with Lynch syndrome and sporadic dMMR/MSI tumors), from 12 different tissue origins, treated with pembrolizumab in chemorefractory disease. In this study, the objective response rate (ORR) was 53% and the disease control rate (DCR) was 77%, providing evidence that MMR status could predict response to immunotherapy regardless of tumor origin [5]. Based on these results, pembrolizumab was approved by the FDA for the treatment of all solid dMMR/MSI advanced tumors who have no satisfactory alternative treatment options.

2.2 Tumor Mutational Burden

As previously described, highly mutated tumors are associated with a high neoantigen load inducing an enhanced immunologic response. However, this immunologic response is rendered inefficient by the expression of inhibitory molecules by immune effector cells of the microenvironment, or by tumor cells [6]. By unleashing this inhibition, immune checkpoint blockers (ICB) can restore an effective antitumoral response. TMB has been associated with favorable outcomes under anti-PD1/anti-PD-L1 therapies in various types of tumors, independently of MSI/MMR status [7, 8]. In the Keynote-158 prospective phase II study, 1066 patients with previously treated advanced tumors received pembrolizumab in monotherapy, and TMB has been assessed for 76% of patients (using the FoundationOne CDx assay). Patients with TMB-high (defined as more than 10 mutations/megabase) tumors (13%) had a better ORR as compared to patients with TMB-low tumors (29% vs. 6%) [9]. The ORR remained promising (23%) even after exclusion of MSI tumors who represented 14% of the population of patients with TMB-high tumors. Based on these results, pembrolizumab was approved by the FDA for the treatment of solid advanced tumors with a high TMB (>10 mutations/megabase) who have no satisfactory alternative treatment options.

Interestingly, in several studies including different tumors locations, a good correlation was found between TMB and mutation rates observed in circulating tumor DNA (ctDNA) [10]. Furthermore, in a retrospective study that included 69 patients with tumors of different origins, a high number of mutations in ctDNA was correlated to good responses and survival rates under immunotherapy [11]. Thus, if its predictive role is confirmed, ctDNA mutation burden assessment might become a routine and non-invasive biomarker for immunotherapy. Of note, in another report, ctDNA mutation burden was higher in patients with dMMR/MSI advanced CRC than in those with proficient (p)MMR/MSS tumor, suggesting that the mutation rate observed in ctDNA could be a surrogate marker for MMR status [12]. Given the very small number of patients included in this study (2 MSI patients), these results must be further confirmed.

However, data on TMB as a predictive biomarker for response to immunotherapy in the context of GI cancers is scarce and several limitations have to be noted. Firstly, as it is a continuous variable, a cutoff value is needed to define patients with high or low TMB. Furthermore, TMB values and shapes of distribution are variable between organs suggesting that different cutoffs according to tumor location might be warranted [13, 14]. Secondly, different techniques of Next Generation Sequencing (NGS) can be used to assess TMB. The first studies were based on Whole Genome Sequencing (WGS) or Whole Exome Sequencing (WES). However, due to their cost and long turnaround time, these techniques are not feasible on a routinely purpose. Different targeted gene panels have been developed for the assessment of TMB, however their correlation with WES is unperfect [15]. Prospective validation of TMB cutoffs in relationship to tumor type and patient outcomes are needed. Furthermore, standardization of TMB assessment across test platforms is important to the successful implementation of TMB in daily practice [16].

2.3 PD-L1 Status

Intratumoral expression of PD-L1 was the first biomarker associated with response to immunotherapy [17, 18]. A correlation between a high PD-L1 expression by tumor cells and a good response and/or survival under ICB have been found in different tumor locations such as urothelial [19], non-small lung [20], and head and neck [21] cancers. Furthermore, for several tumor locations, including GI cancers, expression of PD-L1 by tumor-infiltrating immune cells, notably antigen presenting cells, has been shown to play an essential role in response to ICBs [22]. Based on these findings, different scores combining PD-L1 expression on tumor cells and on immune cells have been established: The Tumor Proportion Score (TPS) assessing PD-L1 expression by tumor cells, the Mononuclear Immune Density Score (MIDS) assessing PD-L1 expression by immune cells, and the Combined Positive Score (CPS) assessing PD-L1 expression by tumor and immune cells (Fig. 1). Multiple immunohistochemistry (IHC) assays to detect PD-L1 expression have been

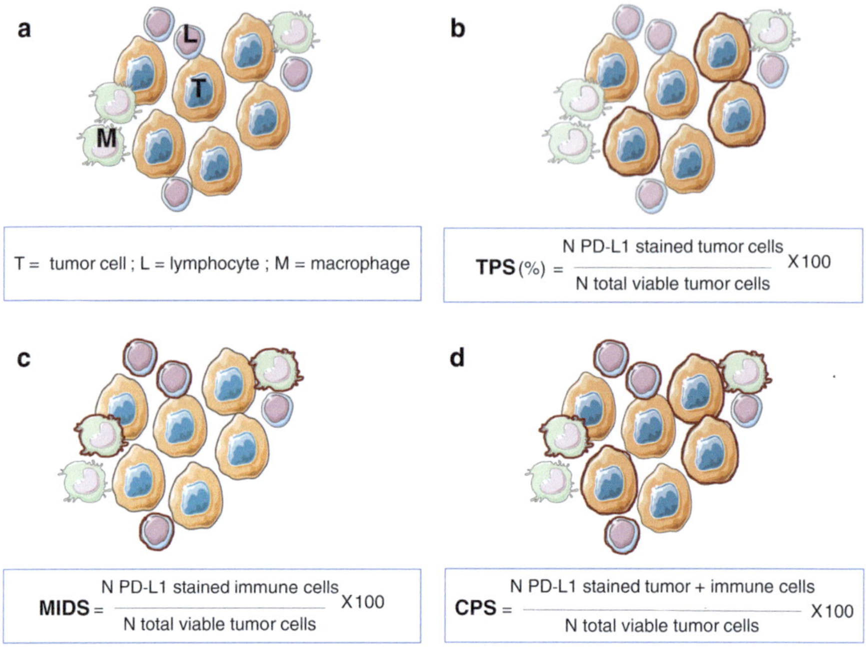

Fig. 1 PD-L1 scores. (**a**) Schematic representation of an epithelial tumor and tumor-infiltrating immune cells. (**b**) Tumor Proportion Score (TPS): Membranous staining of PD-L1 (brown line) on tumor cells is scored. Immune cells remain unscored. (**c**) Mononuclear Immune Density Score (MIDS): membranous and intracellular staining of PD-L1 on immune cells (including all mononuclear cells) is scored. Tumor cells remain unscored. (**d**) Combined Positive Score (CPS): Membranous staining of PD-L1 on tumor cells and membranous/intracellular staining of PD-L1 on immune cells (lymphocytes and macrophages) is scored. Tumor cells must show partial or complete staining to be considered positive, whereas immune cells are scored if any staining is observed

developed and are used in clinical trials to select patients who would benefit from immunotherapy. Several of them have been validated by the Food and Drug Administration (FDA) as a companion diagnostic for ICBs, each test being specific to different tumor location and molecule [23]. Several issues remain unmet such as the optimal cutoff and definition for PD-L1 positivity (percentage of stained cells or intensity of staining) or the assessment of temporal and intratumoral heterogeneity of PD-L1 expression.

3 Colorectal Cancer

3.1 Microsatellite Instability/Mismatch Repair Deficiency

The dMMR/MSI phenotype is observed in 12–15% of localized CRC, which is associated with a good prognosis (especially for stage I–II), and in less than 5% of metastatic CRC [24]. In a phase II trial, Le et al. assessed for the first time the impact of MMR status on response to pembrolizumab (anti-PD1) in metastatic CRC. The ORR was 40% in the dMMR/MSI group (including Lynch syndrome and non-Lynch MSI tumors), and 0% in the pMMR/MSS group. Median overall survival (OS) and progression free survival (PFS) were not reached in the dMMR/MSI cohort and were, respectively, 2.2 and 5.0 months in the pMMR/MSS cohort [4]. This was the first study to establish MMR status as a predictive biomarker of response to pembrolizumab in metastatic CRC. Similar results were observed in patients with dMMR/MSI metastatic CRC treated with nivolumab (anti-PD-1) and with the association of nivolumab and ipilimumab (anti-CTLA4) in the multi-cohort Checkmate 142 phase II study [3, 25]. Based on these results, nivolumab and the combination of nivolumab + ipilimumab were approved by the FDA for the treatment of dMMR/MSI metastatic CRC refractory to chemotherapy. More recently, pembrolizumab was approved by FDA and EMA in first-line treatment of patients with dMMR/MSI advanced CRC based on the Keynote-177 phase III study ($n = 307$ patients) which demonstrated a significant improvement of PFS as compared to chemotherapy [26].

Thus, MMR status appears as a good and validated biomarker for response to immunotherapy in advanced CRC. However, results of the different studies cited above show that not all dMMR/MSI CRC patients benefit from this treatment, underlying the need to identify other biomarkers of response and/or resistance within this specific population. In subgroup analyses of the Keynote-177 trial, the survival benefit of pembrolizumab was conserved in the *BRAF* mutated population but seemed to be abolished in patients with *NRAS* or *KRAS* mutations. Conversely, *RAS* status was not correlated to outcome under nivolumab/ipilimumab in a subgroup analysis of the Checkmate-142 study [25]. Given the relatively small number of patients in these subgroup analyses, the impact of *RAS/BRAF* mutational status on response to immunotherapy deserves to be further explored. Furthermore, several data suggest that TMB could identify dMMR/MSI CRC patients that benefit from immunotherapy. In the phase II study of Le et al. previously cited, patients with dMMR/MSI metastatic CRC responding to pembrolizumab harbored higher TMB than non-responders [5]. In a retrospective cohort of dMMR/MSI metastatic CRC treated with pembrolizumab, a higher TMB (defined as more than 41 mutations/megabase) was associated with a better ORR and a longer PFS [27]. Thus, TMB might be a good biomarker for response to immunotherapy in dMMR/MSI CRC patients.

3.2 Tumor Mutational Burden

As previously described, the impact of TMB on response to immunotherapy in CRC was firstly assessed within the dMMR/MSI tumors, as they are known to be highly mutated [28]. Beyond MSI tumors, Fabrizio et al. identified a subset of patients harboring a high-TMB (defined as more than 11.7 mutations/megabase) in a cohort of 5702 MSS metastatic CRC. This MSS/TMB-high group represented 3% of patients and might benefit from immunotherapy [29]. In a phase II trial comparing durvalumab (anti-PD1) + tremelimumab (anti-CTLA4) versus best supportive care

(BSC) in refractory MSS metastatic CRC patients, elevated TMB (defined as more than 28 mutations/megabase) assessed in circulating cell free DNA was a predictive marker of OS benefit to immunotherapy [30].

However, several limitations have to be noted regarding the published series assessing TMB as a biomarker in CRC such as the limited number of patients included, the different assessment methods and cutoff values and the heterogeneity in the treatment lines evaluated in these trials.

3.3 *POLE* and *POLD1* Mutations

The *POLE* gene codes for the catalytic subunit (exonuclease) of the DNA Polymerase ε, which is involved in DNA replication before cell division [31]. Mutations of this exonuclease proofreading unit, leading to an impaired replication fidelity, have been detected in multiple cancer types, including GI cancers [32–34]. *POLE*-mutated tumors are characterized by a hypermutated phenotype, with an elevated burden of single nucleotide variants (SNVs) [35]. In a large cohort of 6517 CRC, a pathogenic somatic mutation of *POLE* has been found in 1% of patients [36]. In this study, *POLE*-mutated tumors were mutually exclusive from MSI tumors and were associated with increased levels of CD8+ TILs compared with *POLE*-wild type tumors. The same observations were found in a more recent study that assessed the morphological, immunological, and molecular characteristics of 63 patients with pMMR/MSS advanced CRC. In this study, *POLE* mutations were found in 4.8% of tumors and were associated with an increased level of TILs compared to non-mutated tumors [37]. Thus, given their MSI-like characteristics, *POLE*-mutated tumors might be good candidates for immunotherapy although this needs to be demonstrated by larger studies. Two observations have reported sustainable durable responses in patients with a refractory MSS *POLE*-mutated metastatic CRC receiving pembrolizumab monotherapy [37, 38]. If its predictive role is confirmed, *POLE* tumor status might become a routine biomarker assessed in MSS advanced CRC. Moreover, due to the small size of the *POLE* exonuclease domain and the segregation of mutations at recurrent hotspots, detection of *POLE* mutations can be easily achieved by NGS. Furthermore, DNA Polymerase D1 (*POLD1*) germline mutations have also been described, leading to the same hypermutated tumor phenotype [39]. To our knowledge, the impact of *POLD1* mutation on response to immunotherapy has not been assessed yet.

3.4 PD-L1 Status

The overexpression of PD-L1 in IHC varies from 12% to 50% of CRC patients [40–42]. This difference of prevalence might be due to the lack of standardization for the assessment of PD-L1 expression, as discussed previously. PD-L1 overexpression is more frequent in dMMR/MSI than in pMMR/MSS tumors [42–44]. However, as underlined by the recent recommendations by ESMO, the relationship between MMR status and PD-L1 overexpression is complex and one cannot be used as a surrogate marker for the other [45]. In the different cohorts of dMMR/MSI advanced CRC patients treated with nivolumab and nivolumab plus ipilimumab in the CheckMate-142 study (previously described), the PD-L1 status was assessed and was not correlated to survival nor response rates [3, 25]. To our knowledge, the impact of PD-L1 status on response to immunotherapy in advanced MSS advanced CRC has not been assessed in large trials and deserves thus to be further investigated.

Few studies have evaluated the predictive impact of the *PD-L1* copy number amplification on response to immunotherapy in cancer treatment [46]. In a large retrospective cohort that included more than 110,000 patients, an amplification of *PD-L1* was found in less than 1% of CRC [47]. In another study, the prevalence of *PD-L1* amplification in GI tumors was 0.2% [48]. A case report of MSS metastatic CRC harboring *PD-L1* (and *PD-L2*) amplification, without PD-L1 overexpression detected in IHC, showed a sustainable response with nivolumab [49]. This report suggested that though rare, *PD-L1* amplification could be an interesting predictive marker of immunotherapy although these data need to be validated in larger cohorts.

3.5 Tumor-Infiltrating Lymphocytes and Immunoscore

The prognostic role of tumor-infiltrating lymphocytes (TILs) in cancer was initially described in the 1930s and widely studied before the era of immunotherapy. In CRC, the characteristics of the tumor-infiltrating immune cells (including their type, density, and localization within the tumor) were shown to be correlated to prognosis by Galon et al. and others [50, 51]. Later, the same group established a pathological classification based on the evaluation of tumor-infiltrating CD3+ and CD8+ cells. This immunoscore® had a superior prognostic value than the TNM classification to assess the risk of recurrence after surgery [52] and has been validated in two international cohorts [53]. Several studies showed that dMMR/MSI CRC harbored higher levels of CD8+ TILs than pMMR/MSS tumors, whereas correlation between CD4+ TILs and MMR status is controversial [54, 55]. Data on the predictive value of TILs and/or their characteristics for response to immunotherapy in CRC is scarce. In a cohort of 77 patients with dMMR/MSI advanced CRC treated with ICB, a significant improvement of PFS was observed among patient harboring a high number of TILs (65%) (defined as a mean of TILs ≥2.0 within the tumor) as compared to those with TILs-low (35%) (median: not reached vs. 24.8 months; $p = 0.028$) [56]. These data suggested that TILs assessment could select dMMR/MSI advanced CRC patients who would benefit the most from immunotherapy. Interestingly, in the same study, TILs-high was correlated with TMB-high ($r = 0.46$; $p = 0.0429$). Conversely, in a phase II study of Le et al. assessing pembrolizumab in dMMR/MSI metastatic CRC (previously described), CD8+ TILs were not associated with PFS or OS improvement [4]. It is noteworthy that high TILs levels have also been observed in a subset of pMMR/MSS advanced CRC [53, 57], but their predictive impact on response to immunotherapy has not yet been elucidated.

4 Gastric Cancer

4.1 PD-L1 Status

PD-L1 expression status is at this time the main biomarker evaluated for immunotherapy in gastric cancer (GC) (Table 2). The PD-L1 overexpression in IHC has been correlated to an increased tumor response and a prolonged PFS and OS in several trials evaluating ICB in GC [58]. In cohort 1 of the Keynote-059 international phase II study (pembrolizumab in patients with previously treated advanced GC), ORR was 15.5% in PD-L1 positive patients, defined by a CPS $\geq$ 1, and 6.4% in PD-L1 negative patients [59]. In this study, OS was 5.8 and 4.8 months in patients with PD-L1 positive and negative tumors, respectively. Based on these results, pembrolizumab has been approved by the FDA for patients with GC who received at least two previous lines of chemotherapy, and with CPS $\geq$ 1 assessed by the PD-L1 IHC 22C3 pharmDx kit (Dako). In the Keynote-061 study, pembrolizumab failed to increase OS and PFS as compared to the second-line chemotherapy (paclitaxel), even for the patients with PD-L1 positive tumor CPS $\geq$ 1. However, in this trial, ORR was improved in patients with a higher CPS (CPS $\geq$ 10: ORR = 25%; CPS $\geq$ 1: ORR = 16%; CPS < 1: ORR = 2%) [60]. In the phase I/II Checkmate-032 trial (pretreated GC patients receiving: nivolumab 3 mg/kg (arm 1) or nivolumab 1 mg/kg + ipilimumab 3 mg/kg (arm 2) or nivolumab 3 mg/kg + ipilimumab 1 mg/kg (arm 3)), the ORR in PD-L1 positive (defined by a PD-L1 expression on tumor cells $\geq$1%) versus PD-L1 negative tumors were, respectively, 19% versus 12% in arm 1, 40% versus 22% in arm 2, and 23% versus 0% in arm 3 [61]. Conversely, in two large phase III trials (Javelin Gastric 300: avelumab vs. chemotherapy in third-line, and ATTRACTION-2: nivolumab vs. BSC in refractory disease), PD-L1 status was not correlated to response to immunotherapy [62, 63]. Interestingly, in the last two studies cited, PD-L1 positivity was defined by the tumor proportion score (TPS) rather than CPS, raising the question of the implication of PD-L1 assessment method in the results of these trials.

More recently, the international phase III Checkmate-649 study demonstrated that addition of nivolumab to first-line oxaliplatin-based chemotherapy was associated with a significant improvement of PFS and OS in CPS $\geq$ 5 patients [64]. In this study, the improvement of OS correlated to CPS: median OS was 13.8 vs. 11.6 months in the global study population (HR = 0.80; p = 0.0002), 14.0 vs. 11.3 months in patients with CPS $\geq$ 1 (HR = 0.77; p = 0.0001), and 14.4 vs. 11.1 months in tumors with CPS $\geq$ 5 (HR = 0.71; p < 0.0001), which was the primary endpoint. To note, the results for the all-comer population and differences for survival and best response rates in the subgroups for CPS >5 and >1, as well as CPS <5 and <1, will be communicated at ASCO 2021 [65]. Furthermore, on the basis of exploratory subset analyses in Javelin Gastric 100 trial, a trend to better overall survival in favor of avelumab as compared to maintenance first-line chemotherapy was seen in subgroups of patients with no metastatic sites (16.3 vs. 10.7 months), as well as patients with PD-L1 positive tumors based on CPS testing by 22C3 assay (14.9 vs. 11.6 months) [66].

Table 2 PD-L1 assessment in advanced gastric cancer immunotherapy trials

Name, ref	Author, date	Population	Phase	Line	Experimental arm	Control arm	Primary endpoint	Population for primary endpoint	Global study results	Subgroup analysis	Remarks
Immunotherapy in refractory disease											
Keynote-012 [81]	Muro, 2016	World	Ib	2+	Pembrolizumab	None	ORR	PD-L1 ≥ 1% (any scorable cell)	ORR = 22%		
ChecMate-032 [61]	Janjigian, 2018	US and EU	I/II	2+	Nivo3 vs. Nivo1 + Ipi3 vs. Nivo3 + Ipi1	None	ORR	All PD-L1	N3: ORR = 12% N1 + I3: ORR = 24% N3 + I1: ORR = 8%	TPS ≥ 1%	
ATTRACTION-2 [63]	Kang, 2017	Asia	III	3+	Nivolumab	BSC	OS	All PD-L1	Positive	TPS	No impact of TPS on OS
Keynote-059 [59]	Fuchs, 2018	World	II	3+	Pembrolizumab	BSC	ORR	All PD-L1	ORR = 11.6%	CPS ≥ 1	CPS ≥ 1: ORR = 15.5% CPS < 1: ORR = 6.4%
Immunotherapy versus chemotherapy											
Javelin Gastric 100 [66]	Moehler, 2020	World	III	1	Avelumab	Folfox	OS	All PD-L1	Negative	TPS ≥ 1% CPS ≥ 1	Negative for TPS ≥ 1% Exploratory positive signal for CPS ≥ 1
Keynote-061 [60]	Shitara, 2018	World	III	2	Pembrolizumab	Paclitaxel	OS + PFS	CPS ≥ 1	Negative	CPS ≥ 10	
Javelin Gastric 300 [62]	Bang, 2018	World	III	3	Avelumab	Taxane or Irinotecan	OS	All PD-L1	Negative	TPS ≥ 1%	Negative for TPS ≥ 1%

(continued)

Table 2 (continued)

Name, ref	Author, date	Population	Phase	Line	Experimental arm	Control arm	Primary endpoint	Population for primary endpoint	Global study results	Subgroup analysis	Remarks
Immunotherapy in first-line treatment											
Keynote-062 [71]	Shitara, 2020	World	III	1	– Pembrolizumab – Pembrolizumab + FP + cisplatin	FP + cisplatin	OS + PFS	CPS ≥ 1	Negative for superiority (even for CPS ≥10)	CPS ≥ 10	Positive for non-inferiority of pembrolizumab vs. chemotherapy
ATTRACTION-4 [115]	Boku, 2020	Asia	III	1	Nivolumab + S1 or Xeloda + Oxaliplatin	S1 or Xeloda + Oxaliplatin	OS + PFS	All PD-L1	Positive (PFS)	TPS ≥ 1%	No impact of PD-L1
Checkmate 649 [64]	Moehler, 2020	World	III	1	Nivolumab + Xelox or Folfox	Xelox or Folfox	OS + PFS	CPS ≥ 5	Positive (OS + PFS)	CPS ≥ 1 All PD-L1	Positive for CPS ≥ 1 and in all PD-L1

ORR overall response rate, *OS* overall survival, *PFS* progression free survival, *TPS* tumor proportion score, *CPS* combined positive score, *FP* fluoropyrimidine

4.2 Microsatellite Instability/Mismatch Repair Deficiency

The dMMR/MSI tumors account for 5–20% of GC depending on the studies [59, 67, 68]. As previously described, dMMR/MSI status has been shown to predict response to immunotherapy in large tumor-origin agnostic trials that included GC patients [69]. Few studies have addressed the predictive value of MMR status on response to immunotherapy in the specific situation of GC. In a study published by Kim et al., dMMR/MSI advanced GC (representing 11.5% of 61 patients) showed an ORR of 87.5% under pembrolizumab as second or third-line of treatment [70]. Interestingly, in this cohort, a subset of patients with a mixed MSI/MSS tumor phenotype (harboring both MSI and MSS tumor regions) was identified and might be associated with a lower PD-L1 expression (than the homogeneous MSI tumors), and a lower response to pembrolizumab. In the Keynote-059 study (pembrolizumab in advanced GC beyond second-line treatment), ORR was 57% in dMMR/MSI patients (representing 4% of the total population study) versus 9% in pMMR/MSS patients. In the same way, in the Keynote-062 trial (pembrolizumab alone vs. pembrolizumab plus chemotherapy vs. chemotherapy alone in first-line treatment of advanced GC) patients with dMMR/MSI tumors had improved outcomes under pembrolizumab and pembrolizumab plus chemotherapy compared to chemotherapy alone [71]. On the basis of exploratory subset analyses of Javelin Gastric 100 study, positive survival differences with avelumab versus chemotherapy was seen in the subset of patients with MSI phenotype [66].

In a large meta-analysis by Pietrantonio et al. including 1556 patients with resectable GC, the dMMR/MSI phenotype (representing 7.8% of patients) was associated with better disease-free survival (DFS) and OS [68]. Interestingly, in this study, patients with dMMR/MSI tumors did not benefit from neoadjuvant and/or adjuvant chemotherapy, suggesting that dMMR/MSI phenotype may be a predictive marker of resistance to chemotherapy in localized disease and emphasizing the relevance of alternative treatments such as ICB in these patients. A phase II French trial is ongoing to assess the efficacy of nivolumab + ipilimumab in the perioperative setting of dMMR/MSI localized GC [72].

4.3 Epstein–Barr Virus Status

The presence of Epstein–Barr Virus (EBV) is detected in 2–18% of GC, and is usually mutually exclusive with dMMR/MSI phenotype [70, 73]. In a study previously described above, Kim et al. reported for the first time a correlation between EBV status and response to immunotherapy [70, 74]. In this study, EBV-positive patients represented 9.8% of the 61 advanced GC patients included but the percentage of EBV-related GC is probably less frequent in non-Asian populations, even if data remain scarce on this point. In this cohort, all EBV-positive patients exhibited a partial response under pembrolizumab in second and third-line treatment. These results could be explained by the high level of PD-L1 and PD-L2 expression and the strong immune tumor infiltration induced by EBV infection [67, 75]. Studies are ongoing to assess the benefit of immunotherapy in this specific setting of EBV-positive GC (NCT03257163).

4.4 Tumor Mutational Burden

In GC, data regarding the predictive impact of TMB on response to immunotherapy is scarce. In different studies evaluating immunotherapy in advanced GC, TMB-high was either associated with no response to nivolumab [76], or with a survival benefit under pembrolizumab [70, 77] and a better response under toripalimab (anti-PD1) [78]. The role of TMB on response to immunotherapy in the specific situation of GC deserves to be further investigated in larger trials.

4.5 Gene Expression Signatures

In recent studies, gene expression profiling (GEP) has been suggested as a potential biomarker for immunotherapy. Notably, immune gene signatures involved in the IFN-gamma response, or activated T cells, seem to be associated with a good response under immunotherapy in NSCLC and melanoma [79, 80]. In the Keynote-012 phase IB trial (pembrolizumab in advanced PD-L1+ GC), a six-gene IFN-gamma signature was associated with response to pembrolizumab although this association was not significant [81]. In the Keynote-059 trial previously described, the presence of a T-cell inflamed 18-gene signature was associated with response and longer PFS for GC patients treated with pembrolizumab [59]. Lastly, in the Checkmate-032 study, a BMS inflammatory signature was associated with response in GC patients treated with nivolumab ± ipilimumab [82]. Thus, GEP could be an interesting biomarker for immunotherapy in GC although standardization of the assessed signatures is warranted for further investigations.

4.6 Neutrophil-to-Lymphocyte Ratio

A high circulating neutrophil-to-lymphocyte ratio (NLR) reflects an inflammatory state and has been correlated with a worse survival under immunotherapy in melanoma [83] and NSCLC [84]. In a retrospective study based on non-CRC GI cancers, higher baseline NLR (>3) was associated with a reduced OS, independently of MSI or PD-L1 status [85]. The dynamic change in NLR under immunotherapy has also been shown to correlate with survival in 96 GC patients. In this study, patients who experienced a decrease in NLR after 60 days of nivolumab had a better OS compared to those with an increased NLR [86]. Given their retrospective nature, and the relatively small numbers of patients included, these results should be validated in larger trials.

5 Other GI Cancers

5.1 Esophageal Carcinoma

An overexpression of PD-L1 has been reported in 15–83% of tumor cells and in 13–31% of immune cells in esophageal squamous cell carcinomas (ESCCs). In the

Asian phase III Attraction-3 trial, demonstrating the superiority of nivolumab over chemotherapy in second-line treatment of advanced ESCC, the prespecified exploratory subgroup analysis did not find any interaction of treatment effect with PD-L1 expression level [87]. Conversely, in the recently published international Keynote-181 study (pembrolizumab versus chemotherapy in second-line therapy in advanced esophageal cancer, including adenocarcinomas and ESCC), patients with a high PD-L1 expression (CPS $\geq$ 10) had a greater survival benefit from pembrolizumab compared to chemotherapy, in particularly for ESCC and Asian population subgroups. It is noteworthy that this study was not sufficiently powered to evaluate statistically significant differences between histological subtype (squamous cell carcinoma vs. adenocarcinoma) and geographic region (Asia vs. rest of world) in patients with PD-L1 CPS $\geq$ 10 [88]. Based on these results, the FDA approved pembrolizumab as second-line therapy for patients with advanced ESCC with CPS $\geq$ 10. More recently, the first results of the international Keynote-590 phase III trial were communicated at the ESMO meeting 2020 (pembrolizumab plus chemotherapy vs. chemotherapy alone in first-line treatment of advanced esophageal cancer, including ESCC and adenocarcinoma). This study showed a significant improvement of survival in the overall population, but the survival benefit was higher in patients with PD-L1 positive tumor CPS $\geq$ 10 [89]. In the light of these data, PD-L1 expression might be a relevant biomarker of response to immunotherapy in esophageal cancer but needs to be standardized and studied more precisely according to the histological subtype (ESCC vs. adenocarcinoma) and the geographic region of origin (Asian vs. non-Asian countries). Recently, a phase II German AIO trial has been conducted to assess the efficacy of nivolumab + ipilimumab in the second-line setting of ESCC esophageal cancer (Data submitted to ASCO 2021).

5.2 Anal Cancer

Squamous cell carcinoma of the anal canal (SCCA) is a rare malignancy. However, its incidence and mortality have increased by 2–3% per year during the last 10 years [90]. Approximately 90% of SCCA are related to oncogenic human papilloma virus (HPV). This virus-induced tumor has been described as highly infiltrated by TILs and associated with inflammatory responses [91–93]. These observations therefore constitute a strong rationale for the treatment of SCCA by immunotherapy. In a phase II multicenter prospective trial, 39 patients with advanced SCCA who received at least one prior line of chemotherapy were treated with nivolumab [94]. In this study, ORR (primary endpoint) and DCR were 24% and 72%, respectively, while median PFS and OS were 4.1 and 11.5 months, respectively. An interesting anti-tumor activity signal for immunotherapy in advanced SCCA was also observed in the multi-cohort Keynote-028 phase Ib trial (pembrolizumab for PD-L1 positive advanced solid tumors) [95]. For the 24 patients with PD-L1 positive SCAA included in this study, ORR and DCR were 17% and 58%, respectively. Although encouraging, these results suggest that other biomarkers than PD-L1 expression should be assessed to better predict response to immunotherapy. In the nivolumab study, exploratory analyses were conducted in 13 patients with HPV-positive tumors. Responders harbored increased numbers of CD8+ TILs and higher expression of PD-1 by immune cells of the microenvironment compared to non-responders. PD-L1 expression by tumor cells was also higher in responders compared to non-responders. Furthermore in the same study, the tumor mutation rates were low (1.6/megabase), consistent with what has been observed in other studies [96]. Given the small number of patients, these results should be confirmed in larger studies.

5.3 Hepatocellular Carcinoma

Efficacy of immunotherapy in hepatocellular carcinoma (HCC) has been firstly assessed in two phase I/II studies showing interesting anti-tumor activity signals [97, 98]. However, in the Keynote-240 phase III trial, pembrolizumab failed to improve OS and PFS in second-line therapy in comparison to BSC in HCC patients previously treated with sorafenib [99]. In the recently published phase I/II CheckMate-040 randomized multi-cohort trial, patients with HCC previously treated with sorafenib receiving four doses of nivolumab and ipilimumab, followed by a maintenance therapy of nivolumab alone had an ORR of 32%. The median duration of response was not reached [100]. Based on these results nivolumab plus ipilimumab followed by nivolumab was approved by the FDA as a second-line protocol for HCC. In this study, response was not correlated to PD-L1 expression status (defined by an expression of PD-L1 by tumor cells ≥1%) or to HCC etiology (association with HBV or HCV). To note, PD-L1 expression has been associated with aggressive phenotype and worse survival in patients with resected HCC [101, 102]. Interestingly, an exploratory biomarker analysis from another cohort of the CheckMate-040 study (HCC patients receiving nivolumab alone) has reported that tumor response was significantly associated with higher PD-L1 expression by tumor cells, with higher CD3 expression by TILs, and with higher GEP inflammatory signature score [103]. The latter was also associated with a significant improvement of OS ($p = 0.001$). Thus, PD-L1 expression as a predictive marker of response to immunotherapy in HCC deserves to be further explored. Other characteristics such as MSI status and elevated NLR were found to be poor prognostic markers in HCC [104, 105]. To our knowledge, their predictive value for response to immunotherapy has not been investigated yet.

5.4 Pancreatic Adenocarcinoma

The prognosis of pancreatic ductal adenocarcinoma (PDAC) is poor with a 5-year survival rate inferior to 10%, stressing the need to find new therapeutic weapons in this disease. The challenges in PDAC include the physical barrier created by the dense desmoplastic stroma surrounding the tumor, chemokine-mediated exclusion of T cells, relatively low antigenicity, and paucity of infiltrating T cells within the tumor [35, 106, 107]. While outcomes from single agent immunotherapy trials in PDAC were disappointing [108, 109], results from the pivotal KEYNOTE study published by Le et al. have revealed that pembrolizumab demonstrated 62% of ORR in the 8 patients with dMMR/MSI advanced PDAC [5]. However, in one of the cohort of the Keynote-158 trial (pembrolizumab for dMMR/MSI non-CRC), the ORR was "only" 18% among the 22 patients with dMMR/MSI advanced PDAC treated with pembrolizumab [69]. Hence, the value of MMR status as a biomarker of response to immunotherapy in PDAC cancer needs to be further investigated. Furthermore, the rate of dMMR/MSI in PDAC is unclear, several studies having demonstrated a rate of less than 5% [110–112] while others reported a frequency around 10% [113]. Of note, PD-L1 overexpression has been reported in 10–40% of PDAC [44, 114], but its predictive value for response to immunotherapy is undetermined, and several novel vaccine therapies are under investigation to induce T-cell responses and overcome the immune-resistance in PDAC.

6 Conclusion

In the past few years, immunotherapy has emerged as a new therapeutic weapon in GI cancers. In all GI tumor locations, the first published studies have put into light the necessity to find biomarkers of response to select patients who benefit from this treatment. PD-L1 status, MMR status, and high-TMB are the three biomarkers validated by the FDA for the indication of immunotherapy: PD-L1 status in gastric and esophageal cancers, and MMR and TMB status in all solid advanced tumors. However, several questions and limitations remain unmet, such as optimal cutoffs for positivity test, standardization of assessment methods, relevance for different tumors subtypes. Furthermore, as observed in dMMR/MSI advanced CRC studies, these biomarkers might not be sufficient to predict response to ICB and additional parameters are necessary to better select patients who benefit from these treatments. Promising biomarkers such as *POLE* mutational status in CRC or EBV status in GC might be routinely assessed in the future, even if their predictive value has yet to be validated in large trials. Other parameters reflecting the tumor immune contexture (TILs, inflamed GEP) are still under investigation.

Compliance with Ethical Standards

Disclosure of Interests JP has participated in consulting or advisory boards for Amgen and Servier.

JT received honoraria for speaker or advisory role from: Amgen, Baxter, BMS, MSD, Merck, Pierre Fabre, Roche, Sanofi, Servier.

AZ has participated in consulting and/or advisory boards for Amgen, Lilly, Merck, Roche, Sanofi, Servier, Baxter, MSD, Pierre Fabre, Havas Life, Alira Health, Zymeworks.

References

1. Kawakami H, Zaanan A, Sinicrope FA (2015) MSI testing and its role in the management of colorectal cancer. Curr Treat Options in Oncol 16(7):30
2. Llosa NJ, Cruise M, Tam A et al (2015) The vigorous immune microenvironment of microsatellite instable colon cancer is balanced by multiple counter-inhibitory checkpoints. Cancer Discov 5(1):43–51
3. Overman MJ, McDermott R, Leach JL et al (2017) Nivolumab in patients with metastatic DNA mismatch repair deficient/microsatellite instability–high colorectal cancer (CheckMate 142): results of an open-label, multicentre, phase 2 study. Lancet Oncol 18(9):1182
4. Le DT, Uram JN, Wang H et al (2015) PD-1 blockade in tumors with mismatch-repair deficiency. N Engl J Med 372(26):2509
5. Le DT, Durham JN, Smith KN et al (2017) Mismatch repair deficiency predicts response of solid tumors to PD-1 blockade. Science 357(6349):409–413
6. McGranahan N, Furness AJS, Rosenthal R et al (2016) Clonal neoantigens elicit T cell immunoreactivity and sensitivity to immune checkpoint blockade. Science 351(6280): 1463–1469
7. Samstein RM, Lee C-H, Shoushtari AN et al (2019) Tumor mutational load predicts survival after immunotherapy across multiple cancer types. Nat Genet 51(2):202–206
8. Goodman AM, Kato S, Bazhenova L et al (2017) Tumor mutational burden as an independent predictor of response to immunotherapy in diverse cancers. Mol Cancer Ther 16(11):2598–2608
9. Marabelle A, Fakih M, Lopez J et al (2020) Association of tumour mutational burden with outcomes in patients with advanced solid tumours treated with pembrolizumab: prospective biomarker analysis of the multicohort, open-label, phase 2 KEYNOTE-158 study. Lancet Oncol 21(10):1353–1365
10. Schwaederle M, Husain H, Fanta PT et al (2016) Use of liquid biopsies in clinical oncology: pilot experience in 168 patients. Clin Cancer Res 22(22):5497–5505
11. Khagi Y, Goodman AM, Daniels GA et al (2017) Hyper-mutated circulating tumor DNA: correlation with response to checkpoint inhibitor-based immunotherapy. Clin Cancer Res 23(19):5729–5736
12. Kasi PM (2017) Mutational burden on circulating cell-free tumor-DNA testing as a surrogate marker of mismatch repair deficiency or microsatellite instability in patients with colorectal cancers. J Gastrointest Oncol 8(4):747–748
13. Sha D, Jin Z, Budczies J et al (2020) Tumor mutational burden as a predictive biomarker in solid tumors. Cancer Discov 10(12):1808–1825
14. Budczies J, Seidel A, Christopoulos P et al (2018) Integrated analysis of the immunological and genetic status in and across cancer types: impact of mutational signatures beyond tumor mutational burden. Onco Targets Ther. https://doi.org/10.1080/2162402X.2018.1526613
15. Frampton GM, Fichtenholtz A, Otto GA et al (2013) Development and validation of a clinical cancer genomic profiling test based on massively parallel DNA sequencing. Nat Biotechnol 31(11):1023–1031
16. Chalmers ZR, Connelly CF, Fabrizio D et al (2017) Analysis of 100,000 human cancer genomes reveals the landscape of tumor mutational burden. Genome Med. https://doi.org/10.1186/s13073-017-0424-2
17. Topalian SL, Hodi FS, Brahmer JR et al (2012) Safety, activity, and immune correlates of anti-PD-1 antibody in cancer. N Engl J Med 366(26):2443–2454
18. Taube JM, Klein A, Brahmer JR et al (2014) Association of PD-1, PD-1 ligands, and other features of the tumor immune microenvironment with response to anti-PD-1 therapy. Clin Cancer Res 20(19):5064–5074
19. Rosenberg JE, Hoffman-Censits J, Powles T et al (2016) Atezolizumab in patients with locally advanced and metastatic urothelial carcinoma who have progressed following

treatment with platinum-based chemotherapy: a single arm, phase 2 trial. Lancet 387(10031): 1909–1920
20. Gandhi L, Rodríguez-Abreu D, Gadgeel S et al (2018) Pembrolizumab plus chemotherapy in metastatic non-small-cell lung cancer. N Engl J Med. https://doi.org/10.1056/NEJMoa1801005
21. Ferris RL, Blumenschein G, Fayette J et al (2016) Nivolumab for recurrent squamous-cell carcinoma of the head and neck. N Engl J Med 375(19):1856–1867
22. Tang H, Liang Y, Anders RA et al (2018) PD-L1 on host cells is essential for PD-L1 blockade-mediated tumor regression. J Clin Invest 128(2):580–588
23. Gong J, Chehrazi-Raffle A, Reddi S, Salgia R (2018) Development of PD-1 and PD-L1 inhibitors as a form of cancer immunotherapy: a comprehensive review of registration trials and future considerations. J Immunother Cancer. https://doi.org/10.1186/s40425-018-0316-z
24. Koopman M, Kortman GAM, Mekenkamp L et al (2009) Deficient mismatch repair system in patients with sporadic advanced colorectal cancer. Br J Cancer 100(2):266–273
25. Overman MJ, Lonardi S, Wong KYM et al (2018) Durable clinical benefit with nivolumab plus ipilimumab in DNA mismatch repair–deficient/microsatellite instability–high metastatic colorectal cancer. J Clin Oncol 36(8):773–779
26. André T, Shiu K-K, Kim TW et al (2020) Pembrolizumab in microsatellite-instability–high advanced colorectal cancer. N Engl J Med. https://doi.org/10.1056/NEJMoa2017699
27. Tumor mutational burden is predictive of response to immune checkpoint inhibitors in MSI-high metastatic colorectal cancer (2019) Ann Oncol 30(7):1096–1103
28. Campbell BB, Light N, Fabrizio D et al (2017) Comprehensive analysis of hypermutation in human cancer. Cell 171(5):1042–1056.e10
29. Fabrizio DA, George TJ, Dunne RF et al (2018) Beyond microsatellite testing: assessment of tumor mutational burden identifies subsets of colorectal cancer who may respond to immune checkpoint inhibition. J Gastrointest Oncol 9(4):610–617
30. Chen EX, Jonker DJ, Loree JM et al (2019) CCTG CO.26: Updated analysis and impact of plasma-detected microsatellite stability (MSS) and tumor mutation burden (TMB) in a phase II trial of durvalumab (D) plus tremelimumab (T) and best supportive care (BSC) versus BSC alone in patients (pts) with refractory metastatic colorectal carcinoma (rmCRC). J Clin Oncol 37(15_Suppl):3512–3512
31. Pursell ZF, Isoz I, Lundström E-B et al (2007) Yeast DNA polymerase ε participates in leading-strand DNA replication. Science 317(5834):127–130
32. Church DN, Briggs SEW, Palles C et al (2013) DNA polymerase ε and δ exonuclease domain mutations in endometrial cancer. Hum Mol Genet 22(14):2820–2828
33. Muzny DM, Bainbridge MN, Chang K et al (2012) Comprehensive molecular characterization of human colon and rectal cancer. Nature 487(7407):330–337
34. Shinbrot E, Henninger EE, Weinhold N et al (2014) Exonuclease mutations in DNA polymerase epsilon reveal replication strand specific mutation patterns and human origins of replication. Genome Res 24(11):1740–1750
35. Alexandrov LB, Nik-Zainal S, Wedge DC et al (2013) Signatures of mutational processes in human cancer. Nature 500(7463):415–421
36. Domingo E, Freeman-Mills L, Rayner E et al (2016) Somatic POLE proofreading domain mutation, immune response, and prognosis in colorectal cancer: a retrospective, pooled biomarker study. Lancet Gastroenterol Hepatol 1(3):207–216
37. Forgó E, Gomez AJ, Steiner D et al (2020) Morphological, immunophenotypical and molecular features of hypermutation in colorectal carcinomas with mutations in DNA polymerase ε (POLE). Histopathology 76(3):366–374
38. Gong J, Wang C, Lee PP et al (2017) Response to PD-1 blockade in microsatellite stable metastatic colorectal cancer harboring a POLE mutation. J Natl Compr Cancer Netw 15(2):142–147
39. Palles C, Cazier J-B, Howarth KM et al (2013) Germline mutations in the proof-reading domains of POLE and POLD1 predispose to colorectal adenomas and carcinomas. Nat Genet 45(2):136–144

40. Masugi Y, Nishihara R, Yang J et al (2017) Tumour CD274 (PD-L1) expression and T cells in colorectal cancer. Gut 66(8):1463–1473
41. Dong H, Strome SE, Salomao DR et al (2002) Tumor-associated B7-H1 promotes T-cell apoptosis: a potential mechanism of immune evasion. Nat Med 8(8): 793–800
42. Inaguma S, Lasota J, Wang Z et al (2017) Clinicopathologic profile, immunophenotype, and genotype of CD274 (PD-L1)-positive colorectal carcinomas. Mod Pathol 30(2): 278–285
43. Gatalica Z, Snyder CL, Yeatts K et al (2014) Programmed death 1 (PD-1) lymphocytes and ligand (PD-L1) in colorectal cancer and their relationship to microsatellite instability status. J Clin Oncol 32(15_Suppl):3625–3625
44. Salem ME, Puccini A, Grothey A et al (2018) Landscape of tumor mutation load, mismatch repair deficiency, and PD-L1 expression in a large patient cohort of gastrointestinal cancers. Mol Cancer Res 16(5):805–812
45. ESMO recommendations on microsatellite instability testing for immunotherapy in cancer, and its relationship with PD-1/PD-L1 expression and tumour mutational burden: a systematic review-based approach (2019) Ann Oncol 30(8):1232–1243
46. Inoue Y, Yoshimura K, Nishimoto K et al (2020) Evaluation of programmed death ligand 1 (PD-L1) gene amplification and response to nivolumab monotherapy in non-small cell lung cancer. JAMA Netw Open. https://doi.org/10.1001/jamanetworkopen.2020.11818
47. Goodman AM, Piccioni D, Kato S et al (2018) Prevalence of PDL1 amplification and preliminary response to immune checkpoint blockade in solid tumors. JAMA Oncol 4(9): 1237–1244
48. Huang RSP, Haberberger J, Severson E et al (2020) A pan-cancer analysis of PD-L1 immunohistochemistry and gene amplification, tumor mutation burden and microsatellite instability in 48,782 cases. Mod Pathol:1–12
49. Sorscher S, Resnick J, Goodman M (2017) First case report of a dramatic radiographic response to a checkpoint inhibitor in a patient with proficient mismatch repair gene expressing metastatic colorectal cancer. JCO Precis Oncol 1:1–4
50. Galon J, Costes A, Sanchez-Cabo F et al (2006) Type, density, and location of immune cells within human colorectal tumors predict clinical outcome. Science 313(5795): 1960–1964
51. Rozek LS, Schmit SL, Greenson JK et al (2016) Tumor-infiltrating lymphocytes, Crohn's-like lymphoid reaction, and survival from colorectal cancer. J Natl Cancer Inst. https://doi.org/10.1093/jnci/djw027
52. Galon J, Mlecnik B, Bindea G et al (2014) Towards the introduction of the "Immunoscore" in the classification of malignant tumours. J Pathol 232(2):199–209
53. Pagès F, Mlecnik B, Marliot F et al (2018) International validation of the consensus Immunoscore for the classification of colon cancer: a prognostic and accuracy study. Lancet 391(10135):2128–2139
54. De Smedt L, Lemahieu J, Palmans S et al (2015) Microsatellite instable vs stable colon carcinomas: analysis of tumour heterogeneity, inflammation and angiogenesis. Br J Cancer 113(3):500–509
55. Boissière-Michot F, Lazennec G, Frugier H et al (2014) Characterization of an adaptive immune response in microsatellite-instable colorectal cancer. Onco Targets Ther. https://doi.org/10.4161/onci.29256
56. Loupakis F, Depetris I, Biason P et al (2020) Prediction of benefit from checkpoint inhibitors in mismatch repair deficient metastatic colorectal cancer: role of tumor infiltrating lymphocytes. Oncologist 25(6):481–487
57. Kikuchi T, Mimura K, Okayama H et al (2019) A subset of patients with MSS/MSI-low-colorectal cancer showed increased CD8(+) TILs together with up-regulated IFN-γ. Oncol Lett 18(6):5977–5985
58. Coutzac C, Pernot S, Chaput N, Zaanan A (2019) Immunotherapy in advanced gastric cancer, is it the future? Crit Rev Oncol Hematol 133:25–32

59. Fuchs CS, Doi T, Jang RW et al (2018) Safety and efficacy of pembrolizumab monotherapy in patients with previously treated advanced gastric and gastroesophageal junction cancer. JAMA Oncol. https://doi.org/10.1001/jamaoncol.2018.0013
60. Shitara K, Özgüroğlu M, Bang Y-J et al (2018) Pembrolizumab versus paclitaxel for previously treated, advanced gastric or gastro-oesophageal junction cancer (KEYNOTE-061): a randomised, open-label, controlled, phase 3 trial. Lancet 392(10142):123–133
61. Janjigian YY, Bendell J, Calvo E et al (2018) CheckMate-032 Study: efficacy and safety of nivolumab and nivolumab plus ipilimumab in patients with metastatic esophagogastric cancer. J Clin Oncol 36(28):2836–2844
62. Bang Y-J, Ruiz EY, Van Cutsem E et al (2018) Phase III, randomised trial of avelumab versus physician's choice of chemotherapy as third-line treatment of patients with advanced gastric or gastro-oesophageal junction cancer: primary analysis of JAVELIN Gastric 300. Ann Oncol 29(10):2052–2060
63. Kang Y-K, Boku N, Satoh T et al (2017) Nivolumab in patients with advanced gastric or gastro-oesophageal junction cancer refractory to, or intolerant of, at least two previous chemotherapy regimens (ONO-4538-12, ATTRACTION-2): a randomised, double-blind, placebo-controlled, phase 3 trial. Lancet 390(10111):2461–2471
64. Moehler M, Shitara K, Garrido M et al (2020) LBA6_PR Nivolumab (nivo) plus chemotherapy (chemo) versus chemo as first-line (1L) treatment for advanced gastric cancer/gastroesophageal junction cancer (GC/GEJC)/esophageal adenocarcinoma (EAC): first results of the CheckMate 649 study. Ann Oncol 31:S1191
65. Janjigian YY et al (2021) First-line nivolumab plus chemotherapy versus chemotherapy alone for advanced gastric, gastro-oesophageal junction, and oesophageal adenocarcinoma (CheckMate 649): a randomised, open-label, phase 3 trial. Lancet. 398:27–40. https://doi.org/10.1016/S0140-6736(21)00797-2
66. Moehler M, Dvorkin M, Boku N et al (2020) Phase III trial of avelumab maintenance after first-line induction chemotherapy versus continuation of chemotherapy in patients with gastric cancers: results From JAVELIN Gastric 100. J Clin Oncol 39(9):966–977
67. Bass AJ, Thorsson V, Shmulevich I et al (2014) Comprehensive molecular characterization of gastric adenocarcinoma. Nature 513(7517):202–209
68. Pietrantonio F, Miceli R, Raimondi A et al (2019) Individual patient data meta-analysis of the value of microsatellite instability as a biomarker in gastric cancer. J Clin Oncol 37(35):3392–3400
69. Marabelle A, Le DT, Ascierto PA et al (2019) Efficacy of pembrolizumab in patients with noncolorectal high microsatellite instability/mismatch repair–deficient cancer: results from the phase II KEYNOTE-158 study. J Clin Oncol 38(1):1–10
70. Kim ST, Cristescu R, Bass AJ et al (2018) Comprehensive molecular characterization of clinical responses to PD-1 inhibition in metastatic gastric cancer. Nat Med 24(9):1449–1458
71. Shitara K, Cutsem EV, Bang Y-J et al (2020) Efficacy and safety of pembrolizumab or pembrolizumab plus chemotherapy vs chemotherapy alone for patients with first-line, advanced gastric cancer: the KEYNOTE-062 phase 3 randomized clinical trial. JAMA Oncol 6(10):1571–1580
72. Cohen R, Pudlarz T, Garcia-Larnicol M-L et al (2020) Patients atteints d'un cancer gastrique localisé MSI/dMMR, pas de chimiothérapie mais une immunothérapie périopératoire: l'essai de phase II GERCOR NEONIPIGA vient d'être ouvert au recrutement. Bull Cancer (Paris) 107(4):438–446
73. Akiba S, Koriyama C, Herrera-Goepfert R, Eizuru Y (2008) Epstein-Barr virus associated gastric carcinoma: epidemiological and clinicopathological features. Cancer Sci 99(2):195–201
74. Zaanan A, Taieb J (2019) How to better select patients with advanced gastric cancer for immunotherapy. Transl Gastroenterol Hepatol. https://doi.org/10.21037/tgh.2019.01.06
75. De Rosa S, Sahnane N, Tibiletti MG et al (2018) EBV+ and MSI gastric cancers harbor high PD-L1/PD-1 expression and high CD8+ intratumoral lymphocytes. Cancers. https://doi.org/10.3390/cancers10040102

76. Mishima S, Kawazoe A, Nakamura Y et al (2019) Clinicopathological and molecular features of responders to nivolumab for patients with advanced gastric cancer. J Immunother Cancer. https://doi.org/10.1186/s40425-019-0514-3
77. Shitara K, Özgüroğlu M, Bang Y-J et al (2020) The association of tissue tumor mutational burden (tTMB) using the Foundation Medicine genomic platform with efficacy of pembrolizumab versus paclitaxel in patients (pts) with gastric cancer (GC) from KEYNOTE-061. J Clin Oncol 38(15_Suppl):4537–4537
78. Wang F, Wei XL, Wang FH et al (2019) Safety, efficacy and tumor mutational burden as a biomarker of overall survival benefit in chemo-refractory gastric cancer treated with toripalimab, a PD-1 antibody in phase Ib/II clinical trial NCT02915432. Ann Oncol 30(9):1479–1486
79. Auslander N, Zhang G, Lee JS et al (2018) Robust prediction of response to immune checkpoint blockade therapy in metastatic melanoma. Nat Med 24(10):1545–1549
80. Fehrenbacher L, Spira A, Ballinger M et al (2016) Atezolizumab versus docetaxel for patients with previously treated non-small-cell lung cancer (POPLAR): a multicentre, open-label, phase 2 randomised controlled trial. Lancet 387(10030):1837–1846
81. Muro K, Chung HC, Shankaran V et al (2016) Pembrolizumab for patients with PD-L1-positive advanced gastric cancer (KEYNOTE-012): a multicentre, open-label, phase 1b trial. Lancet Oncol 17(6):717–726
82. Lei M, Siemers N, Pandya D et al (2019) Abstract 2673: Association of PD-L1 combined positive score and immune gene signatures with efficacy of nivolumab (NIVO) ± ipilimumab (IPI) in patients with metastatic gastroesophageal cancer (mGEC). Cancer Res 79(13 Supplement):2673–2673
83. Ferrucci PF, Ascierto PA, Pigozzo J et al (2016) Baseline neutrophils and derived neutrophil-to-lymphocyte ratio: prognostic relevance in metastatic melanoma patients receiving ipilimumab. Ann Oncol 27(4):732–738
84. Mezquita L, Auclin E, Ferrara R et al (2018) Association of the lung immune prognostic index with immune checkpoint inhibitor outcomes in patients with advanced non-small cell lung cancer. JAMA Oncol 4(3):351–357
85. Li S, Zou J, Liu C et al (2020) Baseline derived neutrophil-to-lymphocyte ratio as a prognostic biomarker for non-colorectal gastrointestinal cancer patients treated with immune checkpoint blockade. Clin Immunol 212:108345
86. Ota Y, Takahari D, Suzuki T et al (2020) Changes in the neutrophil-to-lymphocyte ratio during nivolumab monotherapy are associated with gastric cancer survival. Cancer Chemother Pharmacol 85(2):265–272
87. Kato K, Cho BC, Takahashi M et al (2019) Nivolumab versus chemotherapy in patients with advanced oesophageal squamous cell carcinoma refractory or intolerant to previous chemotherapy (ATTRACTION-3): a multicentre, randomised, open-label, phase 3 trial. Lancet Oncol 20(11):1506–1517
88. Kojima T, Shah MA, Muro K et al (2020) Randomized phase III KEYNOTE-181 study of pembrolizumab versus chemotherapy in advanced esophageal cancer. J Clin Oncol 38(35):4138–4148
89. Kato K, Sun J-M, Shah MA et al (2020) LBA8_PR Pembrolizumab plus chemotherapy versus chemotherapy as first-line therapy in patients with advanced esophageal cancer: the phase 3 KEYNOTE-590 study. Ann Oncol 31:S1192–S1193
90. Henley SJ, Ward EM, Scott S et al (2020) Annual report to the nation on the status of cancer, Part I: National cancer statistics. Cancer 126(10):2225–2249
91. Heusinkveld M, Goedemans R, Briet RJP et al (2012) Systemic and local human papillomavirus 16-specific T-cell immunity in patients with head and neck cancer. Int J Cancer 131(2):E74–E85
92. Lyford-Pike S, Peng S, Young GD et al (2013) Evidence for a role of the PD-1:PD-L1 pathway in immune resistance of HPV-associated head and neck squamous cell carcinoma. Cancer Res 73(6):1733–1741

93. Partlová S, Bouček J, Kloudová K et al (2015) Distinct patterns of intratumoral immune cell infiltrates in patients with HPV-associated compared to non-virally induced head and neck squamous cell carcinoma. Onco Targets Ther. https://doi.org/10.4161/21624011.2014.965570
94. Morris VK, Salem ME, Nimeiri H et al (2017) Nivolumab for previously treated unresectable metastatic anal cancer (NCI9673): a multicentre, single-arm, phase 2 study. Lancet Oncol 18(4):446–453
95. Ott PA, Piha-Paul SA, Munster P et al (2017) Safety and antitumor activity of the anti-PD-1 antibody pembrolizumab in patients with recurrent carcinoma of the anal canal. Ann Oncol 28(5):1036–1041
96. Morris V, Rao X, Pickering C et al (2017) Comprehensive genomic profiling of metastatic squamous cell carcinoma of the anal canal. Mol Cancer Res 15(11):1542–1550
97. El-Khoueiry AB, Sangro B, Yau T et al (2017) Nivolumab in patients with advanced hepatocellular carcinoma (CheckMate 040): an open-label, non-comparative, phase 1/2 dose escalation and expansion trial. Lancet 389(10088):2492–2502
98. Zhu AX, Finn RS, Edeline J et al (2018) Pembrolizumab in patients with advanced hepatocellular carcinoma previously treated with sorafenib (KEYNOTE-224): a non-randomised, open-label phase 2 trial. Lancet Oncol 19(7):940–952
99. Finn RS, Ryoo B-Y, Merle P et al (2019) Pembrolizumab as second-line therapy in patients with advanced hepatocellular carcinoma in KEYNOTE-240: a randomized, double-blind, phase III trial. J Clin Oncol 38(3):193–202
100. Yau T, Kang Y-K, Kim T-Y et al (2020) Efficacy and safety of nivolumab plus ipilimumab in patients with advanced hepatocellular carcinoma previously treated with sorafenib. JAMA Oncol. https://doi.org/10.1001/jamaoncol.2020.4564
101. Gao Q, Wang X-Y, Qiu S-J et al (2009) Overexpression of PD-L1 significantly associates with tumor aggressiveness and postoperative recurrence in human hepatocellular carcinoma. Clin Cancer Res 15(3):971–979
102. Jung HI, Jeong D, Ji S et al (2016) Overexpression of PD-L1 and PD-L2 is associated with poor prognosis in patients with hepatocellular carcinoma. Cancer Res Treat 49(1):246–254
103. Melero I, Neely J, Sangro B et al (2019) Abstract 2675: Assessment of inflammation biomarkers in relation to clinical outcomes in nivolumab-treated patients with advanced hepatocellular carcinoma in CheckMate 040. Cancer Res 79(13 Supplement):2675–2675
104. Qi X, Li J, Deng H et al (2016) Neutrophil-to-lymphocyte ratio for the prognostic assessment of hepatocellular carcinoma: a systematic review and meta-analysis of observational studies. Oncotarget 7(29):45283–45301
105. Chiappini F, Gross-Goupil M, Saffroy R et al (2004) Microsatellite instability mutator phenotype in hepatocellular carcinoma in non-alcoholic and non-virally infected normal livers. Carcinogenesis 25(4):541–547
106. Bailey P, Chang DK, Forget M-A et al (2016) Exploiting the neoantigen landscape for immunotherapy of pancreatic ductal adenocarcinoma. Sci Rep. https://doi.org/10.1038/srep35848
107. Balachandran VP, Łuksza M, Zhao JN et al (2017) Identification of unique neoantigen qualities in long-term survivors of pancreatic cancer. Nature 551(7681):512–516
108. Brahmer JR, Tykodi SS, Chow LQM et al (2012) Safety and activity of anti–PD-L1 antibody in patients with advanced cancer. N Engl J Med 366(26):2455–2465
109. Royal RE, Levy C, Turner K et al (2010) Phase 2 trial of single agent ipilimumab (Anti-CTLA-4) for locally advanced or metastatic pancreatic adenocarcinoma. J Immunother 33(8):828–833
110. Lupinacci RM, Goloudina A, Buhard O et al (2018) Prevalence of microsatellite instability in intraductal papillary mucinous neoplasms of the pancreas. Gastroenterology 154(4):1061–1065
111. Goggins M, Offerhaus GJ, Hilgers W et al (1998) Pancreatic adenocarcinomas with DNA replication errors (RER+) are associated with wild-type K-ras and characteristic histopathology. Poor differentiation, a syncytial growth pattern, and pushing borders suggest RER+. Am J Pathol 152(6):1501–1507

112. Laghi L, Beghelli S, Spinelli A et al (2012) Irrelevance of microsatellite instability in the epidemiology of sporadic pancreatic ductal adenocarcinoma. PLoS One. https://doi.org/10.1371/journal.pone.0046002
113. Yamamoto H, Itoh F, Nakamura H et al (2001) Genetic and clinical features of human pancreatic ductal adenocarcinomas with widespread microsatellite instability. Cancer Res 61(7):3139–3144
114. Birnbaum DJ, Finetti P, Lopresti A et al (2016) Prognostic value of PDL1 expression in pancreatic cancer. Oncotarget 7(44):71198–71210
115. Boku N, Ryu MH, Oh D-Y et al (2020) LBA7_PR Nivolumab plus chemotherapy versus chemotherapy alone in patients with previously untreated advanced or recurrent gastric/gastroesophageal junction (G/GEJ) cancer: ATTRACTION-4 (ONO-4538-37) study. Ann Oncol 31:S1192

MIX
Papier aus verantwortungsvollen Quellen
Paper from responsible sources
FSC® C105338

If you have any concerns about our products,
you can contact us on
ProductSafety@springernature.com

In case Publisher is established outside the EU,
the EU authorized representative is:
Springer Nature Customer Service Center GmbH
Europaplatz 3, 69115 Heidelberg, Germany

Printed by Libri Plureos GmbH
in Hamburg, Germany